Atlas of
PET/CT
with SPECT/CT

Richard L. Wahl, MD, FACR

Professor of Radiology and Oncology
Henry N. Wagner Jr. Professor of Nuclear Medicine
Director of Nuclear Medicine/PET Facility
Vice Chair for Technology and Business Development
The Russell H. Morgan Department of Radiology and Radiological Sciences
Johns Hopkins University School of Medicine
Baltimore, Maryland

Ora Israel, MD

Director of Nuclear Medicine/PET
Director for Research Operations
Rambam Health Care Campus
Associate Professor
B. Rappaport School of Medicine
Technion—Israel Institute of Technology
Haifa, Israel

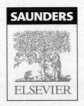

SAUNDERS

ELSEVIER

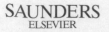

1600 John F. Kennedy Blvd.
Ste 1800
Philadelphia, PA 19103-2899

ATLAS OF PET/CT: WITH SPECT/CT   ISBN: 978-1-4160-3361-5

Notice

Knowledge and best practice in this field are constantly changing. As new research and experience broaden our knowledge, changes in practice, treatment, and drug therapy may become necessary or appropriate. Readers are advised to check the most current information provided (i) on procedures featured or (ii) by the manufacturer of each product to be administered, to verify the recommended dose or formula, the method and duration of administration, and contraindications. It is the responsibility of the practitioner, relying on his or her own experience and knowledge of the patient, to make diagnoses, to determine dosages and the best treatment for each individual patient, and to take all appropriate safety precautions. To the fullest extent of the law, neither the Publisher nor the Editors assume any liability for any injury and/or damage to persons or property arising out of or related to any use of the material contained in this book.

The Publisher

Library of Congress Cataloging-in-Publication Data
Wahl, Richard L.
   Atlas of PET/CT : with SPECT/CT / Richard L. Wahl, Ora Israel.
      p. ; cm.
   ISBN 978-1-4160-3361-5
1. Tomography, Emission—Atlases.   2. Tomography—Atlases.   3. Single-photon emission computed tomography—Atlases.   I. Israel, Ora.   II. Title.
   [DNLM: 1. Positron-Emission Tomography—methods—Atlases.   2. Tomography, Emission-Computed, Single-Photon—methods—Atlases.   3. Clinical Medicine—methods—Atlases.   4. Image Processing, Computer-Assisted—Atlases.   5. Software—Atlases. WN 17 W136a 2008]

RC78.7.T62W34 2008
616.07'57—dc22

                                                          2007004461

Acquisitions Editors: Rebecca Gaertner, Todd Hummel
Developmental Editor: Scott Scheidt
Project Manager: Bryan Hayward
Design Direction: Lou Forgione

Printed in China

Last digit is the print number: 9 8 7 6 5 4 3 2 1

The development and growth of PET/CT and SPECT/CT imaging are the fruits of a dedicated, collaborative effort. We wish to express our heartfelt thanks to our team members and many contributors who participated in this process: our patients, from whom we learn so much; our trainees and medical colleagues who teach us daily; and the physicists, engineers, computer scientists, and technicians who developed and refined these important technologies to provide us with the best tools possible.

We dedicate this work to our spouses—Sandy and Stefan—and our children—Daniel, Mathew, Peter, Katherine, Dalit, Yair, and Harel—who patiently supported us during the long days, nights, and weekends we spent learning these technologies and developing this atlas.

We hope readers will find this volume useful, enjoy reading it, and incorporate hybrid imaging in their daily practice.

Richard L. Wahl, Baltimore, and Ora Israel, Haifa
March 2007

Contributors

Richard L. Wahl, MD, FACR
Professor of Radiology and Oncology
Henry N. Wagner Jr. Professor of Nuclear Medicine
Director of Nuclear Medicine/PET Facility
Vice Chair for Technology and Business Development
The Russell H. Morgan Department of Radiology and Radiological Sciences
Johns Hopkins University School of Medicine
Baltimore, Maryland

Ora Israel, MD
Director of Nuclear Medicine/PET
Director for Research Operations
Rambam Health Care Campus
Associate Professor
B. Rappaport School of Medicine
Technion—Israel Institute of Technology
Haifa, Israel

Rachel Bar-Shalom, MD
Director of PET/CT Unit
Department of Nuclear Medicine/PET
Rambam Health Care Campus
B. Rappaport School of Medicine, Technion
Haifa, Israel

Ahuva Engel, MD
Director of Diagnostic Imaging
Rambam Health Care Campus
B. Rappaport School of Medicine, Technion
Haifa, Israel

Alex Frenkel, PhD
Principal Physicist
Department of Nuclear Medicine/PET
Rambam Health Care Campus
Haifa, Israel

Mehrbod Som Javadi, MD
Research Associate and Resident in Nuclear Medicine
Division of Nuclear Medicine
Department of Radiology
Johns Hopkins University School of Medicine
Baltimore, Maryland

Zohar Keidar, MD, PhD
Deputy Director
Department of Nuclear Medicine/PET
Rambam Health Care Campus
B. Rappaport School of Medicine, Technion
Haifa, Israel

Laura King Dow, CNMT, ARRT
Senior Technologist: PET/CT
Division of Nuclear Medicine
Department of Radiology
Johns Hopkins University School of Medicine
Baltimore, Maryland

Daniela Militianu, MD
Director of Musculo-Skeletal Imaging Unit
Department of Diagnostic Imaging
Rambam Health Care Campus
Haifa, Israel

Preface

Nuclear medicine is, and likely will remain, the major modality translating the promise of "molecular imaging" from research into clinical practice. A growing range of radiotracers are becoming available, aimed at detecting and characterizing an array of biological processes. The high sensitivity of nuclear medicine methods, both positron emission tomography (PET) and single photon emission computed tomography (SPECT), allows for the detection of radiation emitted by small numbers of radioactive molecules from organs and tissues located deep within the patient.

Nuclear medicine imaging with single photon emitters initially evolved as a planar method, and early positron imaging was in the form of linear tomography. At present, advanced nuclear medicine techniques involve tomographic detection and reconstruction approaches designed to trace biological processes with specific radiotracers. The diagnostic value of nuclear medicine as a "stand-alone" approach is clear and proven.

Both SPECT and PET imaging modalities are capable of noninvasively documenting important functional information in an anatomically correct context. The display of morphology and structure, however, is substantially limited to the nontarget uptake in normal tissues. Furthermore, as radiochemistry focuses on developing tracers that become more and more specific for a given process, often only that particular process accumulates a high amount of the radiotracer relative to background, making lesion detection easily possible, but lesion localization a much more approximate undertaking. While achieving the goal of highly specific metabolic and molecular in vivo imaging, precise localization of pathophysiological events and quantitation of the radiotracer accumulation in healthy and diseased tissues remain unifying challenges that must be met to translate targeting into clinical decision making.

For example, highly specific and targeted SPECT agents such as I123 MIBG or In111 pentetreotide accumulate so avidly to lesions that it becomes difficult to determine precisely the anatomic location of the tracer-avid site. Similarly, "hot spot" PET imaging agents such as FDG can demonstrate high avidity for tumors and other highly metabolic processes, but in many instances the precise anatomic localization of these foci is difficult or even impossible because there is not sufficient radiotracer uptake into surrounding normal tissues to define their morphology. The ability to perform highly accurate functional diagnostic imaging is therefore compromised by the lack of anatomic correlative data.

The use of image co-registration, in the form of "anato-metabolic" images for PET fused with magnetic resonance imaging (MRI) or computed tomography (CT), was shown feasible by means of software techniques in early studies of cancer imaging. Although software approaches are quite valuable, they are limited if there is substantial patient motion between studies in nonrigid areas of the body, as well as by the need for sophisticated software and highly skilled teamwork to use it most effectively. These problems can be substantially solved, and most of these limitations are indeed overcome when anatomic and functional images are obtained in close temporal and spatial proximity in the same imaging session using dedicated, in-line hybrid imaging devices such as PET/CT or SPECT/CT.

Over the past 15 years, the two principal authors of this atlas had the opportunity to become involved with fusion imaging at its early stages. Dr. Wahl, while at the University of Michigan, worked with Dr. Chuck Meyer to develop software-based "anato-metabolic" tumor imaging for PET/CT, SPECT/CT, and MRI/PET. After moving to Johns Hopkins, one of the first PET/CT scanners was installed in 2001, and Dr. Wahl and his colleagues have since gained vast experience with the fused PET/CT imaging technology. His institution also invested heavily in the growing area of SPECT/CT imaging, with five SPECT/CT cameras now in clinical and research use. Dr. Israel was involved from the beginning in the clinical development of SPECT/CT technology, with one of the first functioning clinical systems installed at Rambam, in Haifa, Israel. After performing the first clinical studies on a factory prototype in late 2000, her team also received one of the first clinical PET/CT systems, which, coincidentally, was installed the same day in June 2001 at both Johns Hopkins and Rambam. The team at Rambam has developed a vast clinical experience using their four SPECT/CT and PET/CT devices, exploring new clinical indications for the hybrid technology in assessment of infection and inflammation and cardiac imaging beyond the oncologic applications of these modalities.

In late 2001, Dr. Israel proposed to Dr. Wahl the need to develop an atlas dealing with the rapidly emerging new imaging technologies, designed to serve as a quick, anatomically based reference book that could help physicians understand the technology and to facilitate the process of learning how to interpret the studies accurately. Since that time, she and Dr. Wahl have worked to accumulate and highlight key teaching cases from the more than 15,000 studies each of them has supervised, making them suitable for inclusion in a text aimed at practitioners who are just beginning or want to improve their skills on how to interpret either PET/CT or SPECT/CT. Because both editors of this book still feel, 6 years after launching this project, that they "continue learning," the potential readership for this textbook represents a sizable target audience.

Unlike many other books on a similar topic, this atlas is organ site–oriented as opposed to disease type–oriented. This was deliberately selected because the normal variants and the disease processes often occur by "region" of the body and the scans are presented to the interpreting physicians on a "regional" basis. Misregistration due to breathing or movement of the head or increased equivocal foci of radiotracer activity in a single kidney, a dilated renal pelvis, or a healing surgical scar may be encountered in patients with lymphoma, lung cancer, melanoma, or disseminated carcinoid, for example. This is why key normal anatomy, variants, artifacts, and typical and uncommon disease patterns for all regions of the body have been selected.

The introduction of SPECT/CT into routine use has occurred at a somewhat slower pace despite having been introduced as a clinical tool earlier than PET/CT. Foreseeing the more rapid growth that is occurring at present, we predicted that a major need for SPECT/CT educational materials was also clearly present. The SPECT/CT part of the book, though smaller, is organized by scan type as opposed to organ system, as most of these studies are "whole body" in nature.

Because it is our belief that more and more small and large centers will be interested in starting and later expanding hybrid imaging practices, we also provide a brief description of the methods required to produce high diagnostic quality PET/CT and SPECT/CT images. This is based on the experience acquired with daily routine procedures by us and our dedicated staff.

None of us could have envisioned the tremendous development of this technology and its rapid acceptance both by the imaging community and the referring physicians who treat the patients. We are hopeful that this combined atlas, the result of collecting key cases from two busy and experienced clinical services, will prove useful to the imaging community, as we are increasingly called upon to perform and interpret PET/CT and SPECT/CT images. We are grateful to Hermes Medical, which was kind enough to place a substantial number of our cases on DVD so our readers can have a better opportunity for direct interaction with the image sets than is possible with the book pages alone. We are also grateful to the engineers, scientists, and manufacturers of our imaging systems (especially those from General Electric Healthcare and Philips Medical Systems) who have allowed us to deploy this technology as it evolved, for the benefit of our patients.

We are grateful for having been able to work with wonderful, expert, and dedicated teams, some of them joining us every morning for years or even decades. The contributions of our colleagues, including physicians, physicists, and technical and administrative staff, are greatly appreciated. Their work and advice have made this book possible.

Above all, we acknowledge the support of our spouses, Sandy Wahl and Stefan Israel, and our children, without whose patience, encouragement, and understanding this project could not have been completed.

Richard L. Wahl, Baltimore, Maryland
Ora Israel, Haifa, Israel

Contents

Preface   *vii*

SECTION 1

Technical Considerations for
PET/CT and SPECT/CT   *1*

SECTION 2

PET/CT of the Brain   *13*

2.1 Normal Pattern   *14*
    Case 2.1.1 Normal Pattern PET/CT of the Brain and
        Quantitative Analysis   *14*

2.2 Benign Abnormalities   *19*
    Case 2.2.1 Congenital Encephalomalacia
        and Epilepsy   *19*
    Case 2.2.2 Postsurgical Changes   *20*
    Case 2.2.3 Radiation Necrosis   *21*

2.3 Tumors   *21*
    Case 2.3.1 Primary Brain Tumor   *21*
    Case 2.3.2 Brain Metastases and Lung Cancer   *22*
    Case 2.3.3 Residual Tumor and
        Postsurgical Changes   *24*
    Case 2.3.4 Recurrent Tumor and
        Radiation Necrosis   *25*
    Case 2.3.5 Pituitary Adenoma and Stroke   *27*

2.4 Neurological Disorders   *28*
    Case 2.4.1 Epilepsy—Classic Interictal Pattern *28*
    Case 2.4.2 Epilepsy—Interictal Pattern and
        Cerebellar Diaschisis   *30*

    Case 2.4.3 Epilepsy—Interictal Pattern and
        Decreased Cerebellar Uptake   *33*
    Case 2.4.4 Alzheimer's Disease—Diffuse Pattern *35*
    Case 2.4.5 Alzheimer's Disease—Frontal
        Predominance   *37*

SECTION 3

PET/CT of the Head and Neck   *39*

3.1 Normal Pattern   *40*
    Case 3.1.1 Normal Pattern PET/CT of the Head
        and Neck   *40*

3.2 Physiologic Artifacts and Pitfalls   *40*
    Case 3.2.1 Artifact—Misregistration Due to
        Patient Movement   *40*
    Case 3.2.2 Physiologic—Muscle Uptake, Tongue   *41*
    Case 3.2.3 Physiologic—Unilateral Muscle
        Uptake, Mastication   *41*
    Case 3.2.4 Physiologic—Bilateral Muscle
        Uptake, Mastication   *42*
    Case 3.2.5 Physiologic Unilateral Muscle
        Uptake, Neck   *43*
    Case 3.2.6 Physiologic—Unilateral Muscle
        Uptake, Torticollis, and Metal
        Artifact   *44*
    Case 3.2.7 Pitfall—Vocal Cord Paralysis, Left   *45*
    Case 3.2.8 Pitfall—Vocal Cord Paralysis, Right
        and Supraclavicular Nodes   *46*
    Case 3.2.9 Benign—Brown Fat, Neck   *47*
    Case 3.2.10 Benign—Brown Fat, Neck
        and Shoulders   *48*

Case 3.2.11 Benign—Posttreatment Changes in Skin and Subcutaneous Tissue (Surgery and Radiation)   49

Case 3.2.12 Benign—Posttreatment Changes, Reconstituted Lymphoid Tissue and Muscles (Surgery and Radiation)   49

Case 3.2.13 Benign—Postsurgical Changes, Missing Salivary Gland   50

Case 3.2.14 Benign—Posttreatment Changes, FDG-Negative Right Parotid   51

Case 3.2.15 Benign—Postsurgical Changes, Missing Orbit, and Ethmoid, Extraocular Muscular Uptake   52

3.3 Infection and Inflammation   53

Case 3.3.1 Inflammation, Tracheostomy   53

Case 3.3.2 Infection, Acne   54

Case 3.3.3 Infection, Maxillary Sinusitis, Partially Involved   55

Case 3.3.4 Infection, Maxillary Sinusitis, Involvement of Whole Sinus   55

Case 3.3.5 Mucous Retention Cyst in Maxillary Sinus, FDG-Negative   56

Case 3.3.6 Inflammation, Rheumatoid Arthritis, Atlanto-Odontoid Joint   56

3.4 Tumors   57

Case 3.4.1 Tumor of Scalp, Melanoma   57

Case 3.4.2 Tumor of Scalp, Melanoma   58

Case 3.4.3 Tumor of Scalp, Benign, FDG-Negative   59

Case 3.4.4 Tumor of Auditory Canal   59

Case 3.4.5 Tumor of Parotid and Peri-Parotid Nodes   60

Case 3.4.6 Tumor of Parotid   60

Case 3.4.7 Tumor of Nasopharynx, Response to Treatment   61

Case 3.4.8 Tumor of Lip   62

Case 3.4.9 Tumor, Base of Tongue   62

Case 3.4.10 Tumor of Tongue and Level II Nodes   63

Case 3.4.11 Tumor of Tonsil and Level II Nodes   64

Case 3.4.12 Tumor of Pharynx   65

Case 3.4.13 Tumor of Pharynx (Aryepiglottic Fold) and Cervical Nodes   65

Case 3.4.14 Tumor of Larynx, Supraglottic, and Tracheostomy   66

Case 3.4.15 Tumor of Larynx and Destruction of Tracheal Cartilage   67

Case 3.4.16 Tumor of Vocal Cord   68

Case 3.4.17 Tumor of Cervical Esophagus   69

Case 3.4.18 Tumor of Neural Sheath and Brown Fat   70

Case 3.4.19 Tumor of Bone, Vertebral Metastasis   71

3.5 Lymph Node Compartments   72

Case 3.5.1 Level I Lymph Nodes   72

Case 3.5.2 Level I and II Lymph Nodes and Scalene Muscle Uptake   73

Case 3.5.3 Level II Lymph Nodes   74

Case 3.5.4 Level II Lymph Nodes   74

Case 3.5.5 Level II and III Lymph Nodes   75

Case 3.5.6 Level IV Lymph Nodes   76

Case 3.5.7 Level V Lymph Nodes   76

Case 3.5.8 Level VI Lymph Nodes   77

3.6 Thyroid   77

Case 3.6.1 Benign—Thyroiditis   77

Case 3.6.2 Benign—Multinodular, Retrosternal Goiter   78

Case 3.6.3 Benign—Thyroid Adenoma and Distorted Anatomy   79

Case 3.6.4 Tumor—Primary Thyroid Cancer   79

SECTION 4

PET/CT of the Chest   *81*

4.1 Normal Pattern   82

Case 4.1.1 Normal Pattern PET/CT of the Chest   82

4.2 Chest Wall   83

Case 4.2.1 Pitfall—Gynecomastia and Esophageal Cancer   83

Case 4.2.2 Pitfall—Muscular Uptake, Asymmetric   83

Case 4.2.3 Pitfall—Axillary Postinjection Uptake and Breast Cancer   84

Case 4.2.4 Benign—Brown Fat, Shoulder and Upper Chest Wall   85

Case 4.2.5 Benign—Postsurgical Changes   86

Case 4.2.6 Tumor—Chest Wall Recurrence, Breast Cancer   87

4.3 Breast   87

Case 4.3.1 Artifact—Saline Implants, Cold Lesion   87

Case 4.3.2 Pitfall—Seroma   88

Case 4.3.3 Benign—Granuloma and Fracture of Scapula   88

Case 4.3.4 Benign—Postradiation Changes   89

Case 4.3.5 Tumor—Large Primary Breast Cancer   89

Case 4.3.6 Tumor—Primary Breast Cancer and Axillary Nodes   90

Case 4.3.7 Tumor—Recurrent Breast Cancer and Axillary Nodes   91

4.4 Skeleton   92

Case 4.4.1 Benign—Rib Fractures, Varying Ages   92

Case 4.4.2 Benign—Fracture, Sternum   93

Case 4.4.3 Benign—Osteophyte, Thoracic Vertebra   93

Case 4.4.4 Benign—Postradiation "Cold" Vertebrae   94

Case 4.4.5 Tumor—Metastasis, Rib   94

Case 4.4.6 Tumor—Metastasis, Sternum   95

Case 4.4.7 Tumor—Metastases, Thoracic Vertebrae   96

4.5 Pleura   97

Case 4.5.1 Benign—Inflammation, Focal Pattern, Pleurodesis   97

Case 4.5.2 Benign—Inflammation, Diffuse
Pattern, Pleurodesis 98
Case 4.5.3 Tumor—Malignant Effusion and
Tube Insertion 99
Case 4.5.4 Tumor—Pleural Thickening,
Mesothelioma 100
Case 4.5.5 Tumor—Pleural Nodule,
Malignant Implant 101
Case 4.5.6 Tumor—Pleural Masses, Mesothelioma 102

4.6 Lung 103
Case 4.6.1 Pitfall—Misregistration Due to
Respiratory Movement 103
Case 4.6.2 Benign—Postradiation Changes 104
Case 4.6.3 Benign—Pneumonia 105
Case 4.6.4 Benign—Pulmonary Sarcoidosis 105
Case 4.6.5 Benign—FDG-Negative Small
Lung Nodule 106
Case 4.6.6 Benign—FDG-Negative Lung Nodule
and Interval Shrinkage 106
Case 4.6.7 Benign—Single Lung Nodule,
Granuloma 107
Case 4.6.8 Tumor—Single Lesion, Primary
Lung Cancer 107
Case 4.6.9 Tumor—Single Cystic Lesion, Primary
Lung Cancer 108
Case 4.6.10 Tumor—Moderate FDG Avidity,
Bronchioloalveolar Lung Cancer 108
Case 4.6.11 Tumor—Pancoast, Chest Wall
Involvement, and Lung Metastasis 109
Case 4.6.12 Tumor—Response to Treatment,
Primary Lung Cancer with
Nodal Metastases 110
Case 4.6.13 Tumor—Metachronous Lung Cancer 111
Case 4.6.14 Tumor—Recurrent Mesothelioma
and Postsurgical Changes 112
Case 4.6.15 Multiple Lesions, Multifocal Primary
Lung Cancer 113
Case 4.6.16 Tumor—Multiple Lesions, Lymphoma 114
Case 4.6.17 Tumor—Multiple Lesions and
Inhomogeneous Pattern, Lymphoma 115
Case 4.6.18 Tumor—Multiple Lesions, Metastases 116
Case 4.6.19 Tumor—Multiple FDG-Negative
Lesions, Metastases 117
Case 4.6.20 Tumor—Multiple Lesions, Treated
and New Metastases 118

4.7 Thoracic Lymph Nodes 119
Case 4.7.1 Supraclavicular Lymph Nodes 119
Case 4.7.2 Retroclavicular and Pectoralis
Lymph Nodes 119
Case 4.7.3 Axillary and Pectoralis Lymph Nodes 120
Case 4.7.4 Axillary Lymph Nodes 121
Case 4.7.5 Internal Mammary Lymph Node
versus Sternal Lesion 122
Case 4.7.6 Supradiaphragmatic Lymph Nodes 123

4.8 Mediastinal Lymph Nodes 123
Case 4.8.1 Anterior Mediastinal and
Paratracheal Lymph Nodes 123
Case 4.8.2 Prevascular Lymph Nodes,
Normal Size 124
Case 4.8.3 Aortopulmonary Window
Lymph Nodes 124
Case 4.8.4 Pre- and Subcarinal Lymph Nodes 125
Case 4.8.5 Paraesophageal Lymph Nodes 126
Case 4.8.6 Pretracheal, Paratracheal,
Tracheobronchial, and Hilar
Lymph Nodes 127
Case 4.8.7 Retrocaval-Paratracheal, Paraspinal
Lymph Nodes and Response
to Treatment 128

4.9 Mediastinum 129
Case 4.9.1 Pitfall—Brown Fat 129
Case 4.9.2 Pitfall—Blood Clot 130
Case 4.9.3 Benign—Thymus 130
Case 4.9.4 Tumor—Bulky Disease 131
Case 4.9.5 Tumor—Endotracheal Recurrent
Lung Cancer 131

4.10 Esophagus 132
Case 4.10.1 Pitfall—Hiatal Hernia 132
Case 4.10.2 Pitfall—Gastric Pull Up 132
Case 4.10.3 Benign—Esophagitis,
Radiation-Induced 133
Case 4.10.4 Tumor—Cancer of Proximal
Esophagus 133
Case 4.10.5 Tumor—Cancer of Distal Esophagus 134
Case 4.10.6 Tumor—Response to Treatment,
Cancer of Distal Esophagus 135

4.11 Cardiovascular 136
Case 4.11.1 Benign—Takayasu's Aortitis 136
Case 4.11.2 Benign—Coronary Calcifications
and Pericardial Effusion 136
Case 4.11.3 Assessment of Myocardium—Scar 137
Case 4.11.4 Assessment of Myocardium—Viability
and Apical Scar 139
Case 4.11.5 Assessment of Myocardium—
Cardiomyopathy 140
Case 4.11.6 Cardiac PET/CT—Normal Myocardial
Perfusion and Coronary Anatomy 141
Case 4.11.7 Cardiac PET/CT—Ischemia and
Coronary Calcifications
and Narrowing 141

SECTION 5

PET/CT of the Abdomen 143

5.1 Normal Pattern 144
Case 5.1.1 Normal Pattern PET/CT of
the Abdomen 144

5.2 Abdominal Wall   144
  Case 5.2.1 Pitfall—Colostomy   144
  Case 5.2.2 Pitfall—Pararenal Brown Fat   145
  Case 5.2.3 Pitfall—Anterior Abdominal Brown Fat   145
  Case 5.2.4 Pitfall—Paracolic Brown Fat   146
  Case 5.2.5 Benign—Surgical Scar   146
  Case 5.2.6 Benign—Rib Fracture   147
  Case 5.2.7 Tumor—Metastasis   148

5.3 Liver and Spleen   149
  Case 5.3.1 Pitfall—Intracholedocal Stent   149
  Case 5.3.2 Pitfall—Lesions at Liver–Lung Interface   150
  Case 5.3.3 Benign—Chronic Cholecystitis   152
  Case 5.3.4 Tumor—Primary Hepatocellular
              Carcinoma   153
  Case 5.3.5 Tumor—Single Metastasis, Lower Pole
              of Right Liver Lobe   154
  Case 5.3.6 Tumor—Multiple Liver Metastases   155
  Case 5.3.7 Tumor—Liver Metastasis, Recurrence
              at Site of Surgery   155
  Case 5.3.8 Tumor—Single Metastasis in Spleen   156
  Case 5.3.9 Tumor—Multiple Lesions in Spleen
              and Nodal Involvement   156
  Case 5.3.10 Tumor—Splenomegaly and Diffuse
              Involvement by Lymphoma   157

5.4 Pancreas   158
  Case 5.4.1 Tumor—Cancer in Head of Pancreas   158
  Case 5.4.2 Tumor—Cancer in Tail of Pancreas   158
  Case 5.4.3 Tumor and Inflammation—Multiple
              Pancreatic Lesions   159

5.5 Stomach   160
  Case 5.5.1 Physiologic—Gastric Uptake   160
  Case 5.5.2 Tumor—Lymphoma in Distal Antrum   161
  Case 5.5.3 Tumor—Diffuse Pattern, Gastric
              Cancer, and Nodal Metastases   161
  Case 5.5.4 Tumor—Large Gastric Mass,
              Gastrointestinal Stromal Tumor (GIST)   162
  Case 5.5.5 Tumor—Recurrence of Gastric Cancer   163

5.6 Bowel   163
  Case 5.6.1 Benign—Adenoma in Colon   163
  Case 5.6.2 Tumor—Primary Colon Cancer   164
  Case 5.6.3 Tumor—Metastasis in Small Intestine   164

5.7 Peritoneum   165
  Case 5.7.1 Benign—Granulomatotic Nodule   165
  Case 5.7.2 Tumor—Single Nodule, Metastasis   166
  Case 5.7.3 Tumor—Multiple Nodules, Metastases   166
  Case 5.7.4 Tumor—Diffuse Pattern, Peritoneal
              Seeding   168
  Case 5.7.5 Tumor—Peritoneal Masses, GIST, and
              Liver Involvement   169

5.8 Kidneys and Adrenals   170
  Case 5.8.1 Pitfall—Regional Lymphadenopathy
              Near Renal Pelvis   170
  Case 5.8.2 Pitfall—Single Kidney   171

  Case 5.8.3 Pitfall—Ectopic Kidney   172
  Case 5.8.4 Pitfall—Horseshoe Kidney   173
  Case 5.8.5 Pitfall—Distorted Renal Pelvis   173
  Case 5.8.6 Tumor—Single Renal Metastasis   174
  Case 5.8.7 Tumor—Multiple Renal Lesions,
              Lymphoma   175
  Case 5.8.8 Tumor—Single Adrenal Metastasis   176
  Case 5.8.9 Tumor—Bilateral Adrenal
              Involvement, Lymphoma   176

5.9 Lymph Nodes   177
  Case 5.9.1 Gastrohepatic Ligament
              Lymph Nodes   177
  Case 5.9.2 Hepatic Hilum Lymph Nodes and
              Liver Metastases   177
  Case 5.9.3 Splenic Hilum Lymph Nodes   178
  Case 5.9.4 Mesenteric and Retroperitoneal
              Lymph Nodes   178
  Case 5.9.5 Mesenteric Lymph Nodes in Region
              of Root of Mesentery   179
  Case 5.9.6 Para-Aortic Lymph Nodes   179
  Case 5.9.7 Aortocaval Lymph Nodes   180
  Case 5.9.8 Iliac Lymph Nodes   180

5.10 Vascular   181
  Case 5.10.1 Pitfall—Aortic Wall Calcifications   181
  Case 5.10.2 Pitfall—Aortic Aneurysm   182
  Case 5.10.3 Benign Aortic Graft Infection and
              Psoas Muscle Abscess   183

5.11 Bone—Lumbar Spine   184
  Case 5.11.1 Benign—Degenerative Changes in
              Vertebral Body   184
  Case 5.11.2 Benign—Degenerative Changes in
              Articular Facets   184
  Case 5.11.3 Benign—Degenerative Changes of
              Intervertebral Disc   185
  Case 5.11.4 Tumor—Lytic FDG-Avid Metastasis   185
  Case 5.11.5 Tumor—Sclerotic FDG-Negative
              Metastases   186
  Case 5.11.6 Tumor—Bone and Soft Tissue
              Metastasis   187

SECTION 6

PET/CT of the Pelvis   *189*

6.1 Normal Pattern   190
  Case 6.1.1 Male Pelvis   190
  Case 6.1.2 Female Pelvis   190

6.2 Pelvic Wall, Soft Tissues, and Peritoneum   191
  Case 6.2.1 Pitfall—Focal Uptake, Colostomy   191
  Case 6.2.2 Pitfall—Focal Uptake, Inguinal
              Hernia   191
  Case 6.2.3 Pitfall—Focal Uptake, Urinary
              Catheter   192
  Case 6.2.4 Benign—Skin Granuloma   192

Case 6.2.5   Benign—Infection, Pilonidal Sinus   *193*
Case 6.2.6   Benign—Infection, Pelvic Abscess   *194*
Case 6.2.7   Tumor—Presacral Recurrence, Rectal Cancer   *195*
Case 6.2.8   Tumor—Metastasis in Psoas Muscle   *195*
Case 6.2.9   Tumor—Metastasis, Cul-de-Sac Peritoneal Nodule   *196*
Case 6.2.10 Tumor—Metastases, Focal Peritoneal Nodules   *196*
Case 6.2.11 Tumor—Diffuse Peritoneal Involvement   *197*

6.3   Gastrointestinal Tract   *197*
Case 6.3.1   Pitfall—Physiologic, Focal Uptake in Bowel   *197*
Case 6.3.2   Benign—Rectal Polyp   *198*
Case 6.3.3   Benign—Inflammatory Bowel Disease   *198*
Case 6.3.4   Tumor—Primary Rectal Cancer   *199*
Case 6.3.5   Tumor—Primary Rectosigmoid Cancer and Pararectal Nodes   *199*
Case 6.3.6   Tumor—Response to Treatment, Metastatic Rectal Cancer   *200*
Case 6.3.7   Tumor—Recurrence, Rectal Cancer   *201*
Case 6.3.8   Tumor—Recurrence, Rectal Cancer and Iliac Nodes   *202*

6.4   Urinary Tract   *203*
Case 6.4.1   Pitfall—Ectopic Pelvic Kidney   *203*
Case 6.4.2   Pitfall—Renal Transplant   *203*
Case 6.4.3   Pitfall—Focal Uptake in Ureter   *204*
Case 6.4.4   Pitfall—Focal Uptake in Obstructed Ureter   *205*
Case 6.4.5   Pitfall—Dilated Prostatic Urethra   *206*
Case 6.4.6   Pitfall—Bladder Diverticulum   *206*
Case 6.4.7   Pitfall—Bladder Herniation   *207*
Case 6.4.8   Tumor—Carcinoma of Ureter   *210*
Case 6.4.9   Tumor—Carcinoma of Urinary Bladder and Lymphoma of Bone   *211*

6.5   Ovary, Cervix, and Uterus   *212*
Case 6.5.1   Pitfall—Ovulating Ovary   *212*
Case 6.5.2   Pitfall—Menstruation   *212*
Case 6.5.3   Benign—Myoma   *213*
Case 6.5.4   Tumor—Lymphoma in Ovary   *214*
Case 6.5.5   Tumor—Primary Ovarian Carcinoma   *214*
Case 6.5.6   Tumor—Ovarian Carcinoma, Recurrence at Site of Surgery   *215*
Case 6.5.7   Tumor—Primary Cervical Cancer   *215*
Case 6.5.8   Tumor—Primary Cervical Cancer, Inhomogeneous Uptake   *216*
Case 6.5.9   Tumor—Primary Cervical Cancer and Iliac Nodes   *216*
Case 6.5.10 Tumor—Recurrence, Cervical Cancer   *217*

6.6   Prostate and Testis   *218*
Case 6.6.1   Benign—Prostatic Hypertrophy   *218*
Case 6.6.2   Benign—Infection, Orchiepidydimitis   *218*
Case 6.6.3   Tumor—Lymphoma in Testis   *219*

6.7   Lymph Nodes   *220*
Case 6.7.1   Common and External Iliac Lymph Nodes   *220*
Case 6.7.2   Internal Iliac Lymph Nodes   *221*
Case 6.7.3   Internal Iliac Lymph Nodes in Lower Pelvis   *221*
Case 6.7.4   Inguinal Lymph Nodes and Primary Cervical Cancer   *222*
Case 6.7.5   Inguinal Lymph Nodes and Metastatic Melanoma in Gluteal Mass   *222*

6.8   Vascular   *223*
Case 6.8.1   Pitfall—Noninfected Aortobifemoral Bypass   *223*
Case 6.8.2   Benign—Infected Aortic Vascular Graft   *224*

6.9   Bone   *225*
Case 6.9.1   Pitfall—Radiation-Induced "Cold" Sacrum   *225*
Case 6.9.2   Benign—Sacral Fracture   *225*
Case 6.9.3   Benign—Paget's Disease   *226*
Case 6.9.4   Tumor—Metastasis in Sacrum and Epidural Space   *227*
Case 6.9.5   Tumor—Metastasis in Ilium and Soft Tissues   *227*
Case 6.9.6   Tumor—Lymphoma, Involvement of the Ischium   *228*

PET/CT of the Extremities   *229*

7.1   Skin   *230*
Case 7.1.1   Benign—Healing Surgical Scar, Thigh   *230*
Case 7.1.2   Benign—Infected Surgical Scar, Thigh   *230*
Case 7.1.3   Benign—Infected Skin Ulcers, Legs   *231*
Case 7.1.4   Tumor—Malignant Melanoma, Nodules in Thigh and Calf   *232*

7.2   Soft Tissue   *233*
Case 7.2.1   Benign—Abscess, Leg   *233*
Case 7.2.2   Tumor—Subcutaneous Lymphoma, Nodule in Arm   *233*
Case 7.2.3   Tumor—Subcutaneous Melanoma, Nodule in Thigh   *234*
Case 7.2.4   Tumor—Soft Tissue Sarcoma, Hand, with Bone Involvement   *235*

7.3   Joints   *236*
Case 7.3.1   Artifact—Metal-Induced Periprosthetic Activity and Reactive Process, Hip   *236*
Case 7.3.2   Benign—Periarticular Uptake, Trochanteric Bursitis   *237*
Case 7.3.3   Benign—Periarticular Uptake, Synovitis of Knees   *237*
Case 7.3.4   Benign—Tenosynovitis and Tendon Tear, Foot and Distal Leg   *238*
Case 7.3.5   Benign—Low-Grade Infection, Hip   *239*

7.4 Muscles   239
Case 7.4.1 Physiologic—Tense Muscles, Thighs   239
Case 7.4.2 Tumor—Metastasis, Arm   240
Case 7.4.3 Tumor—Metastases, Thigh   240

7.5 Lymph Nodes   241
Case 7.5.1 Epitrochlear Lymph Nodes   241
Case 7.5.2 Popliteal Lymph Nodes   241
Case 7.5.3 Popliteal Lymph Nodes   242

7.6 Vascular   242
Case 7.6.1 Pitfall—Vascular Uptake   242
Case 7.6.2 Benign—Infected Vascular Graft   243

7.7 Bone and Bone Marrow   244
Case 7.7.1 Benign—Osteomyelitis, Phalanx of Foot   244
Case 7.7.2 Tumor—Bone Metastasis, Scapula   245
Case 7.7.3 Tumor—Bone Metastasis, Humerus   245
Case 7.7.4 Tumor—Bone Metastasis, Femur   246
Case 7.7.5 Tumor—Lymphoma, Humerus and Soft Tissues   247
Case 7.7.6 Tumor—Bone Marrow Involvement, Multiple Myeloma, Femur   248
Case 7.7.7 Tumor—Bone Marrow and Soft Tissue Lymphoma, Humerus   248
Case 7.7.8 Tumor—Bone Marrow and Soft Tissue Lymphoma, Tibia and Leg   249

SECTION 8

SPECT/CT

  251

8.1 In111-Pentetreotide SPECT/CT   252
Case 8.1.1 Physiologic—Bowel and Kidney Uptake In111-Pentetreotide SPECT/ Low-Dose CT   252
Case 8.1.2 Pitfall—Uptake in Gallbladder In111-Pentetreotide SPECT/ Multislice CT   252
Case 8.1.3 Tumor—Residual Carcinoid In111-Pentetreotide SPECT/ Low-Dose CT   253
Case 8.1.4 Tumor—Metastatic Carcinoid In111-Pentetreotide SPECT/ Low-Dose CT   253
Case 8.1.5 Tumor—Disseminated Carcinoid In111-Pentetreotide SPECT/ Low-Dose CT   254
Case 8.1.6 Tumor—Vertebral Metastasis, Neuroendocrine Tumor In111-Pentetreotide SPECT/ Low-Dose CT   254

8.2 Iodine131 SPECT/CT   255
Case 8.2.1 Physiologic—Remnant Thyroid I131 SPECT/Multislice CT   255
Case 8.2.2 Physiologic—Bowel Uptake I131 SPECT/Multislice CT   255

Case 8.2.3 Pitfall—Thymic Uptake I131 SPECT/Low-Dose CT   256
Case 8.2.4 Pitfall—Dental and Uterine Inflammatory Process I131 SPECT/Multislice CT   256
Case 8.2.5 Pitfall—Uptake in Ectopic Stomach I131 SPECT/Low-Dose CT   257
Case 8.2.6 Tumor—Mediastinal Nodal Metastasis, Thyroid Cancer I131 SPECT/Low-Dose CT   257
Case 8.2.7 Tumor—Cervical and Supraclavicular Nodal Metastases, Thyroid Cancer I131 SPECT/Multislice CT   258
Case 8.2.8 Tumor—Lung Metastasis, Thyroid Cancer I131 SPECT/Low-Dose CT   258
Case 8.2.9 Tumor—Bone Metastasis, Thyroid Cancer I131 SPECT/Multislice CT   259
Case 8.2.10 Tumor—Bone Metastases, Thyroid Cancer I131 SPECT/Low-Dose CT   259

8.3 Iodine123-Metaiodobenzylguanidine (MIBG) SPECT/CT   260
Case 8.3.1 Physiologic—Cardiac Uptake I123-MIBG SPECT/Low-Dose CT   260
Case 8.3.2 Physiologic—Inhomogeneous Cardiac Uptake, Ischemic Heart Disease and Pheochromocytoma I123-MIBG SPECT/Low-Dose CT   260
Case 8.3.3 Physiologic—Renal Uptake I123-MIBG SPECT/Multislice CT   261
Case 8.3.4 Physiologic—Adrenal Uptake I123-MIBG SPECT/Multislice CT   261
Case 8.3.5 Tumor—Bilateral Pheochromocytoma I123-MIBG SPECT/Multislice CT   262
Case 8.3.6 Tumor—Neuroblastoma and Bone Marrow Involvement I123-MIBG SPECT/Low-Dose CT   262

8.4 Gallium67 SPECT/CT   263
Case 8.4.1 Physiologic—Thymic Uptake Ga67 SPECT/Low-Dose CT   263
Case 8.4.2 Benign—Infection, Osteomyelitis Ga67 SPECT/Multislice CT   263
Case 8.4.3 Benign—Infection, Bone and Soft Tissue, and Bowel Uptake Ga67 SPECT/Low-Dose CT   264
Case 8.4.4 Benign—Infection, Paravertebral Abscess Ga67 SPECT/Low-Dose CT   264
Case 8.4.5 Benign—Infection, Liver Abscess Ga67 SPECT/Low-Dose CT   265
Case 8.4.6 Tumor—Lymphoma Involving the Head and Neck and Mediastinum Ga67 SPECT/Low-Dose CT   265
Case 8.4.7 Tumor—Lymphoma in Pelvic Mass Ga67 SPECT/Low-Dose CT   266

Case 8.4.8 Tumor—Lymphoma in Muscle,
Pitfalls: Rib Fracture and Lung Infiltrate
Ga67 SPECT/Low-Dose CT   267

**8.5 In111 Capromab Pendetide (Prostascint)—
SPECT/CT**   268
Case 8.5.1 Normal Study In111-Capromab
Pendetide SPECT/Low-Dose CT   268
Case 8.5.2 Tumor—Abdominal Lymphadenopathy,
Prostate Cancer In111-Capromab
Pendetide SPECT/Multislice CT   269

**8.6 Tc99m-Methoxyisobutyl Isonitrile (MIBI)
SPECT/CT (Parathyroid Imaging)**   270
Case 8.6.1 Pitfall—Asymmetric Salivary Gland
Uptake and Parathyroid Adenoma
Tc99m-MIBI SPECT/Multislice CT   270
Case 8.6.2 Tumor—Parathyroid Adenoma, Right
Neck Tc99m-MIBI SPECT/Multislice CT   270
Case 8.6.3 Tumor—Parathyroid Adenoma, Left
Neck Tc99m-MIBI SPECT/Low-Dose CT   271
Case 8.6.4 Tumor—Ectopic Parathyroid Adenoma
Tc99m-MIBI SPECT/Low-Dose CT   271

**8.7 Tc99m-Methylene Diphosphonate (MDP)
SPECT/CT**   272
Case 8.7.1 Pitfall—Uptake Related to a Renal
Calculus
Tc99m-MDP SPECT/Low-Dose CT   272
Case 8.7.2 Benign—Facet Joint Disease
Tc99m-MDP SPECT/Low-Dose CT   272
Case 8.7.3 Benign—Osteoarthritis in Hip
Tc99m-MDP SPECT/Low-Dose CT   273
Case 8.7.4 Benign—Fibrous Dysplasia
Tc99m-MDP SPECT/Low-Dose CT   274
Case 8.7.5 Benign—Myositis Ossificans
Tc99m-MDP SPECT/Low-Dose CT   275
Case 8.7.6 Benign—Hematoma at Prior Injection
Site Tc99m-MDP SPECT/Low-Dose CT   275

8.8 In111-Labeled Leukocytes SPECT/CT   276
Case 8.8.1 Diabetic Foot—Osteomyelitis and
Soft Tissue Infection In111–White
Blood Cell (WBC) SPECT/Low-Dose CT   276
Case 8.8.2 Diabetic Foot—Soft Tissue Infection
In111-WBC SPECT/Low-Dose CT   277
Case 8.8.3 Diabetic Foot—Soft Tissue Infection
In111-WBC SPECT/Low-Dose CT   277
Case 8.8.4 Bacteremia—Infected Aortic Plaque
In111-WBC SPECT/Multislice CT   278

8.9 Cardiac SPECT/CT   278
Case 8.9.1 Normal Study SPECT, Myocardial
Perfusion, and CT, Attenuation
Correction Single Isotope (Tc99m-
MIBI), Stress/Rest SPECT/Low-Dose CT   278
Case 8.9.2 Breast Artifact SPECT, Myocardial
Perfusion and CT, Attenuation
Correction Single Isotope (Tc99m-
MIBI), Stress/Rest SPECT/Low-Dose CT   279
Case 8.9.3 Diaphragm Artifact SPECT, Myocardial
Perfusion, and CT—Attenuation
Correction Single Isotope (Tc99m-
MIBI), Stress/Rest SPECT/Low-Dose CT   279
Case 8.9.4 Scar and Ischemia SPECT, Myocardial
Perfusion, and CT—Attenuation
Correction Single Isotope (Tc99m-
MIBI), Stress/Rest SPECT/Low-Dose CT   280
Case 8.9.5 SPECT/CT—Normal Perfusion and
Coronary Anatomy Myocardial SPECT,
Single Isotope (Tc99m-MIBI)
Stress/Rest and 64-Slice CT   281
Case 8.9.6 SPECT/CT—Myocardial Ischemia and
Coronary Lesions Myocardial SPECT,
Single Isotope (Tc99m-MIBI)
Stress/Rest and 64-Slice CT   282

Index   283

Technical Considerations for **PET/CT** and **SPECT/CT**

Richard L. Wahl • Laura King Dow • Alex Frenkel • Ora Israel

PET/CT IMAGING

A positron emission tomography/computed tomography (PET/CT) scanner represents a major financial investment. Because it may be the single most expensive piece of diagnostic imaging equipment in a hospital or outpatient center, administrators as well as users expect that both the PET and CT components of the in-line scanner must be operating properly nearly all of the time. To achieve optimal PET/CT imaging, the PET/CT system must be designed to meet the needs of the individual center.

The approach to choosing a PET/CT scanner for purchase or lease should be a measured and thoughtful one. Several major medical imaging manufacturers market PET/CT systems, which all produce high-quality studies. Although a variety of technical specifications are quoted by each manufacturer, including sensitivity and spatial resolution, we do not advise making the purchase choice on the basis of the manufacturer's stated performance and price alone. The technical specifications are a good place to begin but insufficient to make the final decision. Clinical PET images are generally substantially spatially filtered and thus have considerably lower reconstructed resolution than that quoted by the manufacturers, which is obtained using a Ramp filter. The type of processing that delivers the best resolution may not be at all suitable for routine clinical use because the resulting images contain too much noise, making lesions difficult to detect.

During the decision-making process it is important that clinical images be reviewed at a site that is routinely using the PET/CT system under consideration to determine whether their quality is satisfactory. In the authors' experience, site visits and examining all the images that have been obtained in the 2 days before the site visit can be quite valuable because they likely represent the typical daily range of quality seen in practice. In a well-chosen site, these images will be representative of the spectrum of practice, and are, as a rule, more useful than the best-case studies shown in a sales or marketing demonstration.

The PET Component of the PET/CT Scanner

PET images are of high overall quality. One must be, however, careful not to judge too much from scans of normal patients. Moderately "noisy" images can be better for interpretation than excessively digitally smoothed pictures because smaller tumors may potentially be better detected. A common pitfall is for interpreting physicians to "like" the appearance of a highly smoothed image. Such images may, however, fail to detect small cancer foci. Examination of studies performed in large patients with small tumor foci is a good test of whole body imaging. It is also suggested that images of a variety of areas of the body be examined.

Centers that expect referral of a large number of studies for neurological indications should carefully consider the available options for brain imaging. The challenges of detecting pathology in the brain require acquisition of highest quality, highest resolution images, most commonly using a three-dimensional (3D) protocol. A 3D study acquisition uses events with lines of response (LOR) that are not perpendicular to the principal axis, with the path of the annihilation photons crossing several slices. The major advantage of 3D acquisitions is related to the fact that many more coincidence events are acceptable, and therefore many more counts are collected.

If radiation therapy planning using PET is part of the predicted use in a specific institution, a suitable flat table and appropriate laser systems may need to be part of the purchase considerations. Observation of the specific setups must be made to determine how best to proceed. Additional practical questions can address the size of the bore diameter of the scanner. The size of the bore will determine whether the device will be able to handle large patients and those who are in the treatment position for radiation therapy studies. It should be remembered, however, that, in general, because of angular sampling considerations, the larger the detector ring diameter of the PET scanner, the lower the sensitivity and resolution. Time of flight (TOF) scanners may potentially improve the performance of PET scanners by assisting the tomographic reconstruction algorithm to reduce the statistical noise in the reconstructed image and to increase the capability to resolve structures deep inside large objects. This may help get around the earlier mentioned problem concerning reconstructed resolution. These scanners are at present quite limited in their ability to pinpoint the precise location of an annihilation event based on timing.

The detection issues for myocardial perfusion PET studies are substantially different from those related to the brain or torso. Rb82 imaging is a major challenge because the tracer has a very short half-life of 76 seconds and therefore allows only a short period of time for image acquisition. The tracer must clear from the bloodstream to the myocardium, then be imaged, ideally with enough counts to allow for gating to be performed. Very high count rates early on and low count rates at later times are typical for Rb82 studies. These demands are substantial, and image quality is strongly dependent on the technical performance of the system, including sensitivity, count rate performance, and scatter fraction.

Thus, to achieve high-quality PET/CT studies, the PET component of the PET/CT scanner must be able to handle the type of applications anticipated at the specific center. If a center will perform a large number of cardiac PET studies, the scanner selected should be examined for its suitability to that specific application. Similarly, if brain or tumor imaging is the goal, assessment should also be made based on the worst-case scenarios to be certain image quality is adequate across a wide range of clinical settings; for example, looking at studies performed in small children; small brain lesions; or tumor detectability in the small, medium, and large patients. As discussed later, the specific software for display and analysis is of critical importance.

The CT Component of the PET/CT

Although most PET/CT systems are being used for a larger fraction of their total patient imaging time for PET, the choice of the CT component is also extremely important. A single- or several-slice CT system is likely to meet the diagnostic needs on the CT side for localization of the PET data (if only noncontrast CT scans are done). Such systems can, however, cause stair-step artifacts on the CT coronal images and do not offer optimal CT angiography.

In the United States, where the standard of diagnostic care in imaging is multislice CT, a trend is emerging toward a "one-stop shop" in which a high-quality PET is combined with a diagnostic-quality CT scan for cancer applications. Diagnostic CT is increasingly performed using intravenous contrast, particularly in locations such as the head and neck. Visualization of the vascular anatomy in this area can be helpful to hasten the reading of the study and is likely to improve study accuracy compared with PET alone. Most PET/CT systems are now being offered with multislice scanners, which are more suitable for diagnostic CT studies than the single-slice devices previously used. CT scanners with a range of slice numbers ranging from 1, 2, 4, 6, 8, 16, 40, to 64 and perhaps more including flat-panel detectors are now offered. This range in CT choices is wide, and with more slices come more costs for acquisition and maintenance.

Additional considerations on the CT side include whether the processing software is acceptable for the commonly planned applications. If purchasers plan to use a PET/CT system for a specific application, it is highly reasonable that they observe that functionality in practice. For example, if CT angiography or multiphase contrast studies are considered, these functions must be carefully investigated as a part of the decision-making process.

Increased attention has been paid to radiation absorbed dose from the CT study. This dose can be modulated automatically by many vendors' CT systems. It is suggested that this important feature be considered as one of the major elements in the purchase decision.

The Integrated PET/CT System

Although there are established criteria for assessing the technical performance of both the PET and CT systems, another key issue is the integration level of these two components into the hybrid imaging device. The "workflow" for performing a PET/CT study must be examined, as well as the ease with which the images are reconstructed. If reconstruction is very slow, it may limit the ability of the PET/CT system to generate the workflow required for the system to be cost-effective.

Another issue in workflow assessment is related to image interpretation. During the evaluation process, it is important to assess the ease with which the studies are loaded to the interpreting physician's workstation. Similarly, the ease of interaction to view the diagnostic quality CT, PET, and PET/CT-fused images must be ascertained. PET/CT images should load quickly and scroll rapidly for suitable image assessments. A dedicated workstation should be connected to the PET/CT device to perform this application well enough, even under high workloads.

It is important to understand how older images can be assessed and correlated with the current study. As increasing numbers of PET/CT studies are performed for cancer, we anticipate that there will be a need for more comparisons with previous images. It is important that the software and hardware support of the PET/CT system be able to deal with the clinical demands anticipated in the individual practice setting. Specifically, system support of dual-monitor or large-screen display is desired. Methods for determining simple quantitative parameters such as the standard uptake value (SUV) or SUV normalized to lean body mass should be evaluated as a part of the purchase decision.

When selecting a PET/CT system, consideration with respect to the software choice needs to include assessment of several features. Integrating the image acquisition software with the information system of the radiology department is useful to generate a work list that will eliminate many clerical errors such as misspelling of names and transposition of identification numbers, which can occur with manual study entry. This will avoid difficulties that may occur when trying to retrieve old studies to compare with those currently performed.

The flow of digital data from the workstation to a picture archive and communications system (PACS) is important. For example, decisions on whether to maintain old studies on a PACS system or on an optical disk need to be made. In larger centers, the PACS solution is recommended, and it is critical to verify that the PET/CT system will transmit both the PET and CT files to the PACS system suitably. A reliable archival and transferring system is crucial to the smooth running of the clinic as volumes of studies expand. This assessment must be made in the context of each institution's PACS system. It is important to understand fully how the PET/CT data are transferred to a radiation therapy planning computer workstation. Verifying the network connectivity and the presence and functionality of key image display, and hardware and software is essential and is vendor- and application-dependent. For example if cardiac PET/CT is performed, a much different software analytical package is required compared with the display of static whole body PET images.

A challenge is currently represented by the delivery of images to referring physicians in a format suitable for their viewing of all data, including PET, CT, and fused images. Although ideally it would be best for the referring physician to be able to view the fused studies via PACS, this is not yet commonly available. Other options such as printed films or a CD or DVD burned for each patient can represent potential alternatives. The solution may vary by center, but as volumes grow, cost-effective solutions are critical. Several vendors offer software that will allow the entire study to be transferred to CD. In this format, physicians will be able to view the complete study on their computers. After the initial purchase of the software, this is, in our experience, a cost-effective approach, especially if many of the referring physicians are located at a distance from the PET/CT system and thus do not have access to the PACs system.

Decisions on purchase of expensive devices such as PET/CT are made based on a wide variety of considerations. Purchase price is obviously important, but the history of "uptime," with the PET/CT system in working conditions without breakdown, for a specific scanner is also crucial. The quality of the local service is therefore important, and it is often valuable to determine from a nearby site with the same equipment what its service experience has been. Service contracts can, or at least should, help ensure uptime of the PET/CT device. Pricing for service varies and will be a substantial expense over many years. Many centers choose to have a comprehensive service agreement from the supplier for repairs and routine maintenance, as well as phone support for minor problems. Some centers with extensive on-site expertise may choose to maintain the scanners themselves, possibly only receiving the parts from the vendors through a special service agreement. Price and time of service are critical considerations. High uptime is required for PET/CT to be a reliable and useful technique. Timely service should be available.

Finally, considerations regarding the overall make up of imaging equipment at a specific center must enter into a purchase decision. If all the scanners in the department are brand A and the PET/CT scanner is brand B, this may carry with it some disadvantages as regards pricing and service related to economies of scale. Regardless of the approach chosen for service, a regular preventive maintenance program should be in place including ongoing calibrations of the PET component.

PET/CT Quality Assurance

With the purchase and installation of a PET/CT scanner, a series of "acceptance" tests are performed on the device to ensure it performs properly, with both the CT and PET components being assessed. In addition, the unique software and alignment between the PET and the CT components are evaluated in this early stage.

Although it is beyond the scope of this atlas to discuss the full spectrum of acceptance testing, some of the tests performed on the PET component of the scanner include sensitivity, spatial resolution, count rate performance, scatter fraction, and the performance of a variety of reconstruction methods. For scanners with both two-dimensional (2D) and 3D acquisition capabilities, the availability, accuracy, and processing times of both methods should be assessed. The reader should recall that the resolution of PET scanners is not uniform across the field of view, and resolution is commonly determined in the center of the field of view and off the central axis of the patient.

The American National Electrical Manufacturer Association (NEMA) has described a fairly substantial body of testing that should be performed to ensure that the device performs at the levels specified by the vendor. Because so much PET is now performed for oncology, scatter correction algorithms and scatter fraction measurement using humanlike phantoms are of clinical significance.

The quality control of CT scanners at the time of acceptance testing is well established. The CT scanner delivers a significant amount of radiation to the patient with each image, and it is important that the output of the x-ray tube be carefully validated for proper estimates of radiation energy deposition to patients. Testing the CT scanner includes assessment of resolution and of the quantitative accuracy of the measurement of Hounsfield units in a variety of tissue simulators such as water, air, or bone.

After the PET and CT are shown to be performing properly as individual units, the performance of the entire system is further assessed. Because most modern PET/CT systems depend on the CT scan for attenuation correction, it is critical that both components function properly for the entire system to provide quantitatively accurate results for patient imaging.

A unique aspect of the acceptance testing for a PET/CT system is the need to verify the alignment between the PET and the CT scanner. All currently available PET/CT scanners have the PET and CT components of the scanner offset by 25 cm or more in the axial direction. All degrees of freedom representing the angular relationships of the two scanners must be physically optimized and then electronically aligned, or the images of the same structure on PET and on CT will not be superimposed. In addition to these considerations, the table must be precisely aligned for both devices and travel in a straight line.

Generally, it is not possible to achieve perfection in the PET and CT alignment by mechanical methods alone. Software corrections are typically implemented and may differ by system. Suffice it to say, however, that if the PET and CT are not well aligned, the advantages inherent to PET/CT could be lost. We recommend assessing alignment at several areas on the scanning table with varying weights applied to the table because some can distort or bend under heavy loads. All manufacturers have methods allowing for such assessments, involving acquisition of phantom studies with both radioactive and radioopaque components so that they can be detected by both PET and CT.

In addition to misregistration between lesions on PET and CT images resulting from devices that are not aligned properly, there can also be artifacts and alterations in the quantitative accuracy of PET, which depends on the CT scan for attenuation correction.

Following the intensive quality control performed when a PET/CT is accepted, the high level of initial performance must be maintained. Not uncommonly, PET scanners can slowly drift away from the optimal imaging performance characteristics, as opposed to suddenly failing. This mild drifting can be recognized through implementation of a regular daily and weekly quality control program. The intensity of this type of assessment can vary by center, but a regular quality control program should be in place. Some centers performing only oncology studies may not be concerned with the "absolute sensitivity" of the scanner, but they really should be; absolute sensitivity is required to calculate properly quantitative parameters such as SUV or SUV-lean, increasingly used in lesion characterization and tumor response assessment.

Daily quality control can be brief, limited to checking the uniformity of the CT component and verifying that all modules in the PET scanner are operational. Some centers check camera sensitivity daily, others weekly or slightly less often, depending on the historical performance of the scanner. The sensitivity parameter, expressed as counts/uCi/cc, is important and should be routinely and regularly monitored to guard against variable fluctuating sensitivity. Sensitivity can vary with temperature fluctuations because the detector crystals are somewhat temperature-dependent in their outputs. Thus, proper environmental controls for the scanners are essential to be certain the room temperature does not vary substantially from day to day.

The frequency and kind of recalibrations that are necessary on a routine basis depend on the particular scanner design but may include the following. On a weekly basis, a photomultiplier (PMT) gain calibration should be performed, as well as a coincidence timing calibration (CTC). The PMT gain will fine-tune the high voltage applied to each PET module, readjusting until all modules register the same amount of activity. Even if the daily blank scan appears visually satisfactory, some modules may have drifted, and this procedure will reset their values. The CTC controls which counts will be accepted. This calibration sets the permissible delay between coincident events that will be counted in the image. Once this is complete, a 30-minute or longer blank scan is performed and installed. This correction will be applied to all scans, and thus it is important to repeat this every time the PMT gain is done. The resolution of the CT along with the alignment of the PET and CT systems should be regularly monitored. We believe this determination should be made quarterly or any time there has been a mechanical alteration to the PET/CT scanning system.

Patient Preparation for PET/CT Studies

Although practice varies by center, it is recommended that the supervising or interpreting physician conduct a brief or more detailed history and review of patient records to ascertain the reasons the PET study has been requested. Special attention to recent surgery, infection, chemotherapy, granulocyte colony stimulating factor treatments, and radiation therapy are critical.

For fluorodeoxyglucose (FDG)-PET/CT imaging to detect cancer, optimal images are obtained when serum glucose levels are low. In a nondiabetic patient, this occurs after several hours or even overnight fasting. Blood glucose should be monitored before the PET/CT study and should be under 200 mg/dl, and ideally under 150 mg/dl, to perform the study. High glucose levels can result in a competitive inhibition of FDG uptake in tumors and an artificially low SUV, potentially decreasing tumor visualization. In addition, elevated insulin levels will increase FDG uptake into muscles.

Extensive exercise should be avoided the day before the PET scan is performed to minimize normal muscle uptake of the radiotracer. In our experience, it is important to have a telephone discussion with patients the day before the PET scan to ensure they are fully and appropriately informed of the proper preparations for the PET study.

Additional instructions for preparation are necessary with patients who are diabetic, who have multiple studies, or who are inpatients. Direct communication with the nursing staff is essential. Ideally, there should be no insulin given for several hours before the FDG injection. This is a very basic guideline because large variation exists in patients and the insulin regimen they are using. Patients who use a regular insulin sliding-scale dose often take their last injection the evening before the test. It is preferable that they have a morning appointment to have the blood sugar at the appropriate range, even if it is somewhat elevated. For brittle diabetic patients, it is may be indicated to have them eat some food in the morning, give a dose of short-acting insulin, and then inject at 3–4 hours after insulin dosing. In this way, the blood glucose would be under control, but serum insulin levels would have declined into the normal range. Every diabetic patient is different; it is important to speak with the patients and their physician to get an understanding of their normal blood sugar fluctuations to determine an appropriate examination time.

Patients are often scheduled for more than one test on the same day, and these should be reviewed to avoid any problems. A not uncommon problem is the exercise cardiac stress test. Patients should not have any strenuous exercise the day previous to and certainly not immediately before a PET scan because this will create a great deal of muscle uptake and degrade the images. Another common problem can be CT scanning. If 3D or CT angiography of the abdomen is planned, oral contrast material given as a part of a typical PET/CT preparation may degrade the images of these examinations and make it impossible to segregate out the relevant vessels. An alternative preparation protocol can be instituted; for example, water can be given as an alternative to radio-opaque oral contrast for the PET/CT study. This can allow for subsequent CT angiography to be performed without technical mishap. For these reasons, full knowledge of patients' imaging plans and history are essential.

For inpatients, it is critical that the PET center be in regular contact with the patient care floor to be certain the preparatory instructions are conveyed properly. It is wise to call again in the morning of the scheduled study to be sure that the message was passed to the next shift. All intravenous (IV) drips containing dextrose solution and any total parenteral nutrition should be stopped 4 hours before FDG injection. All patients should be instructed to eat or drink nothing but water (NPO) for 4–6 hours prior to the test.

Several steps should be considered when preparing patients for scanning. The environment, physical preparation, and injection are all important to the final outcome. The room where the patients will spend their uptake phase should be quiet, warm, and dimly lit. A comfortable chair will also assist in keeping the patient still and relaxed. Rooms should be warm and blankets provided to limit the amount of brown fat that is stimulated by the cold environment and thus visualized in the scan. The goal is to keep patients from moving or talking, so it is advisable to keep family and friends out of the room unless the patient is a minor.

For administration of FDG and CT contrast, some centers require an accurate weight estimate to adjust doses accordingly. All patients should be weighed when arriving for the study. Oral contrast may be given to improve the overall quality of the CT. It will help to differentiate some of the abdominal anatomy and localize sites of disease by separating them from normal bowel activity. One recommended protocol is to use a dilute barium solution (1.3% barium sulfate), which will sufficiently fill the bowel yet be fairly well tolerated. A patient who is 150 pounds (~70 kg) or less receives 525 ml before injection and 175 ml at about

two thirds of the way through the uptake period. A larger patient will have 700 ml initially and 350 ml toward the end of uptake time. Other protocols can include using water as the oral contrast medium (negative contrast).

At roughly the same time the patient is drinking the contrast, the IV should be placed. A relatively large-bore IV (22 g) should be used to minimize the occurrence of infiltration and should be flushed immediately before use to ensure its patency.

The FDG injection should be weight based. A dose of 0.22 mCi/kg (0.1 mCi/lb) is a standard dose for whole body scanning at our institutions using a 2D acquisition protocol and a BGO (bismuth germanate) scanner. Lower doses may be suitable for 3D imaging. With this injected dose, an acquisition time of about 4–5 minutes per bed position (15 cm axial field of view) is typical. A patient who requires a scan ranging from head to toe can receive a 30% larger (0.29 mCi/kg) dose to accommodate the increased scan length. This allows the technologist to reduce the field acquisition time because of the increased count rate. Pediatric patients receive 30% less than the normal adult dose to limit their exposure. With 2D scanning, the maximum injected dose should not exceed 25 mCi regardless of patient weight. There are several approaches to dosing. Some institutions use a standard mCi dose, such as 10 mCi. If this is done, longer acquisition times are suggested to provide adequate statistical quality to the images. Weight-based scan duration may be more appropriate for 3D.

An accurate record of the injected dose, along with the residual amount in the syringe, should be kept for entry into the scanner. This information, along with the patient weight, height, and injection and assay times, will be applied to the images to create the SUV measurements. The uptake period begins immediately after injection and typically lasts 50–60 minutes for most whole body oncologic studies. In some centers, even longer uptake times are used, such as 90 minutes to 2 hours, to increase the tumor-to-background ratio. Such times provide suitable images but often have a slightly lower statistical quality than scans begun 1 hour after tracer injection. In a given center, so that sequential studies are quantitatively interpretable, it is recommended that the same duration of uptake time be used in each case. A 45-minute uptake time on the patient's first study and a 2-hour uptake on the second do not represent good clinical choices. Such differences make comparisons difficult.

The previous procedure preparation protocol should be altered for patients who have a head and neck cancer and those who are having a brain-only scan. If the primary focus is in the face or neck, oral contrast may not be given to minimize swallowing and any possible related muscle uptake. Patients performing brain PET with 3D acquisition should receive only 10 mCi of FDG, and the uptake period can be shortened to 30 minutes. A modified protocol may apply for different scanner designs and operating modes. Eye patches and earplugs should be applied to minimize regional brain stimulation. There is not uniform agreement on this point, however, but the uptake methodology should be consistent. No oral contrast administration is required.

Performing the PET/CT Study

After the uptake phase is completed, the patient is ready to be scanned. At this time, the patient should remove all metal accessories and use the restroom to empty the bladder. In most instances, whole body scans should be performed in the caudocranial direction to avoid excessive bladder filling with radioactive FDG during imaging. This protocol may be changed in patients in whom the major pathology is expected in the region of the head and neck, because minor, even involuntary movements can occur over a 15- to 20-minute imaging interval and may impair precise fusion of PET and CT data. Acquisition protocols at our centers differ for head and neck cancer versus whole body imaging for chest or abdomen disease. One option for performing studies in patients with cancer of the head and neck includes a two-part acquisition: first a caudo-to-cranial scan starting at midthigh and extending to the supraclavicular region, with the arms placed above the head to minimize artifacts, and second, an arms-down PET/CT acquisition of the region of the head and neck. This latter acquisition can be followed by a diagnostic-quality CT contrast study to optimize visualization of the head and neck vascular structures and to best separate those structures from small FDG avid lymph nodes. If whole body imaging with contrast is required, a whole body contrast CT scan can also be obtained using the relevant imaging parameters.

Time should be taken to arrange the patient on the bed before imaging to minimize discomfort. This may cut down on the amount of motion artifact that is encountered. Many devices are available to help immobilize the patient. Careful immobilization of the head is required to have the appropriate registration needed for high-quality head and neck cancer imaging.

The use of IV contrast is growing in frequency at many PET centers. It is known that with some systems, IV and high-density oral contrast can cause artifacts of "overattenuation correction," which can degrade PET images substantially. This problem has been addressed to a considerable extent in newer PET/CT systems, but the safest approach to PET/CT imaging with IV contrast, if accurate quantitation is required, remains performing a lower powered CT scan at the outset of the PET study for attenuation correction. After the acquisition of the emission PET component is terminated, the contrast study can be performed for selected relevant areas of the body using the appropriate CT contrast infusion protocol for the region under study. In this way, although radiation dose is increased in the areas that have contrast CT and the low mA noncontrast study, the overall radiation to the patient from CT is probably reduced, because one typically does not need to perform contrast CT scans at high quality in all segments. As far as contrast-induced quantitative artifacts, they are directly related to the Hounsfield Units (HU) of the contrast on the enhanced CT component, if it is used for attenuation correction. The higher the HU of CT, the greater the potential overestimation of activity in the contrast-enhanced area on the PET/CT. This is, however, a controversial issue, and some advocate using the contrast CT for attenuation correction.

Before the patient is discharged from the PET center, it must be determined whether the PET and CT images are of adequate technical quality and whether they have provided the diagnostic information required. Although reimaging is not commonly necessary, if there has been patient motion, or if there remains a concern in separating an FDG-filled ureter from retroperitoneal lymph nodes, repeat imaging of a small or larger portion of the body can be performed. Our most common repeat image is in the abdomen and pelvis, where there is a question of residual urine versus FDG-avid tumor.

SPECT/CT IMAGING

SPECT/CT systems use the same single photon emission computed tomography (SPECT) component as for dedicated nuclear medicine systems—conventional dual-head gamma cameras for planar and tomographic imaging of single-photon emitting radionuclides. First-generation clinical SPECT/CT systems used a low dose, low axial resolution CT detector, whereas recently developed, second-generation SPECT/CT systems incorporate a variety of multislice CT scanners.

SPECT/CT Imaging Devices

The design of SPECT/CT systems is based on separate x-ray and radionuclide devices using a common mechanical gantry to maintain a consistent spatial relationship between the two data sets. Integration of SPECT and x-ray imaging presents challenges that are not met in the design of single modality technologies but that are nearly identical to those of PET/CT. In a dual-modality system, SPECT detectors are offset in the axial direction from the plane of the x-ray source and detector. This offset can be relatively small when a modest x-ray tube is used but can reach more than 60 cm in SPECT/CT systems using a diagnostic CT scanner.

SPECT/CT systems have to enable both detector types to rotate and position accurately for tomographic imaging. Accuracy of translation and angular motion differ among imaging systems. The highest accuracy of motion is required by the CT system, with up to 1000 angular samples acquired for submillimeter accuracy. SPECT has a spatial resolution of a few millimeters, and therefore translation and angular motion can be performed with an accuracy of slightly less than a millimeter for clinical imaging.

In SPECT/CT systems using a low-dose single- or multislice CT, SPECT and CT detectors are mounted on the same rotating platform, and imaging is performed while rotating sequentially around the patient. This concept has the advantage that both imaging modalities can be performed using the same gantry as for a conventional gamma camera. However, this design limits the rotational speed of the dual modality imaging to approximately 20 seconds per rotation. In SPECT/CT systems incorporating diagnostic CT scanners, the gamma camera detectors have to be mounted on a different platform, separated from the high-speed rotating CT device (0.25–0.5 sec/revolution). This design increases the performance of the CT subsystem, while also increasing the complexity of the gantry and the cost of the technology.

The patient scanning table plays an important role in SPECT/CT imaging because tandem x-ray and radionuclide imaging requires longer patient stretchers. These tables are built to support patients weighing up to 500 pounds. They do, however, deflect to some degree while loaded with normal adult patients and extended to accommodate the needs of both components. The extension and degree of deflection of the table can differ for x-ray and SPECT imaging introducing a patient-dependent misregistration between the two types of data. Several solutions to this problem have been implemented. One possibility consists in using a patient table, which is supported on its base at the front of the scanner and has a secondary support at the far end of the x-ray system, thus minimizing the table deflection. Another solution is to use a table fixed on a base, moving on the floor to introduce the patient into the scanner. Because the patient platform is stationary relative to its support structure, the

same deflection of the patient table occurs for both modalities.

SPECT/CT devices incorporate workstations that are responsible for system control, data acquisition, image reconstruction and display, and data processing and analysis. SPECT/CT systems have to calibrate the CT data to obtain attenuation correction maps for the SPECT images. SPECT and CT images are displayed using single or dual screen options in addition to the fused images that represent the overlay of a colored SPECT over a gray-scale CT image. Commercially available software packages perform 3D display and triangulation, allowing the user to locate lesions and sites of interest, by placing the cursor on the CT image and redisplaying its location on registered SPECT and fused SPECT/CT images. Workstations used for SPECT/CT imaging should respond to the same criteria as those previously described for PET/CT. The ease of processing, viewing, comparison with previous studies, PACS archiving and retrieval, as well as transferring images to referring physicians, are all important issues that need to be addressed, as for PET/CT.

SPECT/CT Acquisition Protocols

Data acquisition on SPECT/CT systems is performed in a sequential mode. With devices that have a low-dose CT component, data are typically acquired by rotating the x-ray detector 220 degrees around the patient, with the x-ray tube operated at 120–140 kV and 1–2.5 mA. The CT images that are produced have an in-plane spatial resolution of 2.5 mm and of 5–10 mm in the axial direction. Scan time is of 14 seconds per slice, leading to a total study duration of 5–10 minutes for the entire set of CT data. SPECT/CT systems using diagnostic CT are characterized by faster scanning times, which are, however, also accompanied by higher radiation doses. Reconstruction of CT images are performed "on the fly." While acquiring data from one slice, the former slice is being reconstructed. An attenuation map is created at the end of the CT acquisition time.

A dual-headed, variable-angle sodium-iodide scintillation camera identical to those incorporated in state-of-the-art stand-alone SPECT systems is used. The detectors are placed either in a 180-degree position for imaging of the torso or in a 90-degree position for myocardial perfusion studies. Regardless of the commercial SPECT/CT device used, SPECT acquisition requires the currently routine scanning time of approximately 10–30 minutes, depending on the imaged radiotracer, similar to routine stand-alone SPECT studies. Radionuclide SPECT images are reconstructed using iterative methods such as ordered subset expectation maximization (OSEM), incorporating photon attenuation correction using the x-rays transmission map and also scatter correction. Various novel reconstruction algorithms are currently under investigation in academic centers and the industry. In the near future, these may allow for a shorter SPECT acquisition time of less than 50% of current protocols.

Because x-ray and radionuclide data are not acquired simultaneously, SPECT images are not contaminated by scatter radiation generated during the x-ray image acquisition. Also, because the patient is not removed from the table, both imaging components are acquired with a consistent and identical patient position, allowing accurate image registration if we assume that the relative geometrical locations of both sets of reconstructed data are known and the patient can hold still for the lengthy duration of the SPECT/CT study. CT is usually acquired in matrices of 512×512 with the newer CT scanners or 256×256 in the first-generation devices and has to be resized into slices with the same pixel format and slice width as SPECT. Spatial registration of the CT and SPECT is important because misalignment of the attenuation map relative to corresponding radionuclide images can cause "edge artifacts," expressed as bright and dark "rims" across edges of the problematic regions.

Several challenges may potentially limit the clinical use of SPECT/CT. One well-known problem occurs when the patient moves between the SPECT and CT image acquisitions. Image misregistration or blurring may also occur due to respiration, cardiac motion, and peristalsis. Differences in urinary bladder filling can also lead to erroneous coregistration between SPECT and CT acquisitions. With SPECT/CT devices equipped with low-dose x-ray tubes, CT is performed during shallow breathing, which facilitates image registration. At the same time, however, the longer acquisition time increases the chances for patient motion. With hybrid devices equipped with multislice CT components, transmission data are acquired following breath-hold, during tidal breathing, or during a short part of the respiratory cycle, whereas SPECT data are acquired over several minutes with the patient breathing quietly. This again can lead to misregistration artifacts due to anatomic displacements of the diaphragm and chest wall. In addition to errors in localization, nonregistered attenuation maps can lead to an under- or overestimate of radionuclide uptake in the reconstructed emission data.

The presence of contrast media administered for CT examinations complicates the attenuation correction process because the rescaling of the CT data from x-ray to nuclear medicine energies may not accurately account for the presence of contrast material. Furthermore, high concentrations of intravenous contrast material captured during the CT acquisition may have redistributed by the time the SPECT acquisition is performed. Resulting artifacts are more severe when the administered contrast media is more concentrated, as in the case of abdominal imaging after the patient swallows a bolus of oral contrast. Image segmentation techniques separating different areas inside the images may solve this problem. An alternative approach is a very low-powered noncontrast CT for attenuation correction only, performed before the SPECT scan and the contrast CT study.

SPECT/CT Quality Assurance

After the purchase and installation of a SPECT/CT device, acceptance tests are performed to ensure proper performance of both the CT and SPECT components. The performance assessment tests for SPECT include evaluation of uniformity, resolution and linearity, energy resolution, and count density, performed routinely on every gamma camera according to the NEMA criteria. A full set of tests should be performed at this point to ensure that the device performs at the appropriate level.

Following initial testing, a maintenance program schedule should be put in place for ongoing quality control and calibrations of the scanner. Quality control tests for CT are well established. Because CT delivers a significant amount of radiation energy to the patient with each exposure, it is important that the output of the x-ray tube be carefully estimated.

One of the main issues with installing and operating a SPECT/CT device includes quality control tests that need to be performed routinely to check CT to SPECT registration and verify the accuracy of alignment between the two scanners. The registration tests represent the most important step in the assessment of a SPECT/CT device. One means to determine this is to use a test performed using a special alignment phantom, built from low attenuation material with holes for placing six syringes filled with a radionuclide source, technetium99m (Tc99m) or any other isotope. These sources serve as landmarks for measuring the distance between CT and SPECT data. These values reflect the actual system's performance and are then compared with recommended acceptance limits. If they are within these limits, the CT/SPECT registration is acceptable. Otherwise, the operators must perform the x-ray–to–SPECT calibration procedure. This test must be executed separately for every collimator set that is used on the system. In practice, because it is not possible to achieve a perfect mechanical alignment between the two scanners, electronic corrections are performed. These may differ by system and by vendor. It is recommended to check the alignment at several points on the scanning table, and with varying weights applied, because there are various degrees of bending and distortions with different types of stretchers. All manufacturers provide methods and instructions for this evaluation, which typically involve the use of phantoms with both radioactive and radio-opaque content that can be detected by both SPECT and CT and allow for realignment when needed.

The most important problem, resulting in inaccurate attenuation correction, is count deficiency in transmission data. Comparison of emission images reconstructed using low- and high-count x-ray maps showed differences leading to severe diagnostic errors. Because patients vary significantly in shape and size of the body and of internal organs, artifacts may differ from person to person. It is important that the attenuation maps always be viewed and checked for artifacts before attenuation-corrected images are fully trusted in the diagnostic process.

General Nuclear Medicine SPECT/CT Procedures

The SPECT component of the SPECT/CT procedure is performed using the routine acquisition protocols for the dual-head gamma camera. This device is equipped with collimators adequate for the specific radioisotope in use, such as low-energy, high-resolution parallel-hole collimators for Tc99m, or medium-energy collimators for gallium67, indium111, or iodine131. Imaging is typically performed with the detectors facing each other; 120 projections are typically acquired over a 360-degree orbit, into a 64×64 matrix for the low-count isotopes and 128×128 for Tc99m, using a time per projection of 40–50 seconds.

CT images are obtained immediately following the SPECT acquisition. For the low-dose multislice CT devices, the acquisition parameters include settings at 140 kV, 1–2.5 mA, 14 seconds per slice, 256×256 image matrix, and 5-mm slice thickness and slice spacing. For diagnostic CT acquisitions, the settings are 120–140 kV, 80–300 mAs, 1 second per slice, 512×512 image matrix, 48-cm reconstruction diameter, and 1–5-mm slice thickness and slice spacing. A variety of other settings are possible depending on the specific diagnostic question asked of the CT study. Data are reconstructed using filtered back-projection software and filters provided by the manufacturer.

Coregistered CT and SPECT are acquired by translating the patient from one detector to the other while the patient remains lying on the same table. This allows the CT and radionuclide images to be acquired with a consistent scanner geometry and body habitus and with a minimal delay between the two acquisitions. In none of the commercial systems are SPECT and CT obtained precisely simultaneously.

Cardiac SPECT/CT Procedures

Attenuation correction plays an important role in cardiac imaging. If accurately performed, attenuation correction can help resolve false-positive defects commonly caused by soft-tissue attenuation during myocardial perfusion imaging. Although guidelines of the American Society of Nuclear Cardiology recommend that attenuation correction should be performed in all patients, clearly some patient populations benefit more from this procedure—generally the largest patients. Depending on equipment availability and daily workload, the rest SPECT study is used in some centers as the criterion for triage decisions for performing attenuation correction acquisition.

CT-based attenuation correction is reported as providing the most reliable and accurate high-quality cardiac SPECT images through high-resolution, high-count-rate, and low noise-attenuation maps, resulting in predictable uniform tracer activity in patients with less likelihood of hemodynamically significant coronary artery disease. The CT-based attenuation correction method can be successfully implemented with all clinical cardiac SPECT protocols, including same-day or 2-day, single- and dual-isotope rest–stress procedures.

Cardiac SPECT is performed using a dual-head gamma camera equipped with low-energy, high-resolution parallel-hole collimators, with the detectors at 90 degrees to each other. The acquisition is performed over a 180-degree orbit during a period of 12–20 minutes. Dual-isotope acquisition uses thallium201 (Tl201) for rest and Tc99m methoxyisobutyl isonitrile (MIBI) or tetrofosmin for stress, whereas single-isotope acquisition uses the same isotope Tc99m MIBI or tetrofosmin for both rest and stress. For Tl201, imaging energy windows of 30% and 20% for the peaks of 70 keV and 167 keV, respectively, are being used, whereas the energy window width for Tc99m is 20% for the peak of 140 keV. Both rest and stress SPECT studies are followed by low-dose CT (20–30 mAs, 140 keV for the diagnostic CT, or 1–2.5 mA, 140 keV for a camera-mounted CT) used for correcting the emission data for photon attenuation. The CT-attenuation correction study is performed only over the area of the heart, as defined by the technologist. The patient is asked not to move during study progression to obtain good coregistration between the emission and the transmission scans.

In assessing the probability of significant coronary artery disease, it is important to know whether a mild reduction in the anterior wall tracer activity is due to breast attenuation or coronary disease involving the left anterior descending artery. Similar examples involve decreased uptake in the inferior wall, which may be related to attenuation by the diaphragm or abnormal regional perfusion. Obese patients represent a major group in whom CT-based attenuation correction is recommended. Reliable attenuation correction enhances clinical decision making significantly, decreases morbidity related to invasive procedures, and saves costs related to additional workup induced by equivocal reports.

High-speed multislice coronary CT has a growing impact on assessment of patients with known or suspected coronary artery disease. In the future, combined information with respect to myocardial perfusion data and calcium scoring may enable better stratification of patients with or without ischemic heart disease. In addition, referral algorithms will define patient groups that will benefit from hybrid SPECT/multislice CT imaging of both myocardial perfusion and the anatomy of the coronary tree. SPECT may improve the specificity and positive predictive value of the CT for assessment of the hemodynamic significance of coronary occlusions.

TECHNICAL STAFFING FOR PET/CT AND SPECT/CT

A major tangible asset to the department for proper implementation of novel PET/CT or SPECT/CT procedures is the technologist. In the United States, reimbursement rules have favored outpatient PET/CT imaging over inpatient imaging; thus, many PET centers are no longer hospital based. It is important to take the time to train and educate the technologists so that they can deliver an end product that is of the highest quality. Although it is preferable for the interpreting physician to check technologists' work product directly before the patient leaves the department, in some outpatient settings, technologists must make their own decisions; therefore, they need to be well trained and use robust and reproducible protocols.

In addition to training in nuclear medicine and CT, experience in reviewing scans and being able to identify motion and external artifacts will aid technologists in checking the scan for quality before discharging the patient. Instructing the technologists about pertinent history questions and designing a template to be filled out for each patient will ensure that all of the

clinical information to assist in the reading of the images is available. Training requirements for CT and PET/SPECT technologists differ by state (in the United States) and by country. In some states, less extensive training may be allowed for technologists who perform CT scans for purposes of lesion localization only, whereas full CT training is generally required and appropriate if diagnostic-quality CT scans are being performed that include IV contrast administration as a part of the procedure. In many centers in the United States and Europe, increasing fractions of CT studies are of diagnostic quality and must therefore be performed by personnel well trained in this technology. Under ideal circumstances, a technologist should be fully trained, experienced, and certified in both nuclear and x-ray/CT technologies. Although the risks of contrast reactions are modest, they are nevertheless real, and these procedures should be done when suitably trained physicians are present at the scanning facility.

SUMMARY

A high-quality PET/CT or SPECT/CT scan requires a reliable, well-functioning hybrid scanner that has met acceptance testing criteria and is regularly monitored for quality of performance.

The study must be designed to answer the specific question asked by the referring physician, and the patient must be appropriately educated and compliant with the preparations for the scan, including fasting requirements.

Technical staff must be well trained to perform and monitor the study according to a well-defined protocol that must be carefully followed. The images must be reviewed for technical and diagnostic quality before the patient leaves the department.

Finally, the images must be interpreted by readers skilled in PET or SPECT and CT who are well aware of the clinical history of the patient, using workstations sufficiently optimized to allow integrated viewing of the functional and anatomic data. In this way, a high-quality study can be produced and will consistently provide useful diagnostic information for clinical management and improved patient care. As the quality of CT scanners in PET/CT and SPECT/CT devices improves, it is expected that new applications will emerge in which ever-greater capabilities of the CT component are integrated with PET and SPECT.

PET/CT of the Brain

Richard L. Wahl • Mehrbod Som Javadi

2.1 NORMAL PATTERN

Case 2.1.1 NORMAL PATTERN PET/CT OF THE BRAIN (FIG. 2.1, *A–D*) AND QUANTITATIVE ANALYSIS (FIG. 2.1, *E*)

A

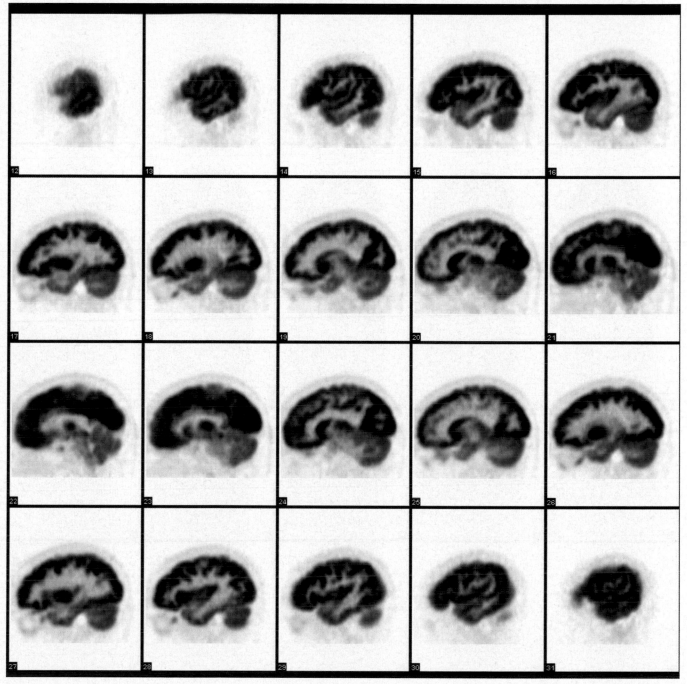

B

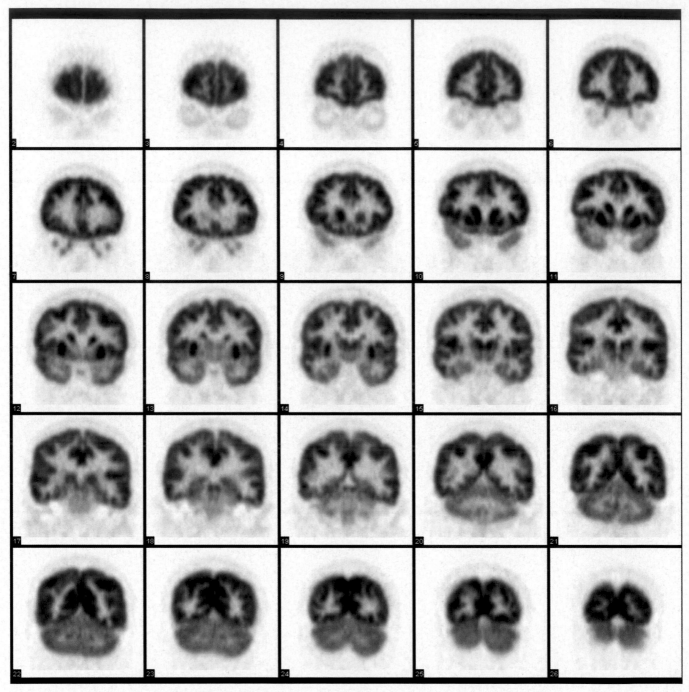

C

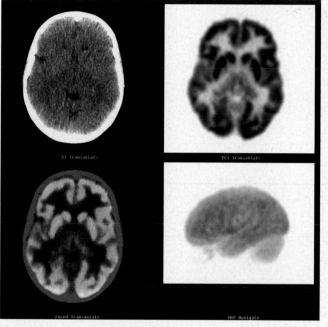

D

Brief History

A 42-year-old patient presented with a history of temporal lobe epilepsy that recently had become difficult to control. Other symptoms included left-sided weakness and headaches, as well as dizziness and loss of balance. There was no evidence of seizure activity before or during the study.

Findings

A–C. Transverse, sagittal, and coronal 2-[18F] fluoro-2-deoxy-D-glucose (FDG) PET images obtained using the three-dimensional (3D) technique show no asymmetry of uptake in the temporal lobes.

D. PET/CT images at the level of the basal ganglia show normal extraocular muscle activity and excellent visualization of the gray matter–white matter interfaces.

E. Quantitative analysis shows an essentially normal map of the brain. The "perfusion defects" at the edge of the brain are not significant and are due to a slight difference in size between a normal brain and the patient's brain.

This is a normal study, as were the correlative CT images.

Main Teaching Points and Summary
1. In this case with normal brain PET images, the major contribution of the CT scan was the attenuation correction.
2. The value of correlative CT imaging is relatively limited in such cases.
3. In patients in whom the brain PET is abnormal, the CT is clearly more contributory to the diagnosis.
4. Coronal images are particularly useful for assessment of the temporal lobes.

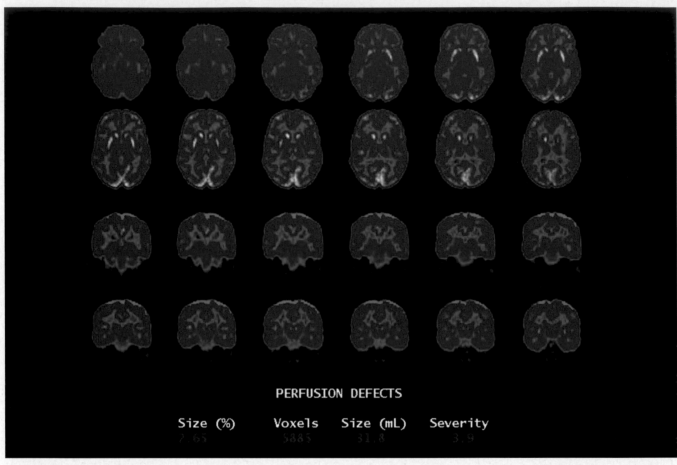

E

2.2 BENIGN ABNORMALITIES

Case 2.2.1 CONGENITAL ENCEPHALOMALACIA AND EPILEPSY (FIG. 2.2.1)

A

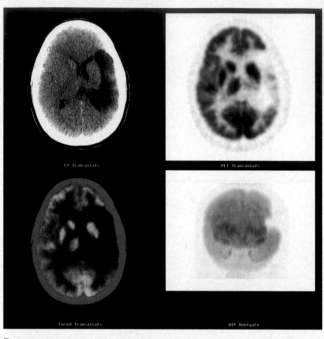

B

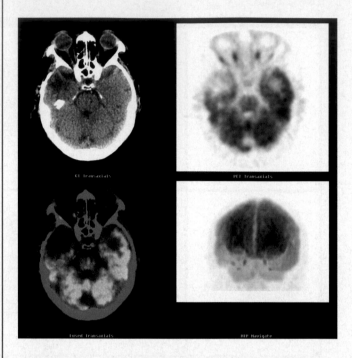

Case 2.2.2 POSTSURGICAL CHANGES (FIG. 2.2.2)

Brief History

A 20-year-old patient had a history of right hemiparesis attributed to intrauterine ischemia and seizures since birth. The seizures had decreased in frequency through childhood after trials with several anticonvulsants. Recently however, the patient has suffered an increase in right-sided jerking and nocturnal seizures.

Findings

A. Multiple transverse PET images show absent FDG activity involving a large part of the left hemisphere. There is also decreased tracer activity in the right temporal lobe, along with a mild reduction in the left cerebellum.

B. PET/CT images demonstrate a large area of absent cortex on CT involving the posterior lateral aspect of left frontal lobe and most of the left parietal lobe, in the distribution of the left middle cerebral artery, and of the left thalamus, which is nearly absent. These anatomic abnormalities also show no FDG uptake. In addition, there is compensatory dilatation of the left lateral ventricle. The findings are consistent with congenital encephalomalacia and interictal right epilepsy.

Main Teaching Points and Summary

1. CT images are extremely helpful for separating anatomic and functional causes of reduced FDG uptake.
2. In this complex case, the reduced right temporal lobe tracer uptake localized the trigger site for seizure activity.
3. The substantial preservation of right cerebellar activity likely reflects plasticity of the central nervous system (CNS) to early birth injury.

Brief History

A 64-year-old patient with a history of lung cancer treated with chemotherapy was diagnosed 18 months later with brain metastases in the right frontal and temporal lobes. Additional chemotherapy was administered, followed by gamma knife radiosurgery. The patient was evaluated for the presence of residual or recurrent cancer.

Findings

PET/CT images show an area of decreased FDG uptake in the region of the right temporal tip, consistent with the site of prior surgical resection and radiation as demonstrated on CT. No residual viable tumor is visualized.

Main Teaching Point and Summary

1. This case is demonstrative of a CT abnormality explaining the reduced FDG uptake.

Case 2.2.3 RADIATION NECROSIS (FIG. 2.2.3)

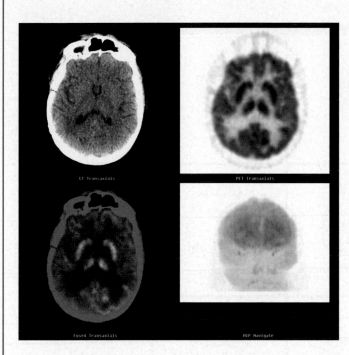

Case 2.3.1 PRIMARY BRAIN TUMOR (FIG. 2.3.1)

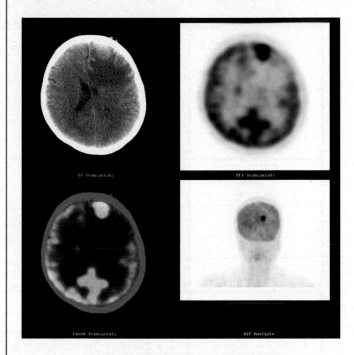

Brief History

A 50-year-old patient underwent resection of a right temporal glioblastoma followed by radiation therapy and adjuvant chemotherapy. Recent brain magnetic resonance imaging (MRI) demonstrates an area of increasing enhancement in the right temporal lobe with surrounding edema. PET/CT was performed to differentiate between radiation necrosis and viable tumor.

Findings

PET/CT images demonstrate mild to moderate decreased FDG activity in the right temporal lobe, in an area corresponding to the site of previous radiation therapy, most likely consistent with postradiation changes. There is also a small, ill-defined area of low attenuation on CT in the site of craniotomy, with corresponding decreased FDG activity.

Main Teaching Points and Summary
1. The findings in this case are most consistent with postoperative changes and radiation necrosis, and not tumor.
2. The abnormal CT indicates that the patient has had a neurosurgical procedure.

Brief History

A 56-year-old patient presented with syncope, headaches, and new-onset aphasia. A recent MRI shows a ring-enhancing mass in the left frontal lobe, as well as contrast enhancement in the left temporal lobe. The patient was referred for whole body imaging in search of a primary tumor.

Findings

PET/CT images show a large area of edema in the left frontal lobe on CT along with a 2-cm radiodense mass in the anterior aspect of this region. There is focal, intense FDG activity in the left frontal lobe mass seen on MRI, associated with decreased tracer activity throughout much of the frontal lobe. The temporal lobe enhancement reported on MRI has no apparent analogous finding on PET.

Whole body PET/CT images (not shown) did not demonstrate any additional foci of abnormal FDG uptake.

Main Teaching Points and Summary
1. This two-dimensional (2D) PET study was part of a whole body examination and is of lower quality than typical 3D brain PET.
2. The patient's blood glucose was elevated at 160, and there was slight patient motion contributing to the lower quality PET brain images seen in this study.

Case 2.3.2 BRAIN METASTASES (FIG. 2.3.2, *A AND B*) AND LUNG CANCER (FIG. 2.3.2, *C*)

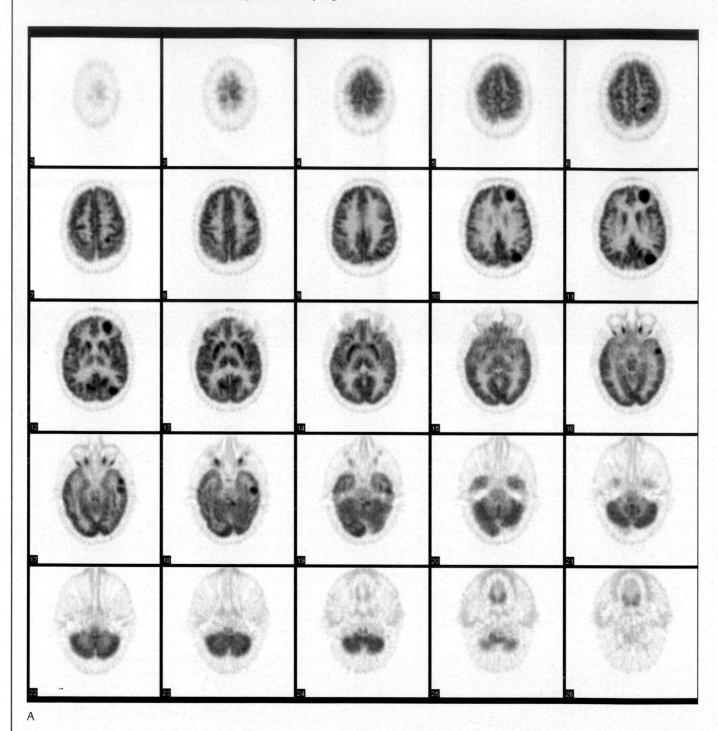

A

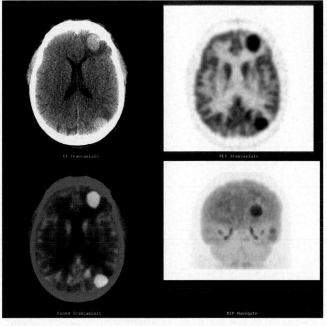

B

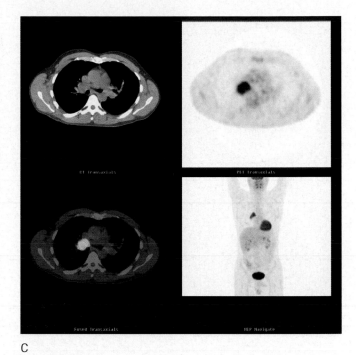

C

Brief History

A 43-year-old patient presented with a history of new-onset seizures. A recent CT study showed multiple round lesions in the brain. CT of the chest showed a 3.5-cm mass in the right hilum along with subcentimeter lymph nodes, suspicious for metastatic lung cancer. PET/CT was ordered for systemic assessment before treatment.

Findings

A. PET images of the brain show multiple foci of increased FDG activity in the left hemisphere.

B. PET/CT images of the brain including noncontrast CT show two hyperdense lesions in the left frontal and occipital lobes, with corresponding foci of abnormally increased FDG uptake.

C. PET/CT images of the thorax demonstrate the presence of an area of intense abnormal FDG activity corresponding to a large right hilar mass, which extends along the right mainstem bronchus, consistent with the primary lung tumor.

Main Teaching Point and Summary

1. Multiple brain lesions on CT and PET strongly suggest metastatic disease or, less likely, disseminated infection.

Case 2.3.3 RESIDUAL TUMOR AND POSTSURGICAL CHANGES (FIG. 2.3.3)

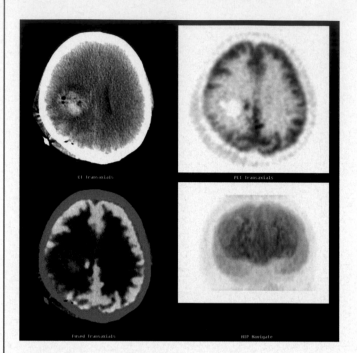

Brief History

A 50-year-old patient recently underwent resection of a 5-cm tumor involving the right parietal lobe of the brain. PET/CT was performed for assessing the presence of residual tumor because it was unclear whether the resection was complete.

Findings

PET/CT images demonstrate a region of soft tissue edema and air, with blood density in the lesion on CT, consistent with the recent postoperative state. On PET there is diffuse reduction of FDG activity in the right parietal lobe and a cold area within the surgical cavity. These findings are consistent with recent postoperative changes. There is a small focus of intense FDG activity along the medial edge of the resection cavity in the parietal lobe, consistent with residual viable tumor at the deep surgical margin.

Main Teaching Points and Summary

1. After surgery, there is little reactive FDG uptake in the brain.
2. Intense FDG uptake at the resection margin of a brain tumor generally represents residual tumor.

Case 2.3.4 RECURRENT TUMOR AND RADIATION NECROSIS (FIG. 2.3.4)

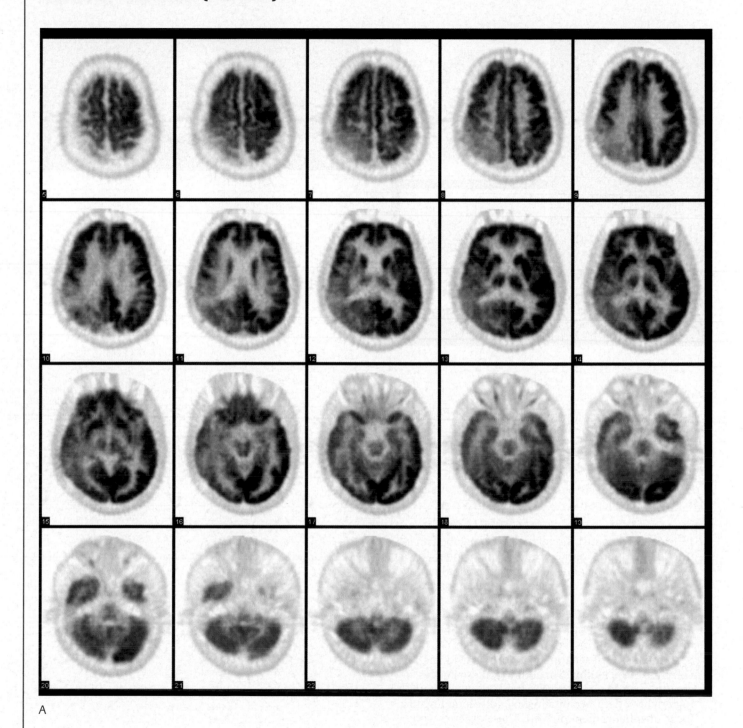

A

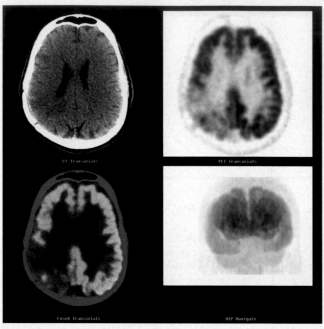

B

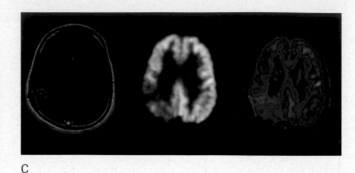

C

Brief History

A 44-year-old patient with a history of astrocytoma of the right parietal lobe underwent resection 5 years before the current PET/CT study. The tumor recurred 1 year pre-PET/CT, and the patient underwent chemotherapy. A recent MRI showed a lesion that could represent recurrence or radiation necrosis, and the patient was referred to make this distinction.

Findings

A. PET images demonstrate relative hypometabolism in the right temporal, parietal, and occipital lobes and in the lateral right thalamus. The left cerebellar hemisphere shows mildly decreased activity compared with the right.

B. PET/CT images show that the right parieto-occipital area of decreased FDG uptake is located in the region of previous tumor resection and craniotomy.

C. Software fusion of separately performed MRI and PET confirms these findings. In addition, these images show a small site of intense metabolic activity in the high right parieto-occipital region corresponding to a focus of enhancement on MRI. These findings were consistent with tumor recurrence and radiation necrosis.

Main Teaching Point and Summary

1. Fusion of MRI and PET/CT component can add certainty to diagnostic results.

Case 2.3.5 PITUITARY ADENOMA AND STROKE (FIG. 2.3.5)

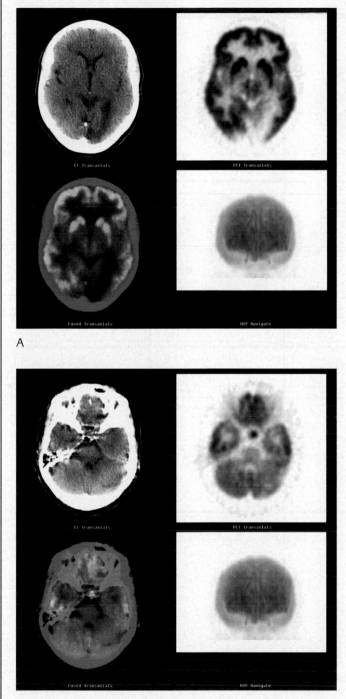

A

B

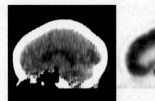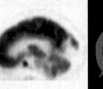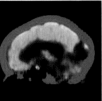

C

Brief History

A 64-year-old patient had recently experienced confusion with no clear etiology. MRI showed encephalomalacia in the occipital lobe and cerebellum consistent with old infarcts. MRI also showed a mass in the midline sella turcica, consistent with a pituitary adenoma. PET/CT was obtained to determine whether there was evidence of Alzheimer's disease versus multi-infarct dementia.

Findings

A. PET/CT images at the level of the basal ganglia demonstrate a hypodense region on CT with corresponding decreased FDG activity in both occipital lobes, more prominent on the left side, representing infarct.

B.–C. Transaxial and sagittal PET/CT images at the level of the base of the skull demonstrate a focus of abnormally increased FDG activity in the region of the pituitary gland, consistent with macroadenoma.

There is no PET/CT evidence of Alzheimer's disease.

Main Teaching Points and Summary

1. In patients with altered mental states, PET/CT can be useful to separate multi-infarct dementia from Alzheimer's disease.
2. Pituitary tumors visible on PET/CT are typically macroadenomas and can be incidental findings on brain studies performed for other clinical indications.
3. A metastasis to the pituitary gland can have a similar appearance to an adenoma on PET.

2.4 NEUROLOGICAL DISORDERS

Case 2.4.1: EPILEPSY—CLASSIC INTERICTAL PATTERN (FIG. 2.4.1)

A

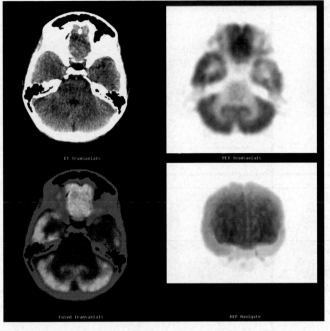

B

Brief History

A 24-year-old patient presented with newly diagnosed intractable complex partial seizures and occasional secondary generalization. Brain MRI (not shown) demonstrated decreased volume in the left hippocampus, suggesting mesial temporal sclerosis. Electroencephalogram (EEG) was suggestive but not diagnostic of a left temporal focus.

Findings

A. PET images show diffusely decreased left anterior and medial temporal FDG activity. There is also minimally decreased activity in the right cerebellum.

B. PET/CT images demonstrate mild left temporal lobe volume loss on CT with a corresponding decrease in FDG activity in this region.

Main Teaching Point and Summary

1. The combination of abnormal MRI, PET, and EEG localization to the left temporal lobe strongly suggests that left temporal lobectomy will help in the management of the patient's seizure disorder.

Case 2.4.2 EPILEPSY—INTERICTAL PATTERN AND CEREBELLAR DIASCHISIS (FIG. 2.4.2)

A

B

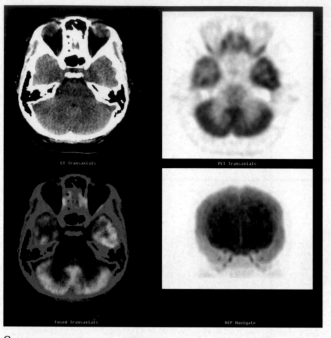

C

Brief History

A 26-year-old patient had a history of complex partial and secondary generalized seizures since early childhood. The last seizure occurred 1 week before PET/CT. MRI 3 months before the PET/CT was normal. MR spectroscopy at the same time showed decreased N-acetyl aspartase signal in the left temporal lobe. EEG performed 1 month pre-PET/CT strongly suggested a seizure focus in the anterior right temporal lobe.

Findings

A.–B. Transaxial and coronal PET images show decreased activity in the right temporal lobe. In addition, there is minimally decreased activity in the contralateral left cerebellum, consistent with crossed cerebellar diaschisis.

C. PET/CT images at the level of the temporal lobes do not demonstrate any CT abnormalities in the region of decreased tracer activity in the right hemisphere.

Main Teaching Points and Summary

1. Decreased right temporal lobe FDG uptake and the contralateral reduction in cerebellar glycolysis on the interictal PET/CT strongly suggest that the epileptogenic focus is located in the right temporal lobe.
2. Cerebellar diaschisis is a useful secondary sign of temporal lobe hypometabolism, but can be subtle.

Case 2.4.3 EPILEPSY—INTERICTAL PATTERN AND DECREASED CEREBELLAR UPTAKE (FIG. 2.4.3)

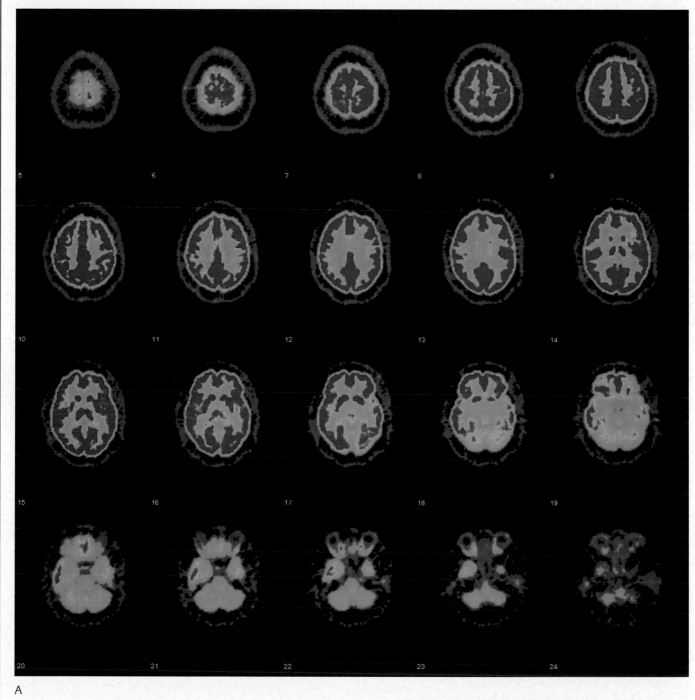

A

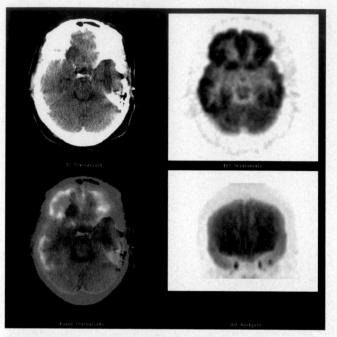

B

Brief History

A 34-year-old patient had a 10-year history of complex partial seizures. EEG suggested a left anterior temporal lobe focus. MRI demonstrated left mesial temporal sclerosis and white matter volume loss in the left anterior temporal lobe.

Findings

A. PET images demonstrate mildly decreased FDG activity in the left temporal lobe compared with the right. In addition, there is symmetrically decreased FDG activity throughout the cerebellum.

B. PET/CT images demonstrate a mild reduction in left temporal lobe volume on CT, corresponding to the area of decreased FDG activity.

Main Teaching Points and Summary

1. The presence of reduction in FDG uptake, MRI volume loss, and abnormal EEG strongly suggest a left temporal lobe origin of epilepsy.

2. Decreased tracer uptake in the cerebellum can be seen with chronic phenytoin therapy.

3. Color PET images can make subtle findings more obvious than black and white images.

Case 2.4.4 ALZHEIMER'S DISEASE—DIFFUSE PATTERN (FIG. 2.4.4)

A

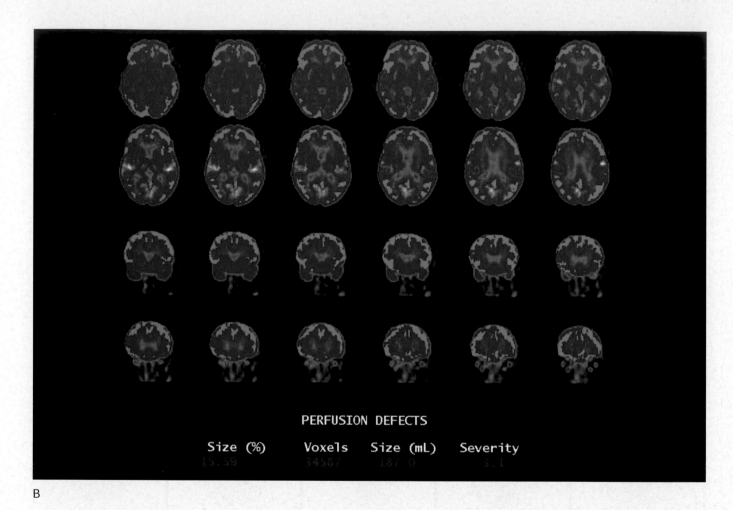

B

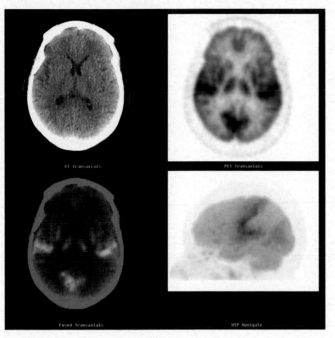

C

Case 2.4.5 ALZHEIMER'S DISEASE—FRONTAL PREDOMINANCE (FIG. 2.4.5)

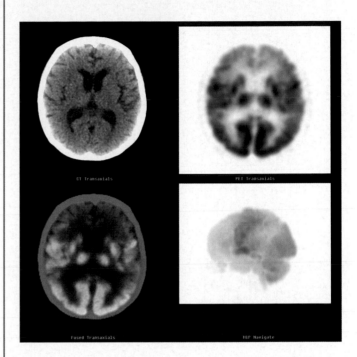

Brief History

A 65-year-old patient had a past history of cerebrovascular accident related to an aneurysm. Recently, the mental status of the patient deteriorated, especially over the 2 weeks before PET/CT. The study was performed to help differentiate between frontotemporal dementia, Alzheimer's disease, and multi-infarct dementias.

Findings

A. PET images demonstrate significantly decreased FDG activity in the frontal, temporal, and parietal lobes bilaterally.
B. Quantitative analysis shows a significant reduction in the FDG activity in the frontal and temporoparietal cortices, as indicated by the green color areas. Over 15% of the brain is affected.
C. PET/CT images show a relatively normal noncontrast CT, whereas on PET there is sparing of FDG activity in the sensorimotor cortex, occipital lobe, and basal ganglia.

Main Teaching Point and Summary

1. These PET/CT findings are classic for advanced Alzheimer's disease and do not suggest the presence of either frontotemporal or multi-infarct dementia.

Brief History

A 63-year-old patient with hypertension and hyperlipidemia had rapidly progressing dementia with severe recent deterioration in mental status. MRI showed mild atrophy and mild ischemic changes. PET/CT was performed in search of the etiology of the patient's mental deterioration.

Findings

PET/CT images show only minimal atrophy with slightly prominent ventricles and sulci on noncontrast CT. FDG activity, however, is significantly decreased in the frontal, temporal, and parietal lobes bilaterally, with sparing of the sensorimotor cortex, occipital lobe, and basal ganglia structures.

Main Teaching Points and Summary

1. These PET/CT findings are typical for moderately advanced dementia of the Alzheimer's type and do not suggest multi-infarct dementia.
2. Frontal involvement is less extensive than would be expected in Pick's disease.
3. Sparing of the temporal lobes weighs against frontotemporal dementia.

PET/CT of the Head and Neck

Richard L. Wahl • Mehrbod Som Javadi

3.1 NORMAL PATTERN

Case 3.1.1 NORMAL PATTERN PET/CT OF THE HEAD AND NECK (FIG. 3.1)

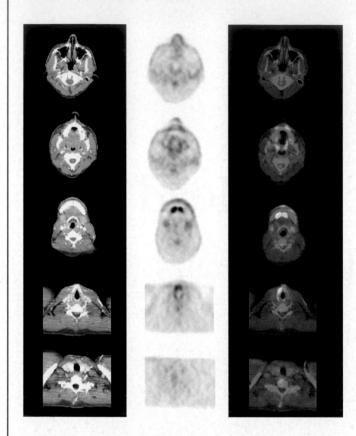

This is an example of a normal PET/CT of the head and neck. This study was performed with intravenous (IV) contrast, which makes it easier to define the location of the blood vessels and separate them from nodal structures. Care must be taken to ensure that there are no PET attenuation correction artifacts induced by very high levels of IV contrast in the vasculature.

In this case, a noncontrast CT scan was first performed (not shown) followed by a contrast CT study. The contrast CT was fused with the emission PET, but the attenuation correction map was generated from the noncontrast CT study.

Normal FDG uptake is identified in salivary glands including the submandibular and sublingual glands, in the genioglossus and cricoarytenoid muscles, lymphoid tissue, and vocal cords. The normal thyroid has only minimal FDG uptake. These normal sites of FDG uptake should not be confused with disease.

3.2 PHYSIOLOGIC ARTIFACTS AND PITFALLS

Case 3.2.1 ARTIFACT—MISREGISTRATION DUE TO PATIENT MOVEMENT (FIG. 3.2.1)

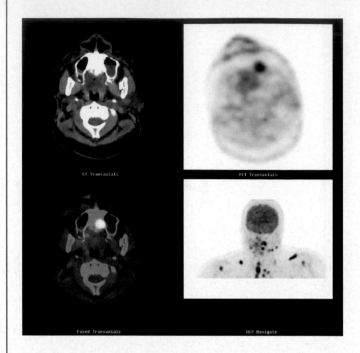

Brief History

A 71-year-old patient with newly diagnosed diffuse large cell lymphoma was referred for PET/CT for staging.

Findings

PET/CT images show increased 2-[18F] fluoro-2-deoxy-D-glucose (FDG) uptake that could represent involvement of the bone in the hard palate. Fused images, however, demonstrate obvious severe misregistration, with the nose on the PET image clearly to the right of CT anatomy due to patient motion. The focus of increased FDG uptake on the left is therefore likely in the maxillary sinus and not in the bone.

Note on maximum intensity projection (MIP): Extensive FDG-avid systemic involvement with lymphoma is seen.

Main Teaching Points and Summary
1. PET/CT is a very good tool for assessment of lymphoma or other malignancies in the region of the head and neck.
2. Precise localization on PET/CT depends on the head being in the same position on both sets of images, sometimes achieved by fixation of the head using a hardware accessory.
3. The head can move in many directions between PET and CT, and misregistration can occur with PET/CT.

Case 3.2.2 PHYSIOLOGIC—MUSCLE UPTAKE, TONGUE (FIG. 3.2.2)

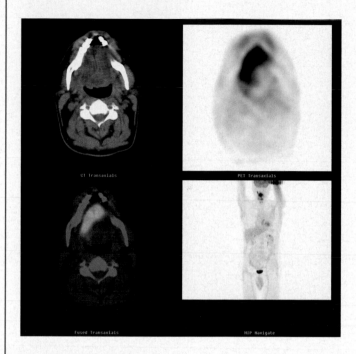

Brief History
A 61-year-old patient with a history of resection for cure of esophageal carcinoma was evaluated for possible recurrence. The patient has a history of continuous lip smacking and tongue movement.

Findings
PET/CT images demonstrate intense FDG uptake in the lips and tongue, especially on the right, localized to muscles that were active during the tracer-uptake phase. The asymmetric increased FDG uptake in the tongue is a result of this patient's continuous muscle contractions during the uptake and imaging phases.

Note on MIP: No evidence for recurrent systemic tumor is seen.

Main Teaching Points and Summary
1. Muscle uptake can be intense and in unusual locations.
2. In this case, PET/CT helped to localize the increased tracer uptake entirely to active muscle contraction and not to the tumor.

Case 3.2.3 PHYSIOLOGIC—UNILATERAL MUSCLE UPTAKE, MASTICATION (FIG. 3.2.3)

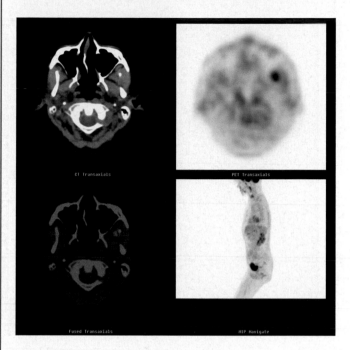

Brief History
A 52-year-old patient with complex medical problems was referred to diagnose potential inflammatory systemic vasculitis or tumor. There was no definite history of cancer.

Findings
PET/CT images show abnormally increased focal FDG uptake localized to the left medial masseter and pterygoid muscles, most likely related to tooth grinding during the uptake phase.

Note on MIP: No evidence of systemic vasculitis or tumor is seen.

Main Teaching Points and Summary
1. Intense FDG uptake in muscles of mastication can be seen as a normal variant, common especially in anxious patients.
2. This patient was quite nervous and had a wide variety of atypical central nervous system symptoms. In some cases, chewing gum can be the cause of mastication muscle uptake that must not be confused with malignancy.

Case 3.2.4 PHYSIOLOGIC—BILATERAL MUSCLE UPTAKE, MASTICATION (FIG. 3.2.4)

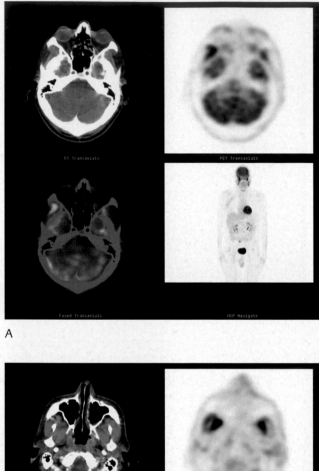

A

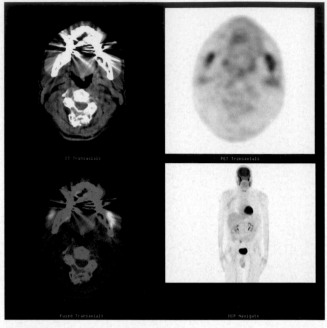

C

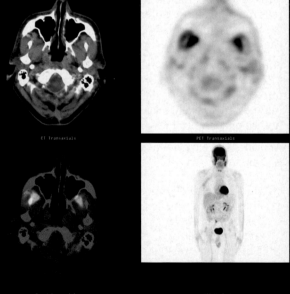

B

Brief History

A 70-year-old patient with metastatic melanoma was referred to PET/CT for whole body evaluation.

Findings

A–C. PET/CT images at various levels show focal-intense FDG uptake localized by fused images to the right temporalis muscle and the muscles of mastication, bilaterally.

Note on MIP: Focal FDG uptake in tumor metastatic to right iliac lymph nodes is evident.

Main Teaching Points and Summary

1. Focal tracer activity in the muscles of mastication can display similar intensity to the metastatic melanoma sites.
2. The physiologic foci can be easily characterized by their CT location as muscles.
3. Instructing the patient not to chew during the uptake phase can minimize increased FDG activity in muscles; however, these findings can be also seen related to involuntary tooth grinding.

Case 3.2.5 PHYSIOLOGIC—UNILATERAL MUSCLE UPTAKE, NECK (FIG. 3.2.5)

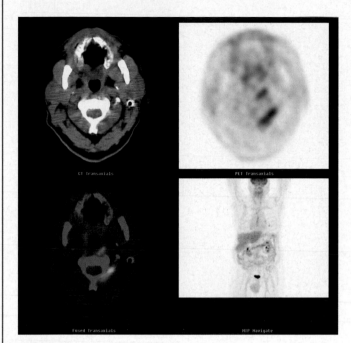

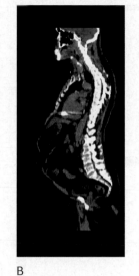

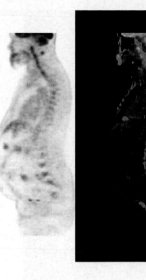

A

B

Brief History

A 57-year-old patient with a history of cardiomyopathy and pulmonary nodules on x-ray and CT was assessed for the suspicion of lung cancer.

Findings

A. Transaxial PET/CT images demonstrate intense FDG activity in the pre- and paravertebral left neck muscles.
B. The sagittal images clearly show the linear pattern of tracer uptake in the neck.

Note on MIP: Intense tracer uptake in a left lung nodule associated with further biopsy-proved primary lung cancer is evident.

Main Teaching Points and Summary

1. Muscle FDG uptake can be intense and easily confused with cancer-related tracer activity.
2. The linear pattern of the tracer uptake, along with its correspondence to muscles on PET/CT images, helps exclude tumor involvement in the head and neck.

Case 3.2.6 PHYSIOLOGIC—UNILATERAL MUSCLE UPTAKE, TORTICOLLIS, AND METAL ARTIFACT (FIG. 3.2.6)

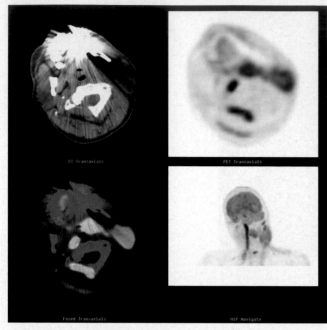

A

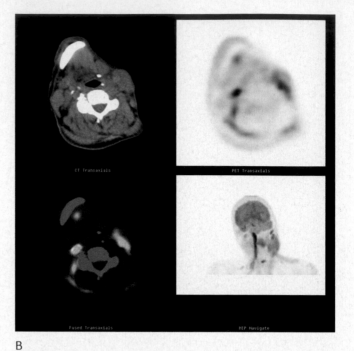

B

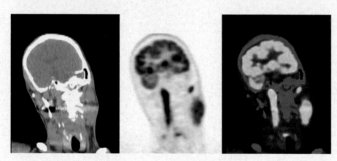

C

Brief History

A 50-year-old patient was recently diagnosed with squamous cell carcinoma of the left neck. The patient had a history of torticollis since childhood. On clinical examination, it was believed that his abnormal neck findings were simply due to the torticollis until a definite mass became palpable. A recent MRI showed the left neck mass to increase in size and demonstrated the presence of enlarged lymph nodes. PET/CT was obtained to assess extent of disease before treatment.

Findings

A. Transaxial PET/CT images show an ill-defined necrotic left neck mass on CT that extends from the left parotid gland to the left palatine tonsil, associated with intense FDG activity. There is also distortion of the CT image by metal hardware in the mouth, with a corresponding cold defect on PET.

B. Transaxial PET/CT images at a lower level show intense FDG activity in the right longus coli, as well as in the paraspinal and posterior neck muscles.

C. Coronal PET/CT images show evidence of torticollis with neck deviation to the right and intense metabolic activity in the left neck mass as well as the right longus coli muscle.

Main Teaching Points and Summary

1. Both malignant lesions and contracting muscles can accumulate FDG. Distinguishing the two processes cannot be always done on the basis of intensity of tracer activity. Assessment of the pattern of uptake and correlation with CT are essential.

2. Intense linear accumulation of FDG in muscles contralateral to the side of the primary tumor is clearly distinct from the typical tumor appearance.

3. Some degradation of technical image quality is caused by the metallic artifacts in the left mandible, which affect mainly the CT component. Use of the non–attenuation-corrected images can be helpful because they are less likely to be affected by artifacts.

Case 3.2.7 PITFALL—VOCAL CORD PARALYSIS, LEFT (FIG. 3.2.7)

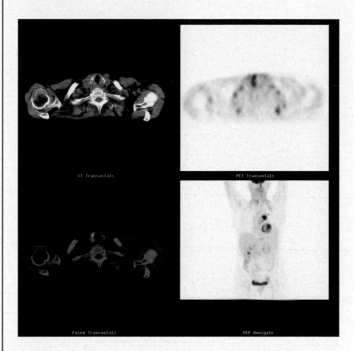

Brief History
An 84-year-old patient with gastroesophageal reflux, mediastinal fullness, hoarseness, and a new left upper lobe nodule on CT was referred with suspicion of malignancy.

Findings
PET/CT images clearly show reduced FDG uptake in the left vocal cord with more intense uptake in the right, consistent with a left vocal cord paralysis. Mild physiologic FDG uptake in brown fat is noted in the posterior neck.

Note on MIP: There is an FDG-avid focus in the left lung as well as a larger mediastinal abnormal FDG-avid focus, both consistent with cancer that has invaded the left recurrent laryngeal nerve.

Main Teaching Points and Summary
1. Not infrequently, a PET study will be the first test to demonstrate the presence of vocal cord paralysis, although the degree of hoarseness can often be quite modest.
2. In patients with thoracic malignant lesions, left vocal cord paralysis is more common than right because the left recurrent laryngeal nerve courses further caudally into the chest than the right.

Case 3.2.8 PITFALL—VOCAL CORD PARALYSIS, RIGHT AND SUPRACLAVICULAR NODES (FIG. 3.2.8)

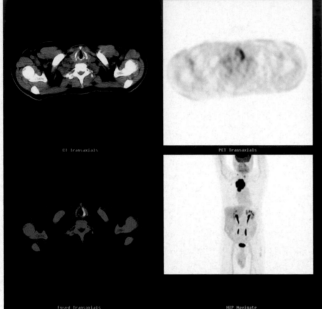

A

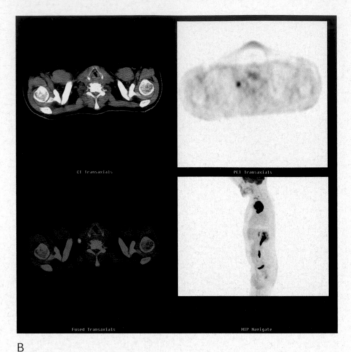

B

Brief History

A 69-year-old patient with hemoptysis and a right paratracheal mass proved to be non–small cell lung cancer was evaluated for initial staging. The patient complained of hoarseness.

Findings

A. PET/CT images show linear intense uptake in the left vocal cord with only minimal uptake on the right, consistent with a right vocal cord paralysis.

B. PET/CT images at a lower level show a focal area of intense tracer uptake in a right supraclavicular Virchow node, consistent with metastatic involvement.

Note on MIP: Intense FDG uptake in a large right upper thoracic mass, consistent with the primary tumor, is seen.

Main Teaching Point and Summary

1. A paralyzed vocal cord typically has low uptake of FDG, whereas intense uptake is seen in the remaining functional vocal cord and the controlling cricoarytenoid muscles.

Case 3.2.9 BENIGN—BROWN FAT, NECK (FIG. 3.2.9)

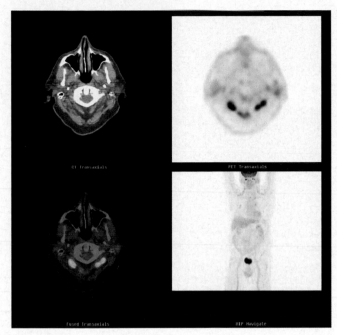

A

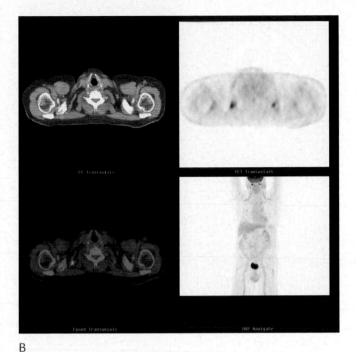

B

Brief History
A 60 year-old patient with history of colorectal cancer diagnosed 6 years before the PET/CT study was referred for a suspicion of recurrent tumor related to elevated serum CEA levels.

Findings
A and B. PET/CT images at the level of the upper (A) and lower (B) neck show foci of intense FDG activity in the neck, which localize to fatty tissue on CT.

Note on MIP: Abnormal tracer uptake in the mediastinum and right lung, consistent with progressive metastatic colon cancer, is seen.

Main Teaching Points and Summary
1. Increased FDG uptake, symmetrically located in the neck and often very intense, can be seen in brown fat and must not be confused with disease. It is a normal variant, known also as brown fat uptake ("USA-fat").
2. A "flowing" pattern is seen on the MIP images, with the increased activity extending downward to the shoulder girdle, and in many cases into the bilateral paraspinal areas and the upper abdomen.

Case 3.2.10 BENIGN—BROWN FAT, NECK AND SHOULDERS (FIG. 3.2.10)

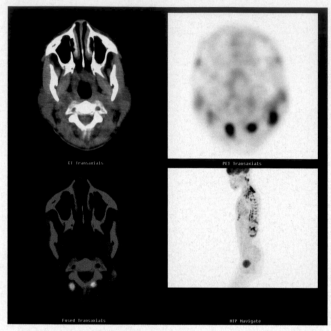

A

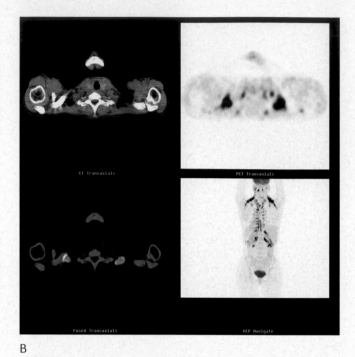

B

Brief History

A 24-year-old patient with history of neurofibromatosis presented with complaints of progressive weakness in the left shoulder. PET/CT was performed in search for malignant transformation.

Findings

A and B. PET/CT images at the level of the neck (A) and shoulders (B) show extensive and intense brown fat FDG uptake. The foci located in the posterior neck could, on PET alone, easily be confused with level V (posterior cervical) lymph nodes. They clearly fuse to CT areas of fat, however.

Note on MIP: The increased FDG uptake clearly extends to the paraspinal region and the upper abdomen, where it surrounds much of the kidneys. There are no abnormalities to suggest FDG-avid malignant neoplasm in this patient with neurofibromatosis.

Main Teaching Points and Summary

1. Brown fat activity is relatively common in young, thin, female patients.
2. Physiologic tracer activity in fatty tissues can be extensive, and although it can mimic nodal tumor involvement, it should not be confused with cancer or malignant transformation of neurofibromatosis.

Case 3.2.11 BENIGN—POSTTREATMENT CHANGES IN SKIN AND SUBCUTANEOUS TISSUE (SURGERY AND RADIATION) (FIG. 3.2.11)

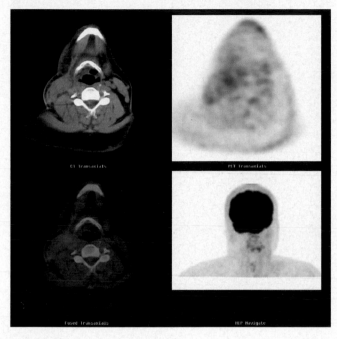

Brief History
A 43-year-old patient with a history of right parotid adenoid cystic carcinoma diagnosed 6 months before this PET/CT study, status post right radical neck dissection and recent radiation to the right neck, was assessed for response to treatment.

Findings
PET/CT images show edema of the skin of the right neck associated with diffuse, mildly intense FDG uptake. These findings were most consistent with treatment-related changes due to previous surgery and radiation, thus excluding recurrent tumor. In addition, there is no visualization of the right submandibular gland.

Major Teaching Points and Summary
1. Recent radiation treatment can lead to increased FDG uptake, which later decreases in intensity.
2. Treatment-related findings can be somewhat variable, and it is therefore critical to be familiar with the recent surgical and radiation history of the patient.

Case 3.2.12 BENIGN—POSTTREATMENT CHANGES, RECONSTITUTED LYMPHOID TISSUE AND MUSCLES (SURGERY AND RADIATION) (FIG. 3.2.12)

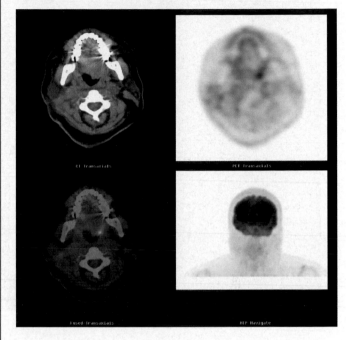

Brief History
A 41-year-old patient with history of T2, N2 squamous cell carcinoma of the tongue, status following post right glossectomy and radiation treatment, was evaluated for possible recurrent tumor 6 months after initial diagnosis and treatment.

Findings
PET/CT images demonstrate focal increased FDG activity at the left aspect of the base of an asymmetric tongue. The possibility of recurrence on the left versus reconstituted lymphoid tissue or asymmetric muscle contraction following radiation (higher radiation doses delivered on the right) was raised.

Follow-up showed no evidence of malignancy. The hypermetabolic area on the left was therefore most likely due to postoperative muscle contraction and lymphoid reconstitution on the left as well as postradiation decrease in tracer uptake on the right.

Major Teaching Points and Summary
1. Head and neck surgery can be complex and include partial removal of organs, often followed by radiotherapy to the same region.
2. Knowledge of the surgical procedure and of the radiation port suggested in this case reconstituted normal lymphoid tissue in an asymmetric residual partial tongue as the cause of uptake.

Case 3.2.13 BENIGN—POSTSURGICAL CHANGES, MISSING SALIVARY GLAND (FIG. 3.2.13)

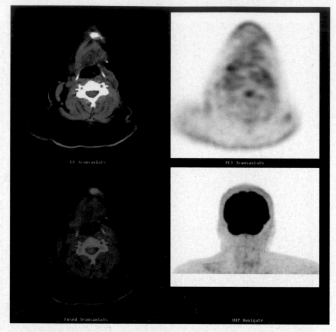

A

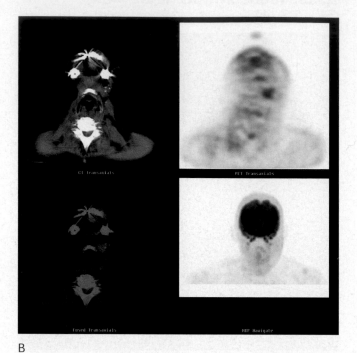

B

Brief History

A 50-year-old patient with a history of squamous cell carcinoma of the left tongue diagnosed 1 year before this PET/CT. The patient had a left neck dissection followed by radiation treatment and was referred with new pain in the right neck for possible recurrent squamous cell carcinoma.

Findings

A. PET/CT images demonstrate a focus of increased FDG uptake in the right neck, suspicious for a right submandibular node. This uptake is actually localized in the normal right submandibular gland, whereas the left submandibular gland is surgically absent (see clips). Mild diffuse FDG uptake is seen throughout the neck due to prior radiation therapy.

B. For comparative analysis: PET/CT images of a similar case following right radical neck dissection demonstrate asymmetric FDG uptake within a remaining normal left submandibular gland due to a missing right gland.

Main Teaching Points and Summary

1. A careful history of surgery and radiation treatment in the region of the head and neck is essential to avoid an incorrect diagnosis on PET/CT studies. Direct discussion with the surgeon and examination of surgical records can be helpful.

2. A missing salivary gland on one side may make the normal remaining gland appear pathologic. This pitfall can be avoided by careful examination of the CT portion of the study and the surgical records.

Case 3.2.14 BENIGN—POSTTREATMENT CHANGES, FDG-NEGATIVE RIGHT PAROTID (FIG. 3.2.14)

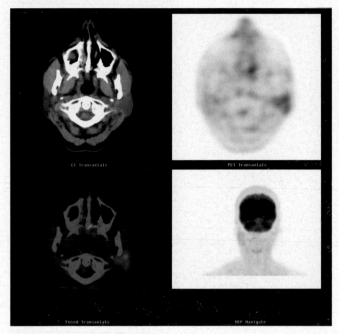

Brief History
A 56-year-old patient with history of squamous cell carcinoma of the right neck 4 years after bilateral neck dissection and radiation treatment to the right neck was referred for restaging of a possible recurrent squamous cell carcinoma in a left neck mass.

Findings
PET/CT images show fatty replacement of the right parotid gland on CT, with very low FDG uptake, most likely due to the prior radiation therapy of the right neck. There is no evidence for recurrent tumor.

Main Teaching Points and Summary
1. Evaluation of PET/CT studies in the region of the head and neck requires precise knowledge of prior therapies to understand the imaging findings.
2. Decreased FDG uptake due to radiation can cause asymmetry and possible misdiagnosis if not recognized.

Case 3.2.15 BENIGN—POSTSURGICAL CHANGES, MISSING ORBIT, AND ETHMOID, EXTRAOCULAR MUSCULAR UPTAKE (FIG. 3.2.15)

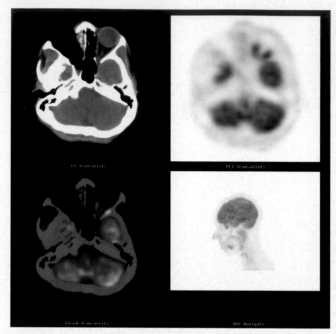

A

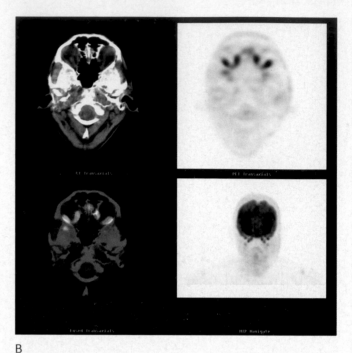

B

Brief History

A 48-year-old patient with history of squamous cell carcinoma of the right ethmoid sinus with tumor spread to the orbit was referred for restaging after radical removal of the whole tumor including the orbit and parts of the ethmoid and sphenoid bones.

Findings

A. PET/CT images demonstrate the absence of the right orbit, extraocular muscles, and parts of the ethmoid and sphenoid bones on CT. A clear wedge-shaped area of decreased FDG uptake corresponds to the large surgical defect. There is no focal FDG uptake to suggest recurrence. Note the asymmetric FDG uptake in normal extraocular muscles on the left.

B. For comparison: PET/CT images in a patient with no pathology in the region of the head and neck shows symmetric FDG uptake in normal extraocular muscles.

Main Teaching Points and Summary

1. The CT portion of PET/CT is key to recognizing postoperative changes.
2. A clear knowledge of the treatment history will help avoid pitfalls in diagnosis.

3.3 INFECTION AND INFLAMMATION

Case 3.3.1 INFLAMMATION, TRACHEOSTOMY (FIG. 3.3.1)

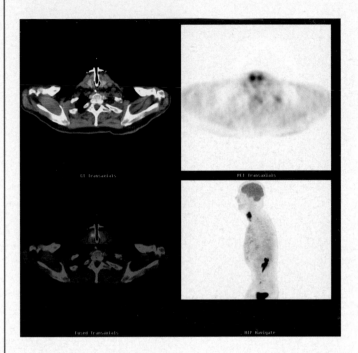

Brief History
A 71-year-old patient with a history of laryngeal papilloma was recently found to have an enlarging laryngeal mass diagnosed as carcinoma. The patient had a tracheostomy placed for airway maintenance 3 days before PET/CT.

Findings
PET/CT images demonstrate moderately increased FDG uptake on either side of the tracheostomy, consistent with benign inflammation.

Note on lateral MIP: Intense abnormally increased FDG uptake is seen in the anterior neck, localized to the laryngeal carcinoma.

Major Teaching Points and Summary
1. Mild to moderately increased tracer uptake due to an inflammatory process can be seen at the edges of the tracheostomy site. This should not be confused with tumor.
2. Laryngeal carcinoma, when large, can lead to airway occlusion and require emergency tracheostomy.

Case 3.3.2 INFECTION, ACNE (FIG. 3.3.2)

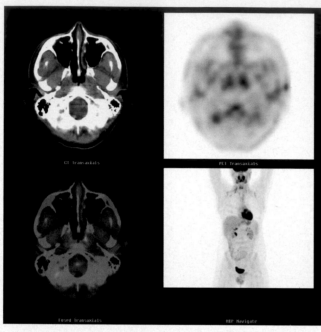

A

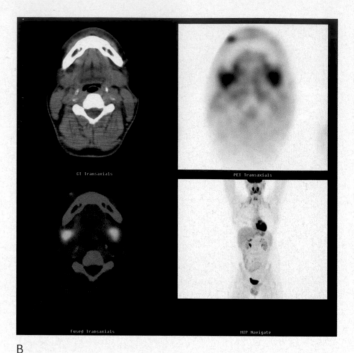

B

Brief History

A 19-year-old patient with history of Hodgkin lymphoma with an excellent clinical response to therapy was evaluated for routine follow-up.

Findings

A and B. PET/CT images at the level of the ears (A) and mouth (B) show focal sites of increased FDG uptake located in the skin, just anterior to the left external auditory canal (A) and in the right chin (B), in foci of active acne. There is no systemic evidence of active lymphoma.

Note on MIP: There is intense physiologic uptake in tonsils and submandibular glands, as well as mild brown fat uptake.

Main Teaching Points and Summary

1. Acne is common in teens and may appear as small foci of cutaneous and subcutaneous FDG uptake.
2. Normal lymphoid tissue and salivary glands can have intense FDG uptake in younger patients but can be characterized by their symmetry and location.
3. Neither of these processes should be confused with malignant disease.

Case 3.3.3 INFECTION, MAXILLARY SINUSITIS, PARTIALLY INVOLVED (FIG. 3.3.3)

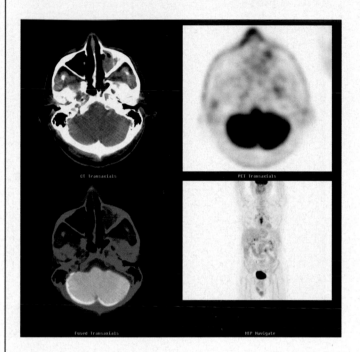

Brief History
A 73-year-old patient with history of esophageal cancer and sinusitis who was clinically stable recently had an abnormal chest radiograph and was evaluated for suspected recurrence.

Findings
PET/CT images demonstrate opacification of most of the left maxillary sinus on CT, and increased FDG uptake is only shown in its most anterior part, consistent with active sinusitis.

Note on MIP: There is intense FDG activity in the mediastinum near the region of the prior resection, raising a strong suspicion for recurrence.

Main Teaching Point and Summary
1. Incidental sinusitis is not an unusual finding on PET/CT and must be distinguished from tumor recurrence in the sinuses.

Case 3.3.4 INFECTION, MAXILLARY SINUSITIS, INVOLVEMENT OF WHOLE SINUS (FIG. 3.3.4)

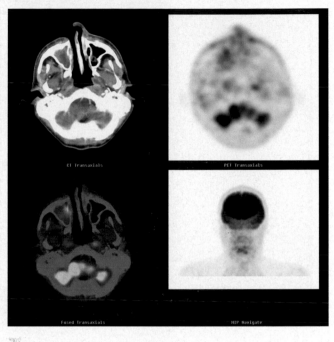

Brief History
A 28-year-old patient with history of nasal lymphoma, who was in remission following chemotherapy, was referred for routine follow-up assessment.

Findings
PET/CT images demonstrate opacification of the right maxillary sinus on CT with mild to moderate FDG accumulation. These findings are in a location separate from the original tumor and are therefore most consistent with maxillary sinusitis. During follow-up, the patient remained free of active lymphoma.

Main Teaching Points and Summary
1. Opacification of the sinuses on CT is not uncommon, but it is generally associated with no or minimal FDG uptake.
2. Mild to moderately intense FDG uptake in the sinuses is most consistent with active sinusitis. Lymphoma would be expected to have considerably more intense FDG uptake.

Case 3.3.5 MUCOUS RETENTION CYST IN MAXILLARY SINUS, FDG-NEGATIVE (FIG. 3.3.5)

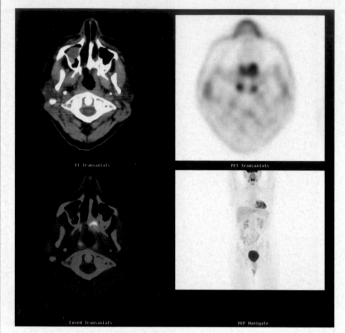

Brief History
A 17-year-old patient with a history of Hodgkin lymphoma was referred to PET/CT during routine follow-up after chemotherapy.

Findings
PET/CT images show partial opacification of the right maxillary sinus on CT, with no increased FDG uptake in this region, consistent with a noninflamed mucous retention cyst.

Note on MIP: No evidence of systemic disease.

Main Teaching Points and Summary
1. Mucous retention cysts are common findings and are typically negative on PET.
2. Large cysts may appear on CT very similar to active sinusitis.

Case 3.3.6 INFLAMMATION, RHEUMATOID ARTHRITIS, ATLANTO-ODONTOID JOINT (FIG. 3.3.6)

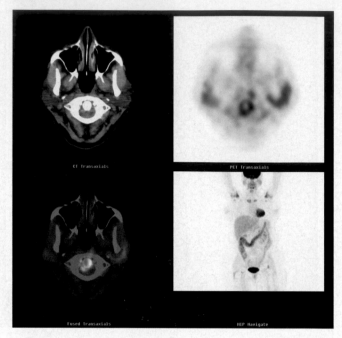

Brief History
A 53-year-old patient with history of ovarian carcinoma presented with rising CA-125 levels suggesting recurrence and was referred to PET/CT. She had a history of active rheumatoid arthritis.

Findings
PET/CT images demonstrate intense FDG uptake surrounding her C1-C2 atlanto-odontoid articulation, consistent with active rheumatoid inflammation in the synovial joint.

Note on MIP: The intense activity in large joints such as the shoulders and sternoclavicular joints is consistent with active systemic rheumatoid arthritis; status post–bilateral hip replacement.

Main Teaching Points and Summary
1. Increased FDG uptake can occur in tumors but is also a potent general and nonspecific marker of inflammation.
2. Inflamed synovial joints in virtually any location can show intense FDG uptake.

Case 3.4.1 TUMOR OF SCALP, MELANOMA (FIG. 3.4.1)

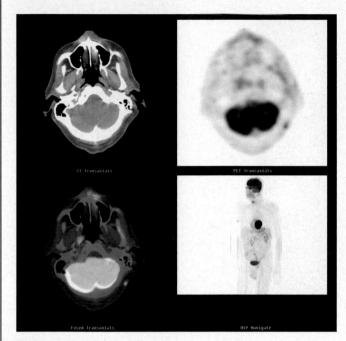

A

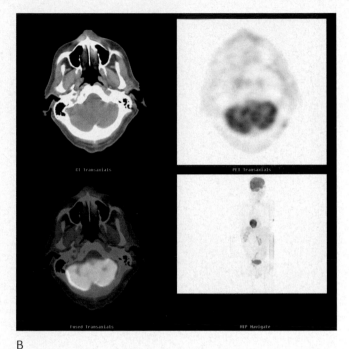

B

Brief History

A 62-year-old patient with history of multiple basal cell carcinomas presented with a newly diagnosed 3-mm-thick melanoma in the posterior scalp. PET/CT was performed to assess extent of disease.

Findings

A. PET/CT images show focal uptake at the site of the primary tumor. No systemic metastases are identified.
B. PET/CT images windowed with FDG intensity appropriate for visualization of the brain showed normal activity in the cerebellum and only faint uptake in the skin lesion.

Main Teaching Points and Summary

1. Small melanomas can be seen as focal FDG uptake on PET (A) in the presence of only minimal or even no abnormality detected on CT.
2. The windowing of PET images to see cutaneous lesions and small nodal metastases will not be the same as the one used to visualize the normal brain (B). Rather, the brain will have to be windowed "brightly" to see these soft tissue abnormalities.

Case 3.4.2 TUMOR OF SCALP, MELANOMA (FIG. 3.4.2)

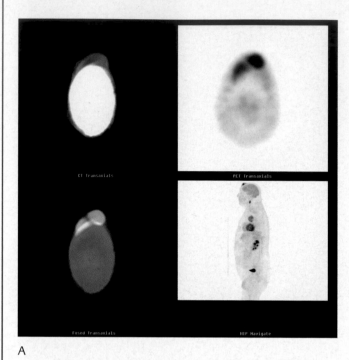

A

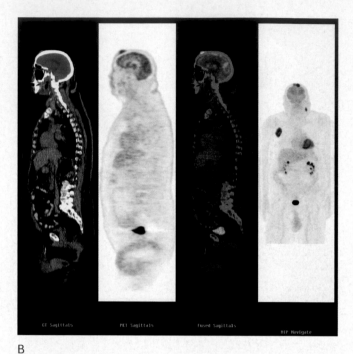

B

Brief History
A 74-year-old patient with a history of melanoma located on the right forearm and scalp 1 year before PET/CT was referred with the clinical suspicion of recurrence in the right axilla and scalp.

Findings
A and B. PET/CT images, transaxial (A) and sagittal (B) planes, show intense FDG uptake in a frontal scalp lesion, consistent with local recurrence.

Note on anterior and lateral MIP: Sites of nodal metastases are seen in the right axilla and left neck.

Main Teaching Points and Summary
1. Melanoma has, as a rule, very high glucose utilization. When occurring in the scalp, proper windowing must be used. In the present case, the melanoma uptake of FDG was greater than that of the normal brain.
2. In patients with known scalp lesions, it is critical to include the entire head in the field of view. In this case, only the most cephalad images show the recurrent primary tumor.

Case 3.4.3 TUMOR OF SCALP, BENIGN, FDG-NEGATIVE (FIG. 3.4.3)

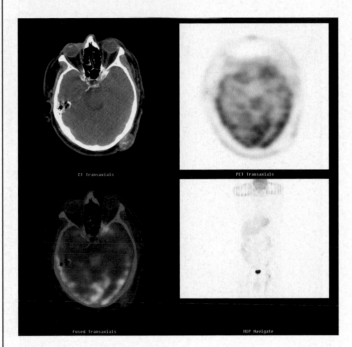

Brief History
A 73-year-old patient with history of liposarcoma of the abdomen and pelvis with a suspicion of recurrence was referred for whole body staging. The patient had a stable lesion on the back of his scalp for 2 years.

Findings
PET/CT images demonstrate a well-circumscribed and partly calcified scalp mass on CT, with no corresponding FDG uptake on PET, considered most likely to represent, clinically and radiographically, a sebaceous cyst unrelated to the primary neoplasm.

Note on MIP: Recurrent tumor in the left hip region.

Major Teaching Points and Summary
1. Masses in the scalp can represent inflammatory processes or tumors such as basal cell carcinoma or melanoma.
2. In this case, the stability over several years, in addition to the lack of FDG uptake, were most suggestive for this finding representing a sebaceous cyst.
3. A sebaceous cyst does not require intervention, in contrast to the life-threatening sarcoma.

Case 3.4.4 TUMOR OF AUDITORY CANAL (FIG. 3.4.4)

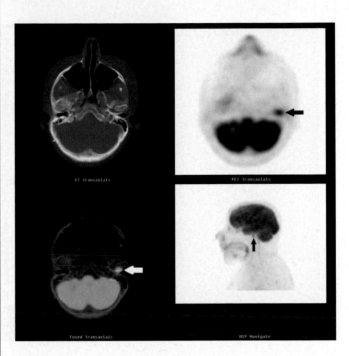

Brief History
A 40-year-old patient with left ear pain and hearing loss was diagnosed to have a lesion in the left auditory canal. Biopsy showed a squamous cell carcinoma and PET/CT was obtained for staging.

Findings
PET/CT demonstrates focal intense FDG activity with no clear corresponding abnormality seen on the CT, localized to the left external auditory canal by fused images (arrow). Incidentally, a VP shunt is demonstrated over the right posterolateral aspect of the skull on CT, due to prior surgery for a frontal meningioma.

Major Teaching Points and Summary
1. Squamous cell carcinomas involving the auditory canal are a diagnostic challenge, difficult to separate from ear infection.
2. The focal uptake in present case is more suggestive of malignancy, with infections often having a diffuse pattern. Biopsy ultimately becomes necessary for clarification of complex clinical cases.

Case 3.4.5 TUMOR OF PAROTID AND PERI-PAROTID NODES (FIG. 3.4.5)

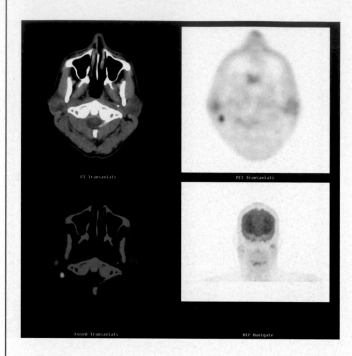

Brief History
A 52-year-old patient with known right parotid adenoid cystic carcinoma was referred to PET/CT for staging.

Findings
PET/CT images demonstrate the presence of a 2 × 1 cm mass with focal calcification in the right parotid gland on CT, showing only minimal FDG uptake. A 9-mm periparotid node, located posterior and adjacent to the gland, demonstrates moderately intense FDG uptake.

Major Teaching Point and Summary
1. FDG-PET imaging is not particularly reliable for detecting parotid tumors nor for the precise characterization of their malignant or benign etiology.
2. Intense nodal uptake, as in this case, is atypical of representing a metastasis from a low FDG avidity malignancy, but this would need to be excluded by biopsy.

Case 3.4.6 TUMOR OF PAROTID (FIG. 3.4.6)

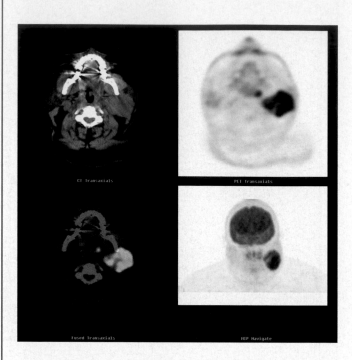

Brief History
A 51-year-old patient with recent left facial swelling and pain was initially diagnosed with apparent parotitis. The symptoms did not resolve, fine-needle aspiration biopsy of the mass showed squamous cell carcinoma, and the patient was referred for PET/CT staging.

Findings
PET/CT images demonstrate a large necrotic nodal mass that has substantially replaced the left parotid gland. In addition, there is focal intense activity in the left tonsillar region. These findings are consistent with squamous cell carcinoma which may have originated in the tonsil and drained to the parotid nodal region. Of note, mild misregistration with the nose is seen on PET but not well defined on CT.

Major Teaching Points and Summary
1. Masses in the parotid area are commonly tumors of salivary gland origin.
2. In this case, the tumor probably did not originate in the parotid but more likely from squamous epithelium such as in the left tonsillar region.

Case 3.4.7 TUMOR OF NASOPHARYNX, RESPONSE TO TREATMENT (FIG. 3.4.7)

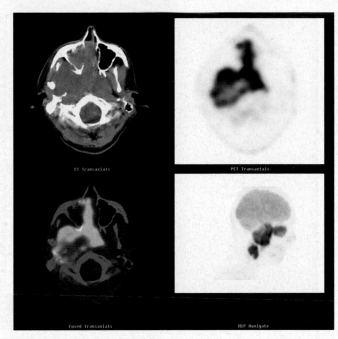

A

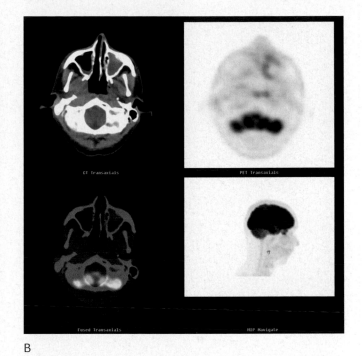

B

Brief History

A 20-year-old patient who had developed nosebleeds was diagnosed with lymphoepithelioma of the right nasopharynx. PET/CT was performed to monitor therapeutic effects. Baseline and post chemotherapy and radiotherapy PET/CT images are shown.

Findings

A. PET/CT images at presentation show a large, intensely FDG-avid mass in the nasopharynx, apparently extending to the right maxillary sinus on CT. The fused image shows that there is abnormally increased tracer activity in the tumor mass. However, the opacification of the right maxillary sinus is mainly FDG-negative, consistent with a blocked sinus.

Note on MIP: Evidence of nodal metastases in the mid and lower neck.

B. PET/CT images after treatment demonstrate complete resolution of the mass on CT and a new opacification of the left maxillary sinus, which appears to have a minimally FDG-avid rim, consistent with sinusitis and not tumor.

All FDG avid cancer-related foci have resolved, including lymph nodes in the neck.

Major Teaching Points and Summary

1. Lymphoepitheliomas are highly responsive tumors to chemotherapy.
2. In patients with extensive tumor, not all abnormalities of the sinuses are due to malignant involvement.
3. PET/CT can help clarify the origin of sinus disease as to whether malignant or benign.

Case 3.4.8 TUMOR OF LIP (FIG. 3.4.8)

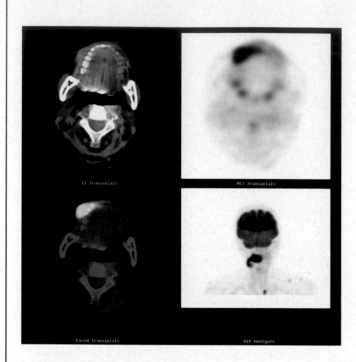

Case 3.4.9 TUMOR, BASE OF TONGUE (FIG. 3.4.9)

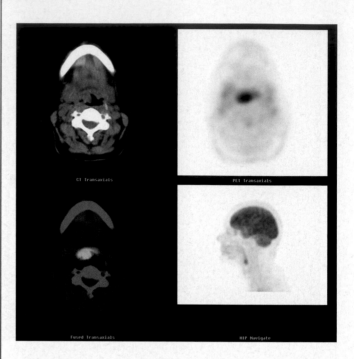

Brief History
A 77-year-old patient had recent swelling in the region of the inner right lip, diagnosed by biopsy as squamous cell carcinoma. The patient was referred to PET/CT for staging.

Findings
PET/CT images show intense focal curvilinear FDG uptake overlying the right inner lip region, corresponding to soft tissue swelling seen on CT.

Note on MIP: There is an additional focus of increased FDG uptake curving posterolaterally from the lesion, consistent with nodal metastases, and focal uptake in a left supraclavicular lymph node.

The patient was found to have extensive metastatic disease and is not a candidate for surgical resection for cure.

Main Teaching Points and Summary
1. Carcinomas of the lip are usually squamous or basal cell in origin. Undiagnosed, they can spread locally to level I nodes and then systemically.
2. Direct examination of the patient is important to ensure that no inflammatory process is responsible for positive PET/CT findings.

Brief History
A 60-year-old patient had a recent MRI showing a mass at the right aspect of the base of the tongue, diagnosed as squamous cell carcinoma. The patient was referred for PET/CT for staging.

Study Findings
PET/CT images demonstrate a right-sided mass in the region of the base of tongue and vallecula, with deviation of the hypopharynx to the left on CT, with corresponding intense FDG activity in the tumor on PET.

Main Teaching Points and Summary
1. Intense FDG uptake is typical for most squamous cell carcinomas of adequate size for detection, as seen in the present case.
2. Tumors located at the base of the tongue often extend to tonsils and hypopharynx.

Case 3.4.10 TUMOR OF TONGUE AND LEVEL II NODES (FIG. 3.4.10)

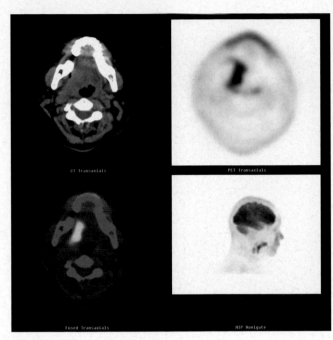

A

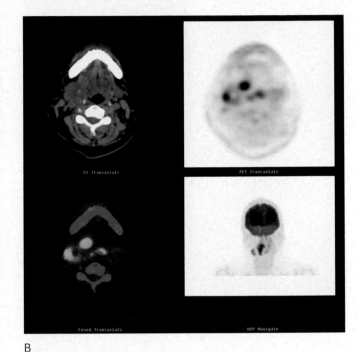

B

Brief History
A 69-year-old patient with a squamous cell carcinoma of the tongue confirmed by biopsy was referred to PET/CT for initial staging.

Findings
A. PET/CT images demonstrate intense tracer activity in an irregular lesion, 4 cm in diameter, in the right lateral tongue, extending to the floor of the mouth and the right lingual/palatine tonsils.
B. PET/CT images at a lower level demonstrate intense activity in a partly necrotic right level II lymph node.

Main Teaching Points and Summary
1. Carcinoma of the tongue is generally squamous cell in origin.
2. These tumors commonly metastasize to regional lymph nodes with levels I and II as the first stations.
3. The tumors are prone to central necrosis, both in the primary lesion and the nodal metastases.
4. Care must be taken to separate tumor in the tongue from altered uptake due to muscle contraction. Lateral MIP and coronal views are helpful in showing the extent of tumor involvement.

Case 3.4.11 TUMOR OF TONSIL AND LEVEL II NODES (FIG. 3.4.11)

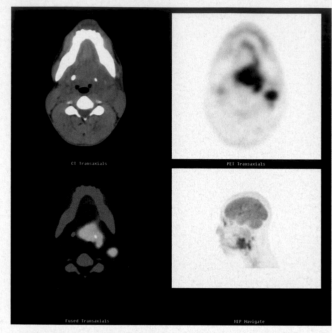

A

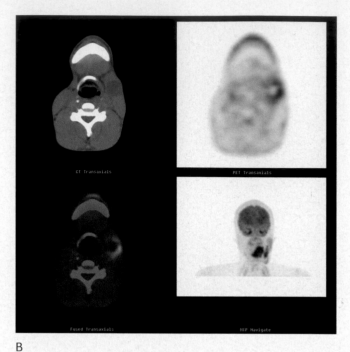

B

Brief History

A 43-year-old patient with squamous cell carcinoma originating in the left tonsil was referred for PET/CT to assess extent of disease before therapy.

Findings

A. PET/CT images show an intensely FDG-avid mass in the left tonsillar pillar extending forward into the left tongue base.

B. PET/CT images also demonstrate solid and necrotic level II lymph nodes caudal to the primary lesion.

Main Teaching Points and Summary

1. Tumors occurring in the palatine tonsillar region can extend to the tongue base and lingual tonsillar area.
2. Metastases to level II, upper jugular lymph nodes, are common. They are frequently necrotic. Not uncommonly, metastatic lesions are larger than the primary tumor.

Case 3.4.12 TUMOR OF PHARYNX (FIG. 3.4.12)

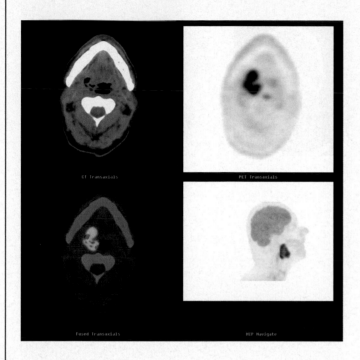

Case 3.4.13 TUMOR OF PHARYNX (ARYEPIGLOTTIC FOLD) AND CERVICAL NODES (FIG. 3.4.13)

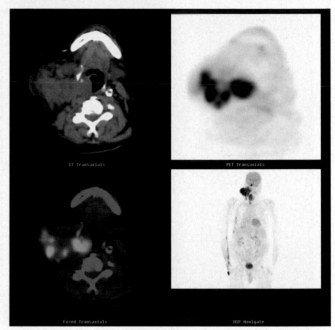

Brief History
A 66-year-old patient with newly diagnosed right para-pharyngeal squamous cell carcinoma was referred to PET/CT for staging.

Findings
PET/CT images demonstrate an area of intense focal FDG activity in a mass that extends from the palate to the base of the tongue and the epiglottic region. No nodal metastases are identified.

Main Teaching Points and Summary
1. PET/CT with FDG is a useful imaging modality to stage head and neck cancer.
2. In this case, the primary lesion is extensive.

Brief History
A 77-year-old patient had an enlarging neck mass for at least 1 year before PET/CT. The patient had a history of smoking and bladder carcinoma.

Findings
PET/CT images demonstrate an agglomeration of FDG-avid lymph nodes in the right neck. There is also markedly increased tracer uptake in the lateral wall of the pharynx and the aryepiglottic region on the right. The precise origin of the mass is difficult to identify, but it is likely from the right aryepiglottic fold.

Note on MIP: Focal increased FDG uptake in the pituitary gland, most likely an unrelated adenoma, is seen.

Main Teaching Points and Summary
1. Malignant cervical tumors if not diagnosed promptly, can result in severe and marked distortion of the neck.
2. At a more advanced stage, they may lead to vascular invasion, bleeding, and death.

Case 3.4.14 TUMOR OF LARYNX, SUPRAGLOTTIC, AND TRACHEOSTOMY (FIG. 3.4.14)

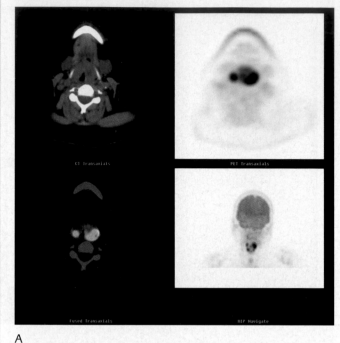

A

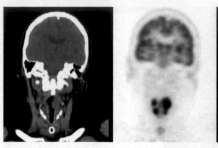
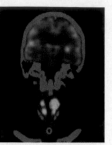

B

History

A 55-year-old patient with newly diagnosed squamous cell carcinoma of the supraglottic larynx was referred for staging. The patient recently had a tracheostomy to ensure airway patency.

Findings

A. Transaxial PET/CT images demonstrate an area of focal intense FDG activity extending from the left hypopharynx to aryepiglottic folds, bilaterally, and to the right false vocal cord.

B. Coronal PET/CT images demonstrate additional mild FDG activity at the tracheostomy site.

Note on MIP: Physiologically increased FDG uptake in the normal right cricoarytenoid muscle.

No distant metastases were identified.

Major Teaching Points and Summary

1. Although typically transverse PET images are examined, coronal and sagittal views may also be useful for determining the precise extent of tumor involvement relative to normal structures or postsurgical changes. In this case, the lesion is more extensive than had been expected.

2. It is critical to recall that normal structures such as the cricoarytenoid muscles can have intense physiologic tracer uptake.

3. Mild to moderate FDG uptake at a tracheostomy site is common.

Case 3.4.15 TUMOR OF LARYNX AND DESTRUCTION OF TRACHEAL CARTILAGE (FIG. 3.4.15)

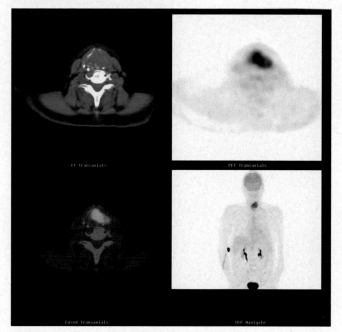

Brief History

A 71-year-old patient with a history of laryngeal papilloma was recently found to have an enlarging laryngeal mass diagnosed as carcinoma. PET/CT was performed for staging.

Findings

PET/CT images demonstrate intense FDG activity in a laryngeal mass, larger than 5 cm in diameter, which has invaded through the left tracheal cartilage and crosses the midline to the right. This tumor has essentially occluded the airway, and the patient had a tracheostomy to maintain the airway open.

Major Teaching Points and Summary

1. Laryngeal carcinomas are typically squamous cell in origin and show intense FDG uptake.
2. Large tumors of the larynx can occlude the airway requiring emergent placement of tracheostomy.

Case 3.4.16 TUMOR OF VOCAL CORD (FIG. 3.4.16)

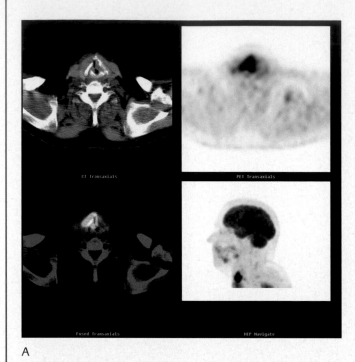

A

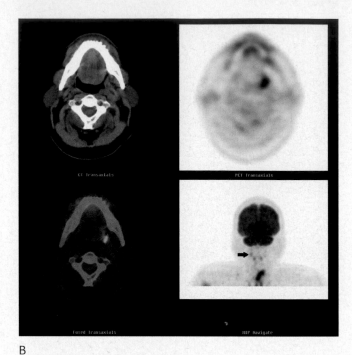

B

Brief History

A 68-year-old patient with a history of a small noninvasive right vocal cord tumor treated previously with external beam irradiation presented with new symptoms of hoarseness and a clinical suspicion of recurrent tumor.

Findings

A. PET/CT images demonstrate intense FDG uptake in the region of the right vocal cord extending through the right thyroid cartilage and the infraglottic soft tissue on the right. The activity does not appear to cross the midline to the left.

B. PET/CT images at an upper level show marked asymmetry of tonsillar uptake, with apparently increased activity in the left tonsil related to previous irradiation of the right tonsil (arrows on posterior MIP image). Right tonsillar activity is reduced.

Major Teaching Points and Summary

1. "Cured" head and neck cancers can recur either at the site of the prior tumor or at a new site.

2. Prior treatment, both radiation and surgery, can result in an altered FDG uptake pattern that may be confused with pathology unless there is a clear understanding of the patient history.

Case 3.4.17 TUMOR OF CERVICAL ESOPHAGUS (FIG. 3.4.17)

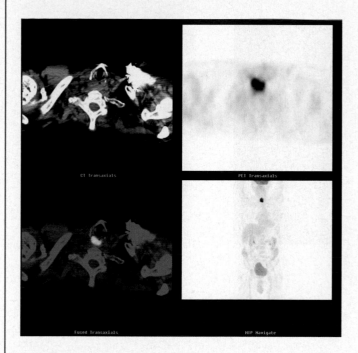

Brief History

A 73-year-old patient presented with painful and difficult swallowing. Direct inspection showed a mass consistent with esophageal carcinoma. PET/CT was performed for staging.

Findings

PET/CT images show intense focal uptake in the proximal third of the esophagus consistent with the location of a primary cancer. Distortion and narrowing of the cervical esophagus by the mass is noted on CT.

Note on MIP: No evidence of systemic metastatic disease.

Main Teaching Points and Summary

1. Esophageal carcinoma commonly occurs in the distal third of the esophagus, associated with gastroesophageal reflux. Less frequently it can also occur anywhere else along the esophagus.
2. When localized in the upper esophagus, squamous cell histology is more common than adenocarcinoma.

Case 3.4.18 TUMOR OF NEURAL SHEATH AND BROWN FAT (FIG. 3.4.18)

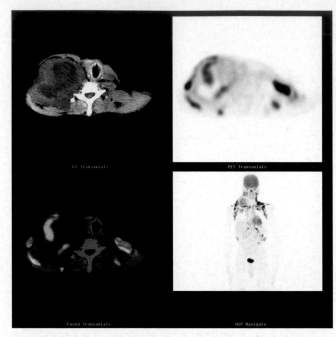

A

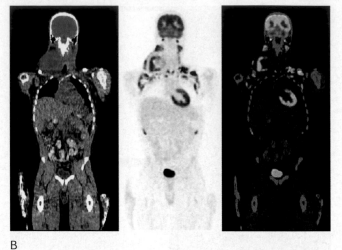

B

Brief History

A 15-year-old patient with a history of neurofibromatosis type I for the previous 8 years was assessed for activity of a known peripheral nerve sheath tumor in the right neck.

Findings

A. Transaxial PET/CT images demonstrate a large mass in the right neck showing inhomogeneous FDG uptake, consistent with the peripheral nerve sheath tumor with central necrosis. There is also increased tracer uptake in regions corresponding to fatty tissues on CT and fused images, as well as in cervical muscles.

B. Coronal PET/CT images show the location, size, and inhomogeneous pattern of the primary tumor and the extension of brown fat uptake to the upper abdomen.

Main Teaching Points and Summary

1. Neurofibromatosis, sarcomatoid in nature, can transform to malignant nerve sheath tumors.
2. FDG-PET can help detect such transformation and differentiate it from plexiform neuroma.
3. In this case, brown fat activity confounds the diagnosis, but PET/CT provides the correct solution.

Case 3.4.19 TUMOR OF BONE, VERTEBRAL METASTASIS (FIG. 3.4.19)

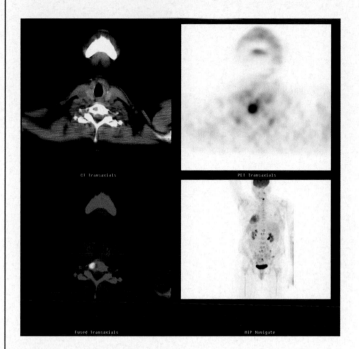

Brief History

A 49-year-old patient with history of breast cancer, diagnosed 1 year before this PET/CT study, complained of back pain and was referred in search of metastatic disease.

Findings

PET/CT images show an area of intense FDG uptake in the right cervicothoracic spinal junction region. This abnormal tracer uptake fuses to a lytic lesion in the right aspect of the C-7 vertebral body, consistent with bone metastases from breast cancer.

Note on posterior MIP: Suspicious foci of FDG uptake in the lower lumbar spine are evident.

Main Teaching Point and Summary

1. Focal uptake in the neck is not invariably due to nodal metastases. In the current case, although PET alone might suggest a paratracheal or retrotracheal node, PET/CT clearly fuses this suspicious focus to a lytic skeletal lesion.
2. Lytic metastases tend to be more FDG-avid than osteoblastic bone lesions.

3.5 LYMPH NODE COMPARTMENTS

There are six named lymph node regions in the head and neck that can be involved with metastatic cancer, depend- *ing, to a substantial extent, on the location of the primary tumor.*

Case 3.5.1 LEVEL I LYMPH NODES (FIG. 3.5.1)

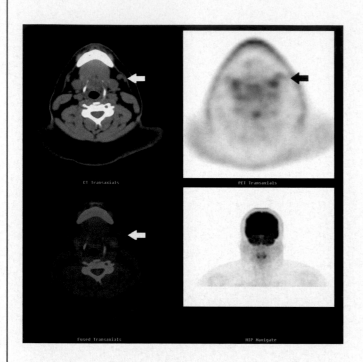

Brief History
A 26-year-old patient with a history of Hodgkin lymphoma in the thorax was being reassessed for possible recurrent tumor.

Findings
PET/CT images demonstrate mild uptake in level I borderline enlarged nodes in the neck (arrow), less than the intensity expected for recurrent lymphoma.

Note on MIP: No evidence for other foci of recurrent Hodgkin lymphoma is seen.

Main Teaching Points and Summary
1. Mild uptake in level I and II nodes is not uncommon in younger patients, mainly because of intercurrent infectious processes. In suspicious cases, histologic confirmation or close follow-up should be attempted.
2. Previous tumor involvement in the same nodal stations can increase the probability that increased FDG uptake in nodes represents recurrent tumor.

Case 3.5.2 LEVEL I AND II LYMPH NODES AND SCALENE MUSCLE UPTAKE (FIG. 3.5.2)

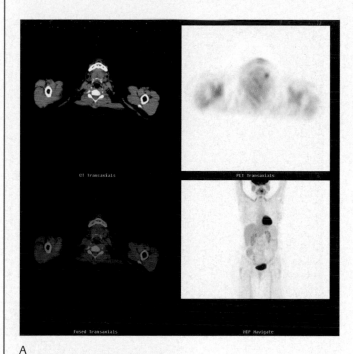

A

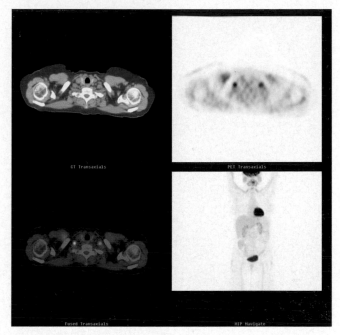

C

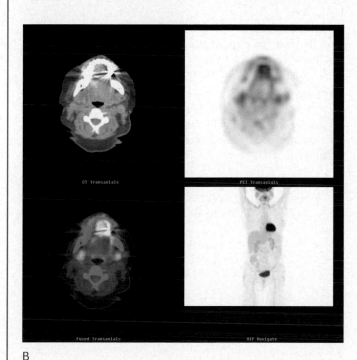

B

Brief History

A 55-year-old patient was diagnosed with low-grade follicular lymphoma 2 years before current study. PET/CT 1 year earlier showed cervical and inguinal node activity, whereas more recent studies were negative. The present study was performed to evaluate for recurrent lymphoma.

Study Findings

A and B. PET/CT images show no significant anatomic findings on CT; however, there is abnormally increased FDG uptake in normal-sized lymph nodes, less than 1 cm in diameter, in a left level I (A) and a left level II (B), concerning for the presence of malignancy.

C. PET/CT images at the level of the lower neck show increased physiologic FDG activity in scalene muscles, likely due to muscle contraction at the time of tracer injection.

Main Teaching Points and Summary

1. Mild-to-moderate level FDG uptake in normal-sized nodes is concerning for recurrent lymphoma.
2. Because of limited count recovery, small nodal structures may show only mild or moderate levels of abnormal tracer uptake.
3. Non-Hodgkin's lymphoma can involve any nodal groups.
4. Scalene muscle uptake could be potentially confused with tumor-involved lymph nodes on transaxial PET-only images but is clearly linear on MIP images.

Case 3.5.3 LEVEL II LYMPH NODES (FIG. 3.5.3)

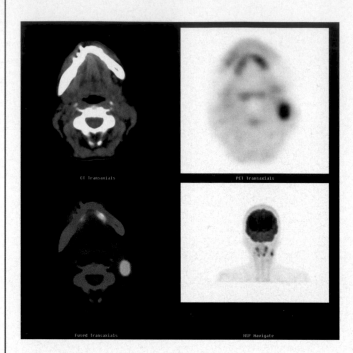

Brief History
A 60-year-old patient presented with a palpable left neck mass. Biopsy performed 2 weeks before PET/CT was positive for squamous cell carcinoma. The current study was performed for staging.

Findings
PET/CT images demonstrate level II lymph node, approximately 2 cm in diameter on CT, corresponding to a focus of intense FDG activity on PET. Smaller level II nodes are present in the contralateral neck on CT but are FDG negative. There is also physiologic activity in the lingual tonsils.

Main Teaching Points and Summary
1. Intense FDG uptake in an enlarged node is typical of metastatic cancer.
2. In this case, the large node was involved with cancer but the primary lesion could not be identified.

Case 3.5.4 LEVEL II LYMPH NODES (FIG. 3.5.4)

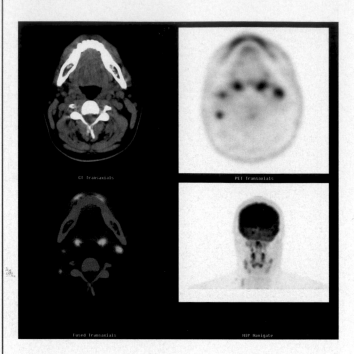

Brief History
A 38-year-old patient had a history of right esthesio-neuroblastoma, a tumor controlled with radiation. PET/CT was obtained to exclude metastases.

Findings
PET/CT images show increased FDG uptake in bilateral, mildly enlarged level II lymph nodes, consistent with metastases. There is also increased tracer activity in the tonsils.

Main Teaching Points and Summary
1. Esthesio-neuroblastoma is a rare tumor that not infrequently metastatisizes to regional lymph nodes.

Case 3.5.5 LEVEL II AND III LYMPH NODES (FIG. 3.5.5)

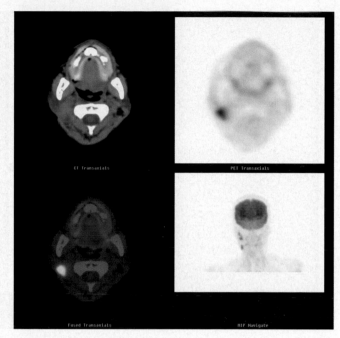

A

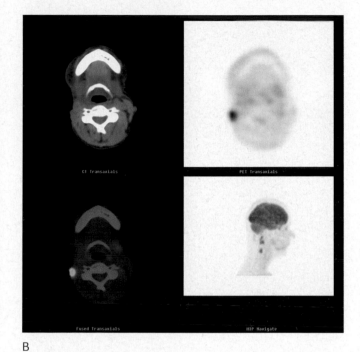

B

Brief History

A 49-year-old patient with history of squamous cell carcinoma of the right tonsil 1 year after chemotherapy and radiation therapy, tonsillectomy, and right neck dissection was referred to assess for recurrent tumor.

Findings

A and B. PET/CT images demonstrate focal intense FDG uptake in level II (A) and level III (B) lymph nodes in the right neck, consistent with regional nodal tumor recurrence. There is loss of normal tissue planes in the right neck due to prior radiation therapy.

Main Teaching Points and Summary

1. The postradiation and postsurgical neck is difficult to assess clinically and by conventional imaging modalities.
2. PET/CT improves substantially the accuracy for diagnosis of cervical tumor recurrences.
3. Level II and III (high and midinternal jugular) nodes are common sites for metastases from tonsillar cancer.

Case 3.5.6 LEVEL IV LYMPH NODES (FIG. 3.5.6)

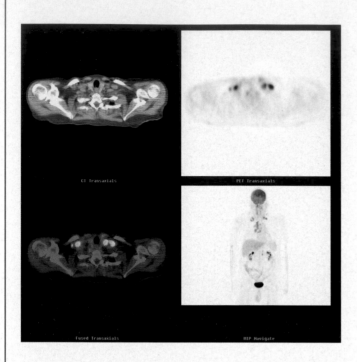

Brief History
A 57-year-old patient with newly diagnosed lung cancer was referred to assess resectability.

Findings
PET/CT images show focal intense FDG uptake in mildly enlarged supraclavicular lymph nodes, which are at the lower limit of neck level IV (including the low internal jugular chain, from the cricoid to the clavicle).

Note on MIP: Abnormal tracer uptake in multiple mediastinal tumor sites is evident.

Main Teaching Points and Summary
1. Interpretation of PET/CT images of the neck requires an understanding of the routes of lymphatic drainage from a variety of locations.
2. Although level IV nodes can be the draining site of head and neck cancers, such nodes can also drain processes in the thorax, especially if central mediastinal lymphatic drainage is obstructed.

Case 3.5.7 LEVEL V LYMPH NODES (FIG. 3.5.7)

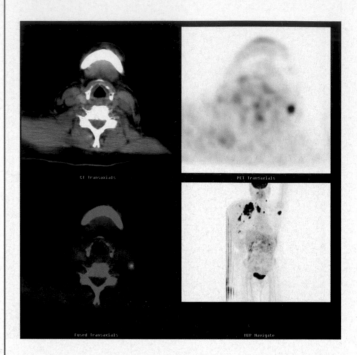

Brief History
A 69-year-old patient with metastatic breast carcinoma who also had lymphedema was referred for assessment of the extent of disease.

Findings
PET/CT images show a level Vb left neck node affected with tumor. This node is posterior to the sternocleidomastoid muscle and caudal to the cricoid cartilage.

Note on MIP: Extensive metastatic disease.

Main Teaching Points and Summary
1. Although in this case, the disease is extensive and precise nodal nomenclature is not clinically critical, it illustrates clearly the typical location of a level Vb node, in contrast to level Va nodes, which are cephalad to the cricoid cartilage.
2. Level V nodes are also referred to as the spinal accessory nodal chain.

Case 3.5.8 LEVEL VI LYMPH NODES (FIG. 3.5.8)

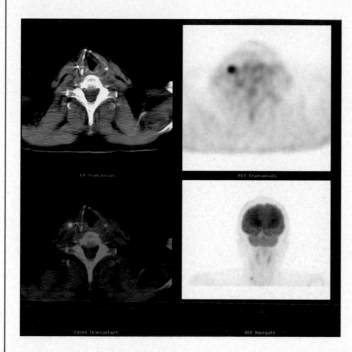

Case 3.6.1 BENIGN—THYROIDITIS (FIG. 3.6.1)

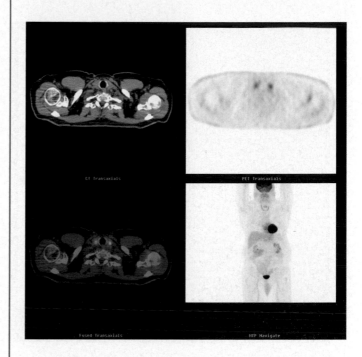

Brief History

A 62-year-old patient with a history of papillary thyroid carcinoma, status following three treatments with radioactive iodine, now has a negative radioiodine scan but rising serum thyroglobulin levels, suspicious of recurrent thyroid carcinoma.

Findings

PET/CT images show focal intense uptake in the anterior cervical, level VI lymph node in the right neck, adjacent to the site of prior surgery.

This was further biopsy proven to be recurrent thyroid cancer.

Main Teaching Points and Summary

1. Anterior cervical nodes represent a site of drainage for thyroid and vocal cord tumors.
2. There are three subgroups of anterior nodes: anterior-midline prelaryngeal, Delphian paratracheal, and pretracheal.
3. Anterior nodes can drain directly into the upper mediastinum.

Brief History

A 62-year-old patient with a history of a large B-cell non-Hodgkin's lymphoma, currently in clinical remission. PET/CT was performed for routine follow-up.

Findings

PET/CT images demonstrate mild to moderate diffuse FDG activity in both lobes of the thyroid consistent with thyroiditis.

No focal lesions are seen to suggest lymphoma recurrence systemically.

Main Teaching Point and Summary

1. Mild to moderate FDG uptake in the thyroid is not unusual and is likely due to subclinical thyroiditis and not to lymphomatous infiltration of the thyroid.
2. Patients showing this finding as a rule do not have clinical symptoms related to the thyroid.
3. It is important to recognize that these findings border on the range of normal variants and should not be confused with active lymphoma or other tumors.

Case 3.6.2 BENIGN—MULTINODULAR, RETROSTERNAL GOITER (FIG. 3.6.2)

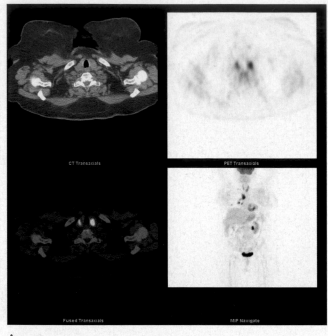

A

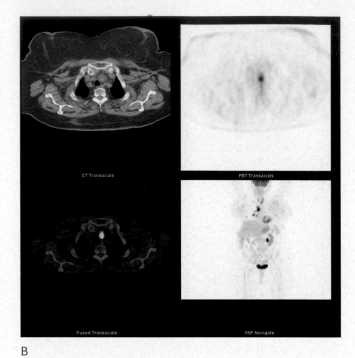

B

Brief History

A 72-year-old patient with a history of a breast cancer and rising tumor markers was referred for suspected tumor recurrence.

Findings

A and B. PET/CT images demonstrate moderately intense inhomogeneous FDG uptake in both lobes of the thyroid, consistent with a known multinodular goiter. The left lobe of the thyroid is enlarged (A) and reaches the superior mediastinum, posterior to the manubrium (B).

Note on MIP: Multiple foci of abnormally increased FDG uptake involving a right lower lobe pulmonary nodule, as well as mediastinal and right supraclavicular lymph nodes, is evident, consistent with disseminated metastatic breast cancer.

Main Teaching Points and Summary

1. As a rule, inhomogeneous FDG uptake in an enlarged thyroid is suggestive of multinodular goiter.
2. The differential diagnosis of increased FDG uptake in the anterior upper mediastinum should include retrosternal thyroid tissue and thymus.

Case 3.6.3 BENIGN—THYROID ADENOMA AND DISTORTED ANATOMY (FIG. 3.6.3)

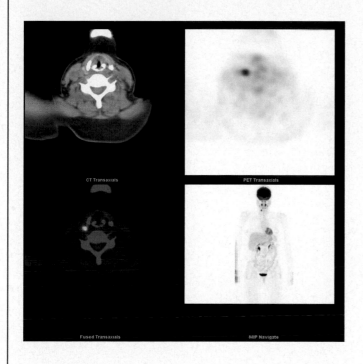

Brief History
A 53-year-old patient with recurrent aggressive non-Hodgkin's lymphoma was assessed to determine response to second-line chemotherapy.

Findings
PET/CT images demonstrated a focal area of abnormally increased FDG uptake in the right neck, localized to the upper pole of an enlarged right lobe of the thyroid (note iodine content on the CT). This activity is positioned posterior and lateral to the thyroid cartilage.

Note on MIP: No evidence for residual active lymphoma.

PET/CT-guided biopsy diagnosed a benign follicular adenoma.

Main Teaching Points and Summary
1. Although in a significant fraction of patients a single FDG-avid thyroid nodule is of malignant etiology, the presence and intensity of increased tracer uptake in such nodules cannot reliably differentiate between malignant and benign lesions.

Case 3.6.4 TUMOR—PRIMARY THYROID CANCER (FIG. 3.6.4)

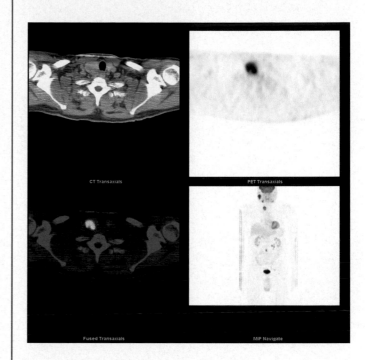

Brief History
A 64-year-old patient with MALT non-Hodgkin's lymphoma of the parotid gland was assessed for staging.

Findings
PET/CT images demonstrate intense inhomogeneous FDG uptake in a large right thyroid nodule.

Note on MIP: Multiple sites of abnormally increased FDG uptake involving the right parotid gland, right cervical, and retroperitoneal lymph nodes, are consistent with lymphomatous involvement.

The etiology of the intrathyroidal lesion could not be established based on PET alone. PET/CT-guided biopsy diagnosed a second primary papillary thyroid cancer.

Main Teaching Points and Summary
1. Focal FDG uptake in a thyroid nodule represents malignancy in a significant fraction of patients.
2. Focal FDG uptake in a thyroid nodule in a patient with known cancer does not necessarily define the lesion as metastatic, even in the presence of additional FDG-avid foci.
3. Biopsy is required for definitive diagnosis.

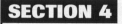

SECTION 4

PET/CT of the Chest

Richard L. Wahl • Mehrbod Som Javadi

4.1 NORMAL PATTERN

Case 4.1.1 NORMAL PATTERN PET/CT OF THE CHEST (FIG. 4.1)

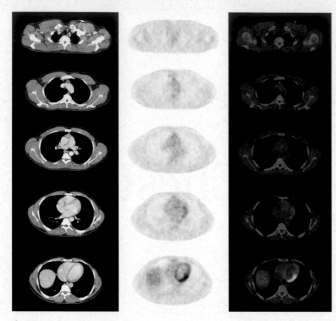

A

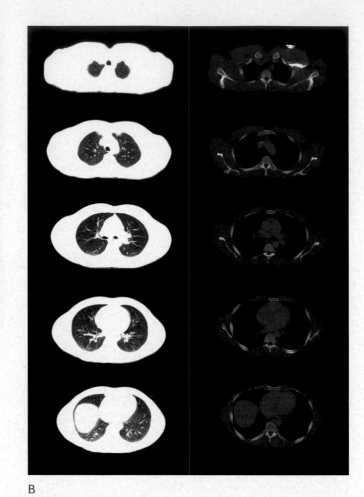

B

This is an example of a normal PET/CT of the thorax. This study was performed following administration of intravenous (IV) contrast, which facilitates the separation of blood vessels and the heart from nodal or other anatomic structures and from pathologic findings. The CT component of the hybrid imaging study is visualized with multiple windows including soft tissue (A) as well as lung and bone windows (B).

Normal low-intensity 2-[18F] fluoro-2-deoxy-D-glucose (FDG) uptake is identified in the mediastinum and heart. Non–attenuation-corrected PET images (not shown) demonstrate diffuse increased tracer uptake in the lungs, which is not seen on corrected images, where the lungs appear FDG negative. While reviewing PET/CT images of the chest, special attention needs to be given to respiration-related misregistration due to short duration CT image acquisition time versus the longer duration of PET image acquisition during shallow breathing.

4.2 CHEST WALL

Case 4.2.1 PITFALL—GYNECOMASTIA AND ESOPHAGEAL CANCER (FIG. 4.2.1)

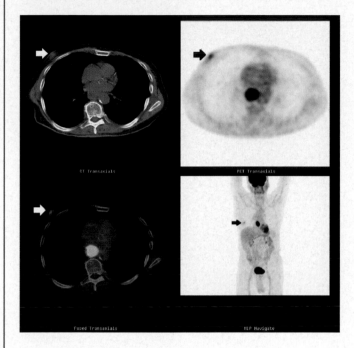

Case 4.2.2 PITFALL—MUSCULAR UPTAKE, ASYMMETRIC (FIG. 4.2.2)

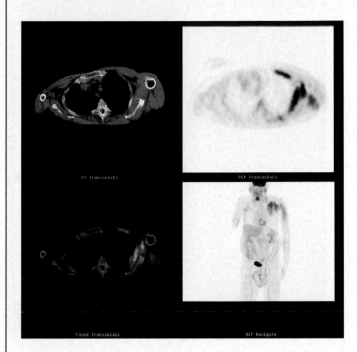

Brief History

A 78-year-old patient with history of chest pain and vomiting was diagnosed with esophageal carcinoma and was referred for preoperative staging. The patient was also receiving hormone deprivation therapy for prostate carcinoma.

Findings

PET/CT images show a moderately intense focus of FDG uptake in the glandular tissue of the right breast consistent with gynecomastia (arrows), which developed following the hormone deprivation therapy for prostate cancer.

Note on MIP: The distal esophageal primary cancer.

Main Teaching Point and Summary

1. Gynecomastia can develop relatively soon after hormone blockade therapy for prostate cancer and present as asymmetric foci of findings with FDG avidity.
2. Knowledge of patient history is of value for interpretation of this study. Had there not been recent hormonal therapy, this imaging pattern could raise concern for a new male breast cancer requiring more examinations, at times invasive, to confirm or exclude this possibility.

Brief History

A 59-year-old patient with history of obstructive airway disease was referred for further assessment of newly diagnosed pulmonary nodules. The patient also had congenital birth injury and Erbs palsy with profound weakness of the right arm.

Findings

PET/CT images show increased FDG uptake in the hypertrophied left shoulder girdle musculature and atrophy of the muscles on the right, related to the known Erbs palsy.

Main Teaching Points and Summary

1. FDG muscle uptake can be intense.
2. In this case, there is compensatory hypertrophy on the left and only minimal musculature on the right, accounting for the marked asymmetry.

Case 4.2.3 PITFALL—AXILLARY POSTINJECTION UPTAKE AND BREAST CANCER (FIG. 4.2.3)

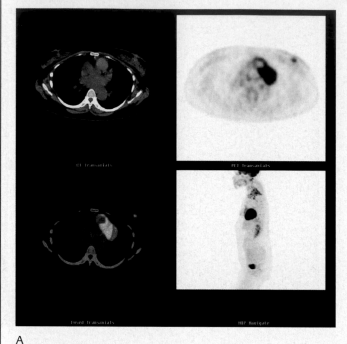

A

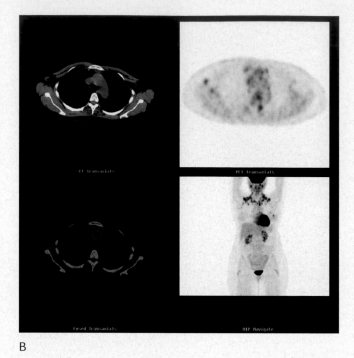

B

Brief History

A 56-year-old patient with newly diagnosed left breast cancer was believed, on an outside PET-only study, to have left subpectoral and axillary nodal involvement.

Findings

1. PET/CT images show focal intense FDG activity in a nodular density seen on CT in the left breast, consistent with the primary tumor.
2. PET/CT images at a cephalad level show mild FDG uptake in a normal-sized lymph node with a hypodense center in the right axilla.

Of note: The patient was injected in the right arm, possibly causing the tracer uptake in the right axillary node. There is no evidence for metastases on PET/CT.

Note on MIP: Substantial brown fat activity in the supra-clavicular region.

Main Teaching Points and Summary

1. This case illustrates how PET/CT can prevent false-positive interpretations of FDG-avid foci such as axillary lymph nodes.
2. The right axillary increased tracer activity, mimicking nodal metastases fused to normal nodes draining the injection site, a common potential cause of false-positive uptake.

Case 4.2.4 BENIGN—BROWN FAT, SHOULDER AND UPPER CHEST WALL (FIG. 4.2.4)

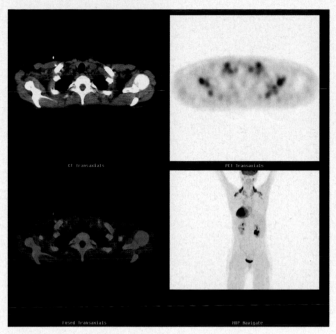

A

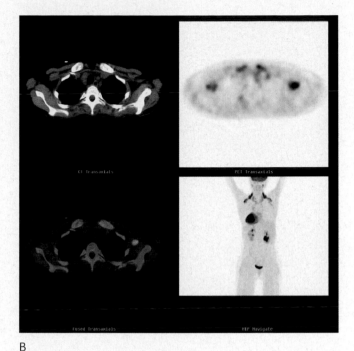

B

Brief History

An 18-year-old patient with history of Hodgkin's lymphoma, status post–bone marrow transplantation, achieved complete response and was evaluated as part of an early posttransplant surveillance program.

Findings

A and B. PET/CT images show extensive FDG uptake in a linear and nodular pattern bilaterally in the neck and upper thorax. This activity fused to fatty tissue on CT.

Note on posterior MIP: Increased tracer activity in fatty tissues in supraclavicular regions and axillae.

On follow-up, there was no evidence of active lymphoma.

Main Teaching Points and Summary

1. In younger patients, especially females, brown fat activity is common and intense on FDG-PET. Correlation with CT is critical to ensure that active lymphoma is not present in addition to the brown fat uptake.
2. Warming the patient or administration of beta-blockers or reserpine before tracer injection may reduce this uptake.

Case 4.2.5 BENIGN—POSTSURGICAL CHANGES (FIG. 4.2.5)

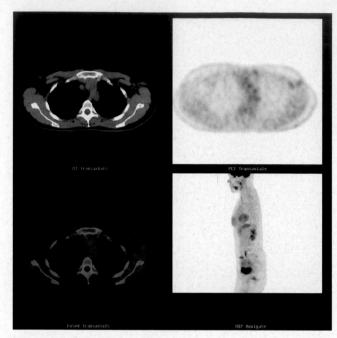

A

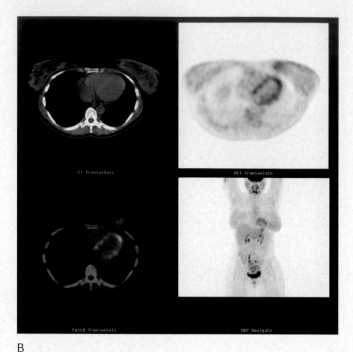

B

Brief History

A 42-year-old patient with a history of left breast cancer treated by lumpectomy and left axillary dissection 2 months before PET/CT was referred for restaging before definitive therapy because microscopic tumor had been found in one sentinel node.

Findings

A. PET/CT images demonstrate mild focal linear uptake at the site of a healing left axillary dissection. Minimal FDG uptake is seen in axillary nodes.
B. PET/CT images at a lower level show moderately increased tracer uptake in the medial aspect of the left breast, at the site of the lumpectomy (which had negative surgical margins).

The findings are most consistent with postoperative changes. No evidence of gross active tumor is identified.

Main Teaching Points and Summary

1. Surgical procedures can cause mildly increased tracer uptake at the surgical site.
2. Knowing the time elapsed from the procedure until PET/CT imaging is important because postsurgical changes often resolve within several months.

Case 4.2.6 TUMOR–CHEST WALL RECURRENCE, BREAST CANCER (FIG. 4.2.6)

Case 4.3.1 ARTIFACT–SALINE IMPLANTS, COLD LESION (FIG. 4.3.1)

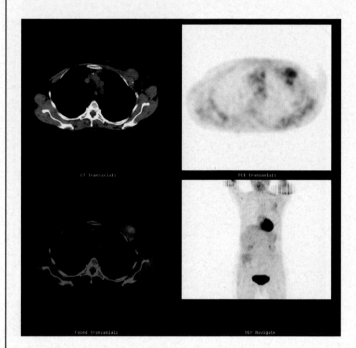

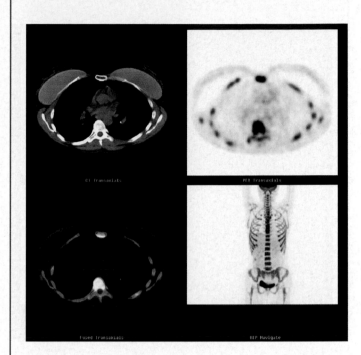

Brief History
A 57-year-old patient with a 1-year history of breast cancer, treated with mastectomy, had clinical signs suggesting recurrence and was referred to PET/CT for further assessment.

Findings
PET/CT images demonstrate focal intense FDG activity in a soft tissue mass situated in immediate proximity to the pectoralis major muscle. An additional deeper nodule with a clip within it is located in the pectoralis minor muscle and shows increased FDG uptake. The findings are consistent with recurrent metastatic cancer.

Main Teaching Points and Summary
1. Recurrent breast cancer can be challenging to detect and separate from treatment-related changes in the chest wall or remaining breast tissue.
2. PET/CT can be helpful in such instances and direct biopsies to the relevant areas.

Brief History
A 38-year-old patient with breast cancer who recently received chemotherapy was assessed in search of residual active tumor. The patient had received pegfilgrastim 1 week before the PET/CT scan and had bilateral saline breast implants.

Findings
PET/CT images show that the saline implants are photo-penic on FDG-PET.

Note on MIP: Intense treatment-induced FDG uptake throughout the bone marrow.

Main Teaching Points and Summary
1. Saline implants are photopenic on PET in contrast to their radiodense appearance on mammograms.
2. Pegfilgrastim increases marrow uptake of FDG and can easily mask tumor involvement.

Case 4.3.2 PITFALL–SEROMA (FIG. 4.3.2)

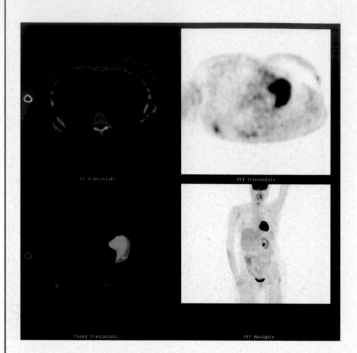

Brief History
A 49-year-old patient with recently diagnosed breast cancer, status post-lumpectomy with negative surgical margins, was referred for staging.

Findings
PET/CT images show a rectangular-shaped radiodensity in the region of the surgical resection site in the right breast on CT. This lesion is devoid of FDG uptake except for minimal activity at the edges of the density, in a region of corresponding mild thickening of the skin, consistent with seroma and not tumor.

Note on MIP: FDG-avid nodal metastases in the high right axilla.

Main Teaching Points and Summary
1. Large FDG-negative densities in the postoperative breast are generally not malignant.
2. Seroma and hematoma are typically FDG negative, with the exception of minimal uptake at the lesion edges likely due to inflammatory reactions.

Case 4.3.3 BENIGN–GRANULOMA AND FRACTURE OF SCAPULA (FIG. 4.3.3)

Brief History
A 50-year-old patient with history of sebaceous breast carcinoma underwent left mastectomy with implant 18 months before PET/CT and was evaluated for possible recurrent breast cancer and metastases. The patient recently sustained a major fall.

Findings
PET/CT images demonstrate the patient to be status post–left mastectomy, with the implant in place. Focal FDG upta]ke is evident in the upper external quadrant of the left breast, at the site of a previous biopsy performed approximately 4 months before the PET/CT. There is also focal tracer uptake fused to the right scapula, corresponding to a known fracture.

Biopsy of the lesion in the breast showed a foreign body granuloma with giant cell formation, with no evidence of malignancy.

Main Teaching Points and Summary
1. Focal FDG uptake in breast and bone in a patient with a history of breast cancer is concerning for tumor.
2. CT adds specificity to PET, avoiding false positive readings, but biopsy is still sometimes essential. In this case, biopsy confirmed the benign etiology of the left breast focus.
3. Correlation with CT and clinical history of previous trauma indicated recent fracture as the cause for the FDG avid focus in the scapula.

Case 4.3.4 BENIGN—POSTRADIATION CHANGES (FIG. 4.3.4)

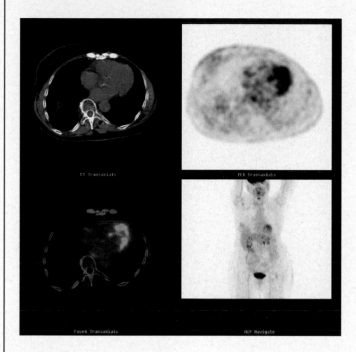

Brief History
An 83-year-old patient treated for breast cancer (hormone receptor negative invasive ductal tumor) by lumpectomy and radiation 14 years before the current study presented with borderline elevated serum CEA levels and was being assessed by PET/CT for possible recurrent tumor.

Findings
PET/CT images show mildly increased FDG uptake through most of the right breast, and in the skin overlying the breast, most likely due to radiation-induced changes.

Main Teaching Points and Summary
1. Inflammatory skin changes after radiation therapy are not unusual and can demonstrate mildly increased FDG uptake.

Case 4.3.5 TUMOR—LARGE PRIMARY BREAST CANCER (FIG. 4.3.5)

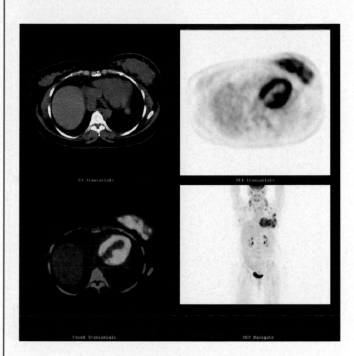

Brief History
A 39-year-old patient with a large tumor in the left breast and a right breast mass, both biopsy-proven as breast cancer, was referred for a baseline evaluation before chemotherapy.

Findings
PET/CT images show intense tracer uptake in the left breast, consistent with the known large malignant tumor.

Note on MIP: Intense uptake in the left axilla, consistent with metastatic lymphadenopathy, a small focus of FDG uptake in the right breast, in the known second primary tumor, and brown fat tracer activity in the supraclavicular and neck regions.

Main Teaching Points and Summary
1. Intense FDG uptake is typically present in aggressive breast cancers.
2. Tumors with lobular histology may demonstrate low FDG uptake levels.
3. Brown fat activity must be distinguished from metastatic nodal involvement.

Case 4.3.6 TUMOR–PRIMARY BREAST CANCER AND AXILLARY NODES (FIG. 4.3.6)

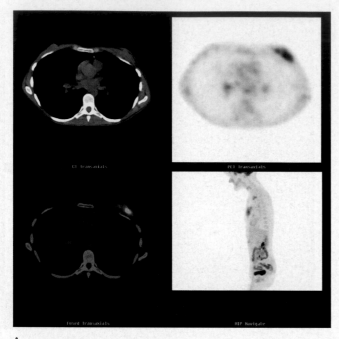

A

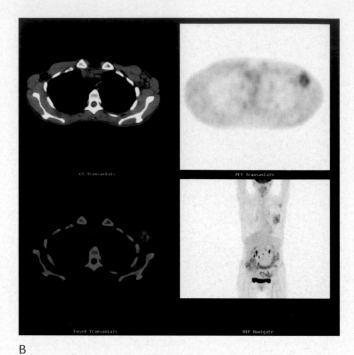

B

Brief History
A 34-year-old patient had recently noticed a left breast lump. Biopsy showed invasive ductal carcinoma. The patient was evaluated for extent of disease and for suitability for mastectomy.

Findings
A. PET/CT images show focal intense FDG uptake in a mass located in the left breast.
B. PET/CT images at a cephalad level show mildly enlarged, FDG-avid lymph nodes in the anterior aspect of the left axilla, consistent with metastases.

Main Teaching Points and Summary
1. Intense uptake in the breast and multiple foci in the axilla are highly predictive of locoregional breast cancer involvement.

Case 4.3.7 TUMOR—RECURRENT BREAST CANCER AND AXILLARY NODES (FIG. 4.3.7)

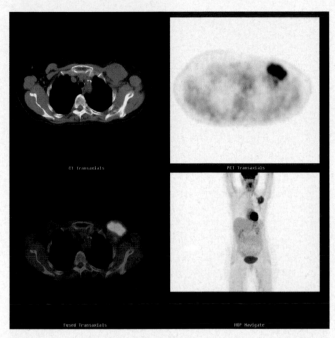

A

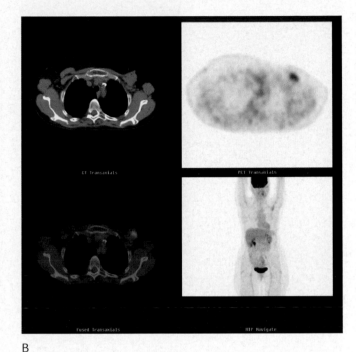

B

Brief History
A 66-year-old patient with a history of left breast cancer diagnosed in 1986 developed a left chest wall mass 14 years later and was referred for characterization and restaging.

Findings
A. PET/CT images demonstrate intense focal FDG uptake in an approximately 5-cm diameter mass in the left chest wall. A small axillary lymph node is identified deep and adjacent to the chest wall mass. These findings are consistent with recurrent breast cancer and nodal metastasis.

B. PET/CT images after the patient received chemotherapy demonstrate a substantial, although incomplete reduction in tumor glycolytic activity, which is greater than the reduction in tumor size. The nodal metastasis has disappeared. Based on PET/CT, there is evidence of residual active tumor after treatment.

Main Teaching Points and Summary
1. Recurrent breast cancer can be hard to diagnose and difficult to manage.
2. In this case, PET/CT demonstrates and easily localizes recurrent tumor and metastasis and also documents the partial response to therapy.

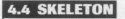

4.4 SKELETON

Case 4.4.1 BENIGN—RIB FRACTURES, VARYING AGES (FIG. 4.4.1)

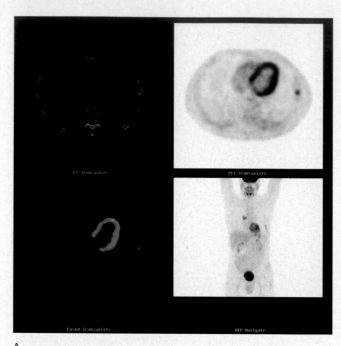

A

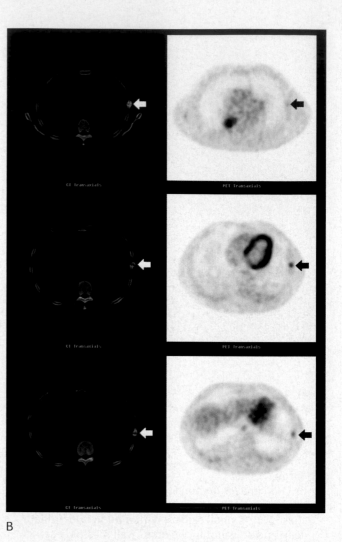

B

Brief History
A 54-year-old patient presented with pneumonia. A lung mass and enlarged lymph nodes were demonstrated on CT. PET/CT was performed to determine whether malignancy was present and for whole body staging.

Findings
A. PET/CT images show focal FDG uptake in the left chest wall, fusing precisely to a rib fracture.
B. Corresponding PET and CT images at other selected levels show variable degrees of FDG uptake (none, mild, or intense) in rib fractures of varying ages (arrows).

Note on MIP: A right hilar mass, consistent with lung carcinoma

Main Teaching Point and Summary
1. Recent rib fractures have intense tracer uptake, which tends to fade as the fracture heals, though at a slower pace for pathologic fractures, if untreated.
2. With complete healing, FDG uptake disappears in most nonpathologic rib fractures.

Case 4.4.2 BENIGN—FRACTURE, STERNUM (FIG. 4.4.2)

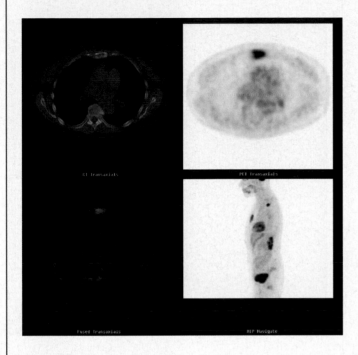

Brief History
An 81-year-old patient with chest pain was referred to characterize a new pulmonary nodule seen on CT. The patient had a recent accident with direct trauma to the sternum.

Findings
PET/CT images demonstrate intense FDG uptake through the distal part of the sternum, corresponding to a fracture seen on CT.

Note on lateral MIP: Intense FDG uptake in the apex of the lung, consistent with a new lung cancer.

Main Teaching Point and Summary
1. Sternal fractures can show intense tracer uptake, mainly within the first few weeks after they have occurred.
2. Careful clinical history of a traumatic event and examination of corresponding x-rays help avoid inadvertently confusing this tracer uptake with tumor involvement.
3. The extent of FDG uptake may exceed the size of the fracture during the healing process.

Case 4.4.3 BENIGN—OSTEOPHYTE, THORACIC VERTEBRA (FIG. 4.4.3)

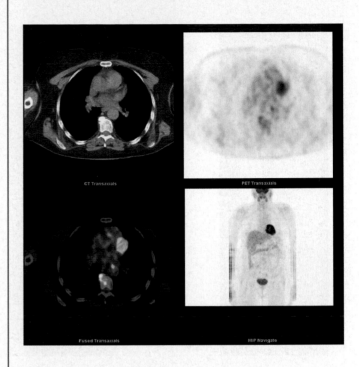

Brief History
A 68-year-old patient with follicular low-grade non-Hodgkin's lymphoma involving multiple abdominal nodal sites was assessed for response to treatment. The patient also complained of back pain.

Findings
PET/CT images demonstrate a focus of mild FDG activity in the posterior mid-mediastinum fused to an osteophytic lesion in the anterior right aspect of a midthoracic vertebral body.

Note on MIP: No evidence of active lymphoma.

Main Teaching Point and Summary
1. Degenerative changes and osteophytes can show mild to moderately increased tracer uptake in 15%–20% of cases.
2. PET/CT locates suspicious foci to the spine and based on the benign CT pattern of the skeletal lesions it excludes the presence of malignancy.

Case 4.4.4 BENIGN—POSTRADIATION "COLD" VERTEBRAE (FIG. 4.4.4)

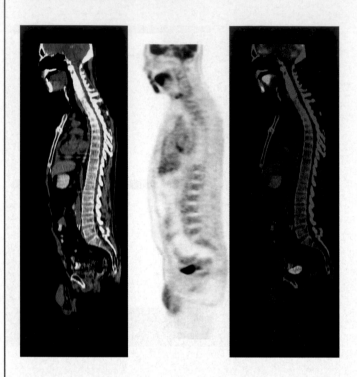

Brief History
A 61-year-old patient with a history of esophageal carcinoma diagnosed 18 months before PET/CT had been treated with chemotherapy and radiotherapy to the primary tumor. The patient was referred for suspicion of recurrence.

Findings
PET/CT images, sagittal planes, show markedly decreased FDG uptake in the midthoracic spine, corresponding to the radiation treatment port on CT associated with decreased density in the marrow of these vertebral bodies.

Note also increased tracer uptake in the tongue; the patient had excessive tongue motion and lip smacking at the time of tracer injection.

Main Teaching Point and Summary
1. Decreased FDG uptake in radiation ports is common on PET/CT studies performed after treatment.
2. Although not usually a diagnostic challenge, care must be taken not to mistake the normal tracer activity in bone marrow above or below the port for malignant involvement.

Case 4.4.5 TUMOR—METASTASIS, RIB (FIG. 4.4.5)

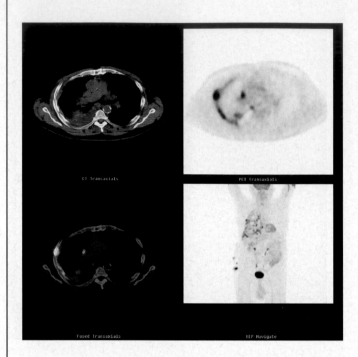

Brief History
A 77-year-old patient with weight loss, nausea, anorexia, and general malaise presented with a right pleural effusion of uncertain etiology. PET/CT was performed in search of systemic malignancy.

Findings
PET/CT images show intense focal FDG uptake in the lateral aspect of the right chest wall, corresponding to a mixed lytic and blastic lesion in the rib, most consistent with metastases. In addition, there is mild FDG uptake in right medial and lateral pleural nodules. A posterior cold area in the right hemithorax is due to the presence of pleural fluid. Non–small cell lung cancer was proven histologically although mesothelioma could be considered based on PET alone.

Note on MIP: Diffuse FDG uptake throughout the right hemithorax in a nodular pattern that parallels the pleural space is evident. Modest urinary contamination is seen in the lateral aspect of the right upper thigh.

Main Teaching Points and Summary
1. The differential diagnosis of a FDG-positive rib lesion includes recent fracture or metastasis.
2. The presence of lytic and blastic changes on CT indicates the malignant etiology of this uptake.

Case 4.4.6 TUMOR–METASTASIS, STERNUM (FIG. 4.4.6)

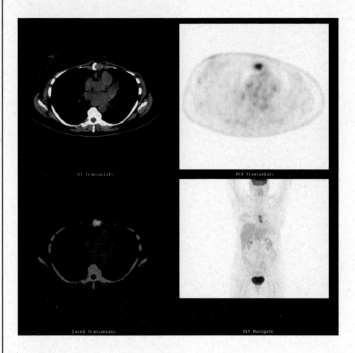

Brief History
A 52-year-old patient with breast cancer diagnosed 8 years before PET/CT had a history of trauma to the chest and an abnormal MRI, worrisome for tumor involvement in the sternum.

Findings
PET/CT images show intense FDG uptake in a lytic lesion in the left aspect of the sternum. No clear fracture was identified. The patient is status post–left mastectomy.

Main Teaching Point and Summary
1. Focal uptake in the sternum in women with breast cancer can be a metastatic site.
2. Direct invasion from internal mammary lymph node metastases is likely responsible for the malignant involvement of the sternum.
3. In this case, the history of trauma delayed diagnosis because symptoms were initially thought to be related to the trauma.

Case 4.4.7 TUMOR–METASTASES, THORACIC VERTEBRAE (FIG. 4.4.7)

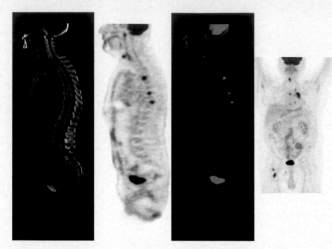

A

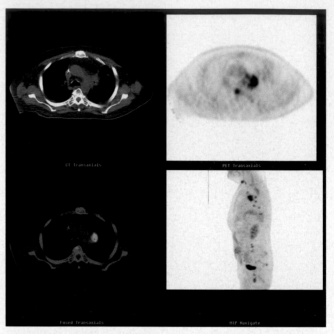

B

Brief History
A 71-year-old patient with newly diagnosed lung cancer complained of severe cough and back pain. PET/CT was performed for staging.

Findings
A. PET/CT images, sagittal slices, show several FDG-avid lesions in vertebral bodies, most of which do not show obvious CT abnormalities.
B. PET/CT images, transaxial slices at the level of the midthorax show a focus of abnormally increased FDG uptake which on PET alone appears located in the posterior mediastinum. On fused images, this intense lesion is localized to a thoracic vertebra. In addition, there is a large left hilar mass (10L and 11L nodes) showing intense abnormal FDG uptake, consistent with metastatic lymphadenopathy.

Note on anterior and lateral MIP: A focal lesion is seen in the right femoral neck and is suspicious for metastasis. The focus of increased uptake in anterior lower neck is localized by PET/CT (not shown) to asymmetric vocal cord activity because of paralysis on the left.

Main Teaching Points and Summary
1. FDG-avid bone metastases may present without obvious CT abnormalities.
2. PET/CT can define the specific localization of a malignant focus.
3. In this case, the close proximity of posterior mediastinal nodes and the thoracic vertebrae demonstrates why PET/CT is essential to differentiate a skeletal from nodal lesion.
4. Diagnosis of bone metastases upstages the patient and spares unnecessary surgery.

4.5 PLEURA

Case 4.5.1 BENIGN–INFLAMMATION, FOCAL PATTERN, PLEURODESIS (FIG. 4.5.1)

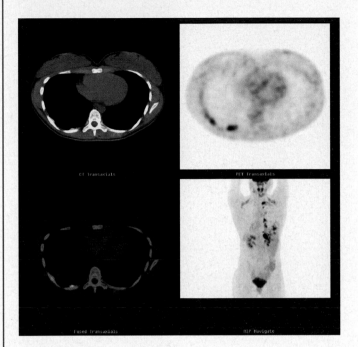

Brief History

A 21-year-old patient with a history of diffuse large B cell non-Hodgkin's lymphoma associated with effusions in the right pleural space had received a full eight cycles of rituximab and chemotherapy with marked improvement. He also underwent a talc pleurodesis of the right chest 1 year before PET/CT. The study was performed to search for residual active lymphoma.

Findings

PET/CT images show discrete focal densities in the posterolateral aspect of the right pleural space, with corresponding foci of intense FDG uptake, consistent with talc-induced inflammation in the right hemithorax. These findings were stable for a 9-month period without treatment.

Note on posterior MIP: Moderate tracer uptake in supra-clavicular brown fat.

Main Teaching Points and Summary

1. Clinical history is critical for proper interpretation of this study.
2. The differential diagnosis of this imaging pattern includes mesothelioma or pleural lymphoma versus posttreatment inflammatory changes.

Case 4.5.2 BENIGN—INFLAMMATION, DIFFUSE PATTERN, PLEURODESIS (FIG. 4.5.2)

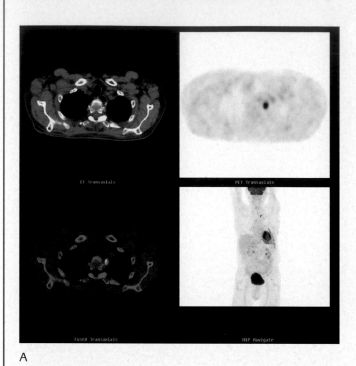

A

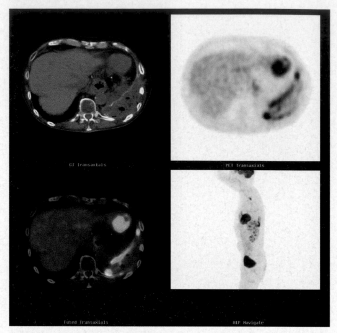

B

Brief History

A 63-year-old patient, status post–esophagectomy (for carcinoma) and gastric pull-up procedure, developed a chronic left pleural effusion treated by a lung decortication procedure with instillation of talc in the pleural space, 2 months before this examination. PET/CT was performed in search of metastatic dissemination.

Findings

A. PET/CT images at the level of the upper thorax show a lesion, located in the medial pleural space adjoining the mediastinum on the left, with high density on CT and intensely increased FDG uptake on PET.

B. PET/CT images at the level of the lower thorax demonstrate intense FDG uptake in the pleural space corresponding in part to the dense material seen on CT with mild uptake in the compressed lower lung. These findings are all consistent with an inflammatory reaction to talc.

There is mild physiologic FDG activity in the stomach (B), which has been pulled up into the chest, and intense abnormal uptake in the bowel in the left anterior abdomen.

Main Teaching Points and Summary

1. Pleurodesis is a procedure designed to generate an intense inflammatory process in the pleural space to minimize or eliminate the accumulation of pleural effusions.
2. Talc is both radiodense and highly inflammatory.
3. Talc pleurodesis can induce intense FDG uptake outlining the pleural spaces in corresponding areas of high Hounsfield units (HU) on CT, persisting for years after the procedure.
4. Talc in the pleural space can mimic the appearance of asbestos-induced calcified pleural plaques and FDG-avid mesothelioma unless the interpreting physician is aware of the patient's clinical history.

Case 4.5.3 TUMOR–MALIGNANT EFFUSION AND TUBE INSERTION (FIG. 4.5.3)

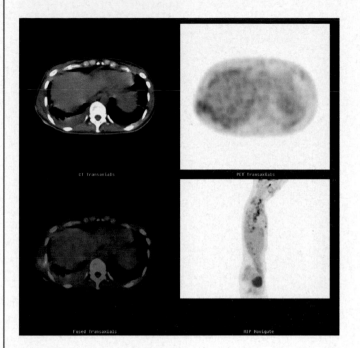

Brief History
A 40-year-old patient with biopsy-proven adenocarcinoma showing multiple pulmonary nodules on CT was referred for initial staging.

Findings
PET/CT images demonstrate mildly increased FDG uptake in a right pleural effusion. In addition, there is moderately increased FDG uptake in a site of recent right chest tube insertion.

Note on lateral MIP: Multiple hypermetabolic malignant foci are evident in the lungs.

Main Teaching Points and Summary
1. Pleural effusions with increased FDG uptake are usually exudative, related to inflammatory or malignant processes, and not typical for transudates.
2. The history of chest tube placement explains the right chest wall uptake.

Case 4.5.4 TUMOR—PLEURAL THICKENING, MESOTHELIOMA (FIG. 4.5.4)

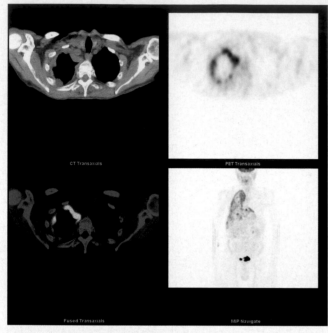

A

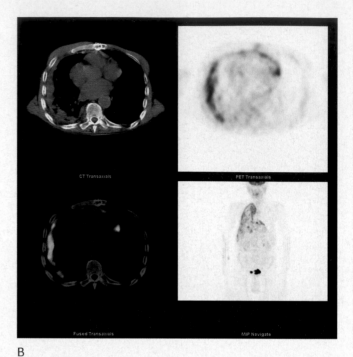

B

Brief History

A 78-year-old patient with pleural thickening, diagnosed as mesothelioma on biopsy, was referred to assess extent of disease and for planning the therapeutic strategy.

Findings

A. PET/CT images at an upper level show abnormally increased FDG uptake in circumferential, irregular pleural thickening in the right hemithorax.

B. PET/CT images at a lower level show abnormally increased FDG uptake in circumferential, irregular pleural thickening in the right hemithorax and in the anterior paracardiac aspect of the left mediastinal pleura.

All findings are consistent with mesothelioma extending into the pleura on both sides, more prominent on the right.

Main Teaching Point and Summary

1. PET/CT findings of mesothelioma can affect the contralateral lung and the peritoneal cavity.
2. Patient history is important to differentiate active tumor from iatrogenic pleural inflammation induced by treatment with drugs or talc.

Case 4.5.5 TUMOR–PLEURAL NODULE, MALIGNANT IMPLANT (FIG. 4.5.5)

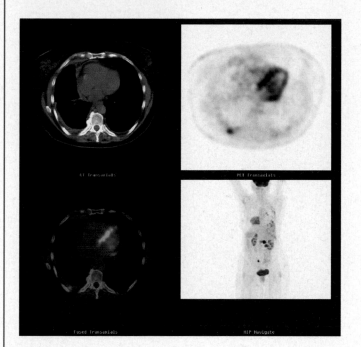

Brief History
A 64-year-old patient with history of primary peritoneal carcinoma diagnosed 5 years before PET/CT was evaluated in search of progressive cancer.

Findings
PET/CT images demonstrate the presence of pleural thickening and a focal area of increased FDG uptake, consistent with a solid pleural implant of adenocarcinoma.

Note on posterior MIP: Multiple foci of increased FDG uptake are evident in the right hemithorax, including the mediastinal nodal uptake. Several tumor foci are also apparent in the abdomen.

Main Teaching Point and Summary
1. A highly robust sign of a malignant pleural effusion is the presence of focal accumulation of FDG in a nodule in the pleural space.

Case 4.5.6 TUMOR—PLEURAL MASSES, MESOTHELIOMA (FIG. 4.5.6)

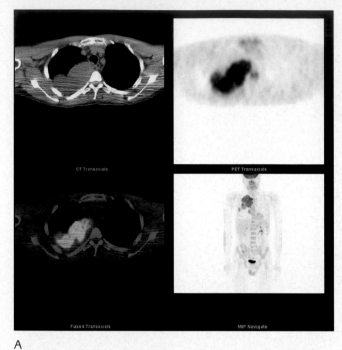

A

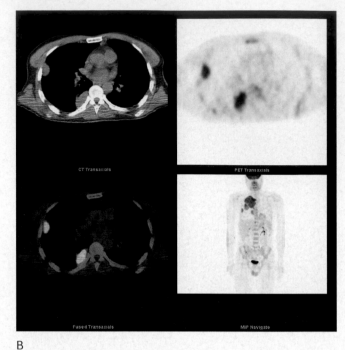

B

Brief History

A 46-year-old man with newly diagnosed mesothelioma involving the right pleura was referred for assessment of the extent of disease.

Findings

A. PET/CT images at an upper level of the chest show highly abnormal, inhomogeneous FDG uptake in large lobulated pleural masses in the posterior aspect of the right hemithorax.

B. PET/CT images at a lower midmediastinal level demonstrate abnormally increased FDG uptake in two pleural masses in the lateral and posterior paravertebral right hemithorax.

All findings are consistent with extensive right pleural mesothelioma.

Main Teaching Point and Summary

1. FDG-avid pleural masses must be considered mesothelioma unless proved otherwise.
2. Other processes that can cause similar findings include non–small cell lung cancer and, rarely, thymoma.
3. History of asbestos exposure is common but not always present in patients with mesothelioma.

Case 4.6.1 PITFALL—MISREGISTRATION DUE TO RESPIRATORY MOVEMENT (FIG. 4.6.1)

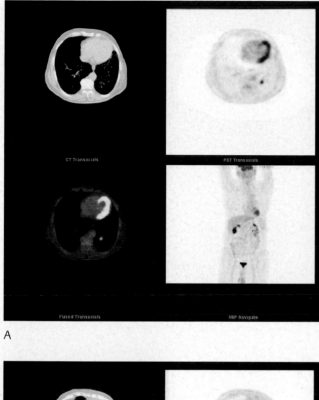

A

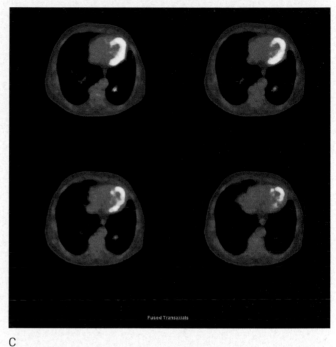

C

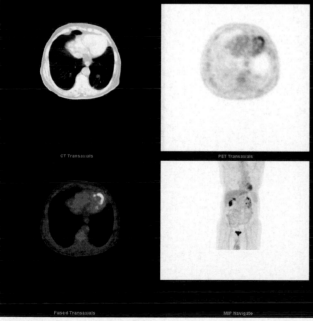

B

Brief History

A 75-year-old patient with left lung cancer, 16 months after surgery, complained of pain in the left chest wall. On CT, there was a new nodule in the left lower lobe, 15 mm in diameter.

Findings

A. PET/CT images show a small, moderate-intensity focus of FDG uptake in the left lower lobe with no anatomic lesion seen on the corresponding CT slice.

B. PET/CT images at a lower level demonstrate the presence of a pulmonary nodule in the left lower lobe on CT, with no associated abnormal FDG uptake.

C. Serial transaxial PET/CT images demonstrate the 4.5-mm-thick (one-slice) misregistration between the FDG-avid lesion on PET and the pulmonary nodule seen on CT.

A second non–small cell lung cancer was diagnosed and removed at surgery.

Main Teaching Point and Summary

1. Misregistration of lesions on PET and CT can occur, most commonly in the lungs, because of respiratory motion and image acquisition during different parts of the respiratory cycle between PET and CT.

2. Misregistration is encountered more often with lesions located at the base of the lungs, where respiratory artifacts are more accentuated.

3. PET/CT image acquisition with respiratory gating can potentially overcome this pitfall.

4. To avoid misreading of thoracic PET/CT images, several slices from below and above the lesion on CT must be sequentially examined for the presence of abnormalities corresponding to PET findings.

Case 4.6.2 BENIGN—POSTRADIATION CHANGES (FIG. 4.6.2)

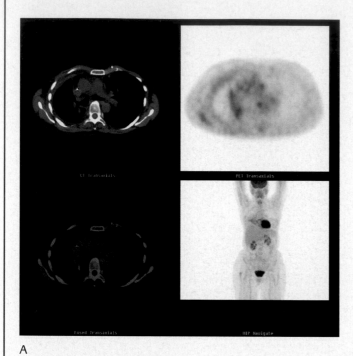

A

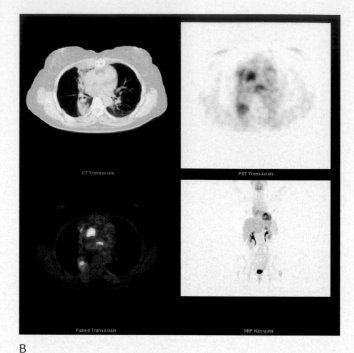

B

Brief History

A 57-year-old patient with a history of right lung cancer, status post–lower lobectomy 7 years before PET/CT, had recently received radiation treatment to recurrent mediastinal disease. The patient was restaged with PET/CT for disease activity.

Findings

A. PET/CT images demonstrate a geographically shaped region of increased FDG uptake of moderate intensity in the right paramediastinal region, consistent with radiation-induced inflammation, without evidence of residual cancer. FDG uptake in the marrow is low.

B. For comparison: PET/CT images in another patient show radiation-induced increased FDG uptake in the right paramediastinal region, visualized with lung windows on CT, also following the geographic shape of radiation portals. FDG uptake in marrow is low due to radiation.

Main Teaching Points and Summary

1. Increased FDG uptake in the lungs due to radiotherapy is characterized by its shape, which is similar to the radiation port, and diffuse pattern.
2. Assessment of the CT component with both soft tissue and lung windows can identify the inflammatory changes and their characteristic pattern.
3. Reduction in FDG uptake in the spinal marrow post irradiation is common.

Case 4.6.3 BENIGN—PNEUMONIA (FIG. 4.6.3)

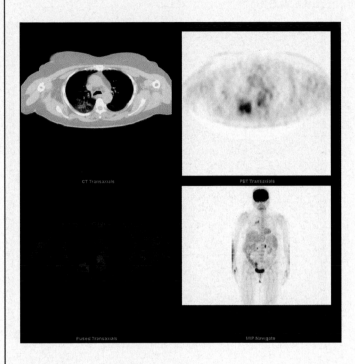

Brief History
A 71-year-old patient with relapsed mucosa-associated lymphatic tissue (MALT) lymphoma, status postchemotherapy, was assessed to monitor response to treatment.

Findings
PET/CT images show an infiltrate in the right upper lobe on CT, with a moderate degree of FDG uptake, consistent with pneumonia.

The patient's clinical history and physical examination suggested recent respiratory tract infection.

Note on MIP: Increased tracer activity in residual para-aortic and retroperitoneal nodal lymphoma is noted.

Main Teaching Points and Summary
1. Moderately increased FDG uptake in a pulmonary infiltrate in a patient with lymphoma, especially after treatment, should raise the suspicion of an infectious process, although differential diagnosis with lymphoma of the lungs can be difficult.
2. Clinical history can be helpful in establishing the final diagnosis.

Case 4.6.4 BENIGN—PULMONARY SARCOIDOSIS (FIG. 4.6.4)

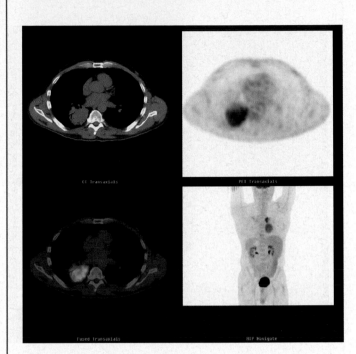

Brief History
A 63-year-old patient with history of pulmonary sarcoidosis presented with a round mass and consolidation in the right lower lobe. PET/CT was obtained to evaluate the metabolic activity of the process.

Findings
PET/CT images show a density, nearly 6 cm diameter, in the right lower lobe on CT, with air bronchograms crossing parts of this lesion, with moderately intense associated FDG uptake.

Note on posterior MIP: Increased FDG uptake in central mediastinal lymph nodes is evident.

Biopsy and follow-up indicated that all findings were due to active sarcoidosis.

Main Teaching Points and Summary
1. Intense FDG uptake distal to a central FDG-avid nodal mass is often obstructive pneumonia distal to a central tumor.
2. Tissue confirmation remains necessary for the differential diagnosis with cancer or other FDG-avid processes, such as sarcoidosis in this case.
3. Air bronchograms on CT suggest a process that does not have extensive secretions (i.e., is not pneumonia) and are often encountered in pulmonary sarcoidosis or lymphoma.

Case 4.6.5 BENIGN—FDG-NEGATIVE SMALL LUNG NODULE (FIG. 4.6.5)

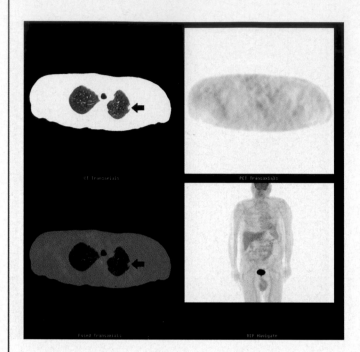

Brief History
A 79-year-old patient with a history of left lower lobectomy for lung cancer had a new peripheral left lung nodule on follow-up CT. PET/CT was performed for the suspicion of recurrent lung carcinoma.

Findings
PET/CT images demonstrate a left apical lung nodule, 1 cm in diameter, located near the chest wall on CT (arrows), with no increased FDG uptake in the lesion.

On follow-up, there was no evidence of tumor recurrence.

Main Teaching Points and Summary
1. Lack of FDG uptake in pulmonary nodules 1 cm in diameter and larger, excludes the presence of malignancy with high probability.
2. Follow-up in such cases is essential to identify occasional false-negative studies.

Case 4.6.6 BENIGN—FDG-NEGATIVE LUNG NODULE AND INTERVAL SHRINKAGE (FIG. 4.6.6)

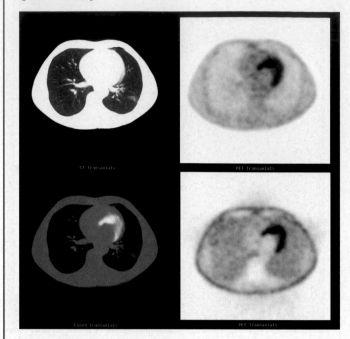

Brief History
A 51-year-old patient with history of Crohn's disease recently had a resection of the terminal ileum. CT at the time of surgery was reported to show a 2.4-cm left lower lobe lung lesion. The patient was referred to PET/CT to assess this nodule 2 months later, after recovering from surgery.

Findings
PET/CT images show a 1 × 1.5–cm opacity in the left lower lobe, of moderate tissue density on CT with no corresponding FDG uptake on attenuation corrected (upper right) or noncorrected (lower right) images.

The interval shrinkage of the lesion since the prior CT and the lack of tracer uptake on PET suggest a benign lesion. No malignancy was found for a period of nearly 2 years of follow-up.

Main Teaching Points and Summary
1. Not uncommonly, the size of lesions on the CT component of the PET/CT is smaller than that observed on the previously performed chest x-ray or CT studies that triggered the current study. This is typical for benign pulmonary lesions.
2. A non–attenuation-corrected PET image of the thorax should also be examined in such cases because it may improve the ability to resolve increased FDG uptake in small lesions. The non-attenuation-corrected image (lower right) was negative in this case.

Case 4.6.7 BENIGN–SINGLE LUNG NODULE, GRANULOMA (FIG. 4.6.7)

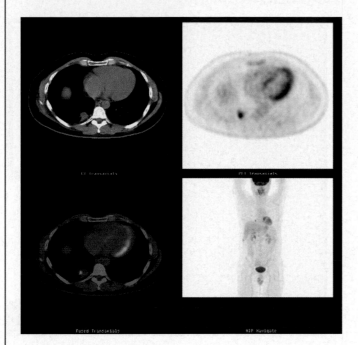

Brief History
A 42-year-old patient with history of hydatid cysts, status post–surgical resection of thoracic lesions 25 years before PET/CT, had a new lung nodule detected on CT. The patient was referred for PET/CT to determine whether the nodule was of malignant etiology.

Findings
PET/CT images demonstrate a 2.5-cm diameter pleural-based right lung lesion with intense FDG uptake, considered highly suspicious for active infection or tumor.

At surgery, this lesion was diagnosed as a granuloma, which had developed around a retained suture from previous surgery.

Main Teaching Point and Summary
1. Intense FDG uptake in a pulmonary lesion is highly suggestive of cancer, but tissue confirmation remains essential because of the wide range of causes for false positive FDG uptake.

Case 4.6.8 TUMOR–SINGLE LESION, PRIMARY LUNG CANCER (FIG. 4.6.8)

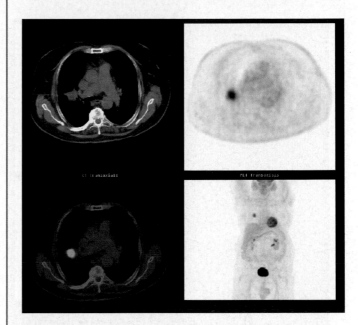

Brief History
An 80-year-old patient with history of bladder carcinoma presented with a new pulmonary nodule. PET/CT was obtained to determine whether the nodule represented malignancy (either lung cancer or metastasis) or another process.

Findings
PET/CT images demonstrated intense FDG uptake in a right perihilar mass, more than 3 cm in diameter on CT.

A second lung cancer was diagnosed at surgery.

Main Teaching Points and Summary
1. In patients with a history of malignancy, single focal hypermetabolic lesions can represent either primary or metastatic cancer.
2. The intense FDG activity in the pulmonary lesion indicated the need for biopsy and/or surgical resection.
3. Large single pulmonary lesions are more commonly related to new primary tumors than to metastases, as in this case.

Case 4.6.9 TUMOR—SINGLE CYSTIC LESION, PRIMARY LUNG CANCER (FIG. 4.6.9)

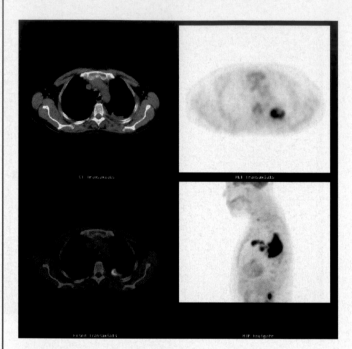

Brief History

A 67-year-old patient with a 60 pack-year cigarette use history and recent weight loss had a 6-cm mass detected on chest x-ray in the superior segment of the left upper lobe, highly suspicious for carcinoma. PET/CT was ordered to stage presumed lung cancer.

Findings

PET/CT images demonstrate a cavitary lesion in the superior segment of the left lower lobe, with a thick posterior rim of intense FDG uptake in most of the periphery of the lesion.

Note on lateral MIP: FDG-avid mediastinal lymphadenopathy is evident.

Cytology diagnosed squamous cell lung carcinoma.

Main Teaching Points and Summary
1. Cystic lung lesions, if very thin rimmed, are often benign. This lesion has a thicker posterior rim and intense FDG uptake that is highly suggestive of cancer. Infectious or inflammatory processes can have a similar appearance.
2. Squamous cell lung cancers are particularly prone to central cavitation and necrosis.

Case 4.6.10 TUMOR—MODERATE FDG AVIDITY, BRONCHIOLOALVEOLAR LUNG CANCER (FIG. 4.6.10)

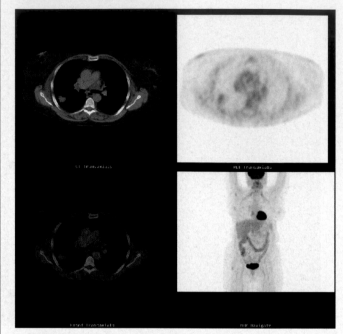

Brief History

A 60-year-old patient with a history of smoking had a 2-cm right upper lobe lung nodule detected on CT obtained as a part of a screening program.

Findings

PET/CT images demonstrate a 2-cm well-delineated right upper lobe lesion on CT. FDG uptake in this lesion is similar in intensity to blood pool activity (standardized uptake value [SUV] of 2.5). The lesion was reported as concerning for lung cancer.

Diagnosis at surgery indicated a bronchioloalveolar carcinoma.

Main Teaching Points and Summary
1. The intensity of FDG uptake in this right upper lobe lung lesion is not as high as typically seen in lung cancer but is comparable to mediastinal blood pool and thus concerning.
2. Bronchioloalveolar carcinoma often has lower FDG uptake than lung cancer of other histology and may be less biologically aggressive.

Case 4.6.11 TUMOR—PANCOAST, CHEST WALL INVOLVEMENT, AND LUNG METASTASIS (FIG. 4.6.11)

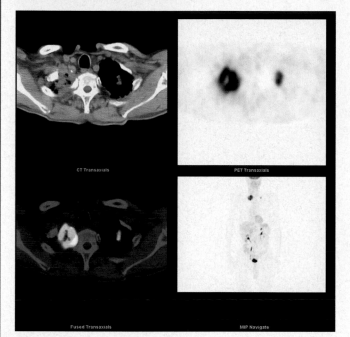

A

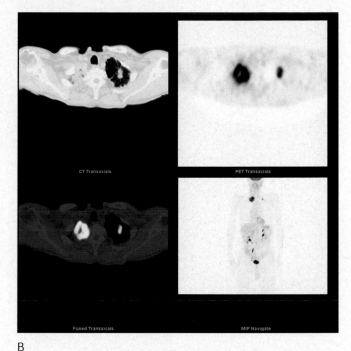

B

Brief History

A 70-year-old patient with a history of smoking was referred for further assessment of a right upper lung mass, 5 × 4 cm, detected on CT performed for assessment of severe neck and shoulder pain.

Findings

A. PET/CT images demonstrate highly intense FDG uptake in a large, inhomogeneous mass in the apex of the right lung, involving the posterior aspect of the chest wall, with erosion of the posterior arch of the first right rib, consistent with a Pancoast tumor.

B. PET/CT images at the same level, with CT displayed using lung windows, localize an additional focus of abnormally increased FDG uptake to an irregular lesion at the apex of the left lung, later confirmed as a synchronous metastasis from the lung cancer on the right.

Main Teaching Points and Summary

1. The intensity and localization of the right lung mass are characteristic of a Pancoast tumor.
2. Involvement of the chest wall, including the ribs, is easily demonstrated on PET/CT images, with further impact on the planning of the surgical procedure.
3. Diagnosis of a second malignant focus in the left lung defined the patient in this case as nonresectable.

Case 4.6.12 TUMOR—RESPONSE TO TREATMENT, PRIMARY LUNG CANCER WITH NODAL METASTASES (FIG. 4.6.12)

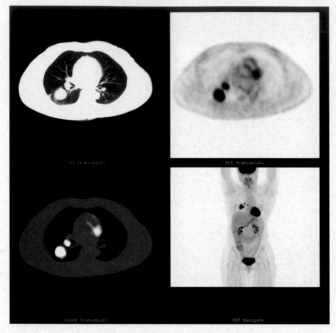

A

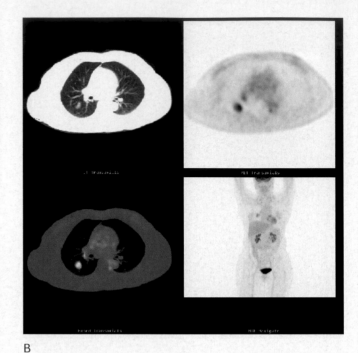

B

Brief History

A 55-year-old patient with known adenocarcinoma of the right lung was assessed before and at the end of neo-adjuvant chemotherapy and radiotherapy to restage disease activity prior to possible surgery.

Findings

A. PET/CT images at baseline demonstrate intense FDG uptake in the primary right lower lobe lung lesion and in a hilar nodal metastasis.

B. PET/CT images after treatment demonstrate that both the lung and nodal lesions have shrunken substantially but still show some degree of increased FDG uptake in the residual mass, consistent with residual active tumor.

The patient showed tumor progression a few months later.

Main Teaching Points and Summary

1. PET/CT can effectively demonstrate response to chemotherapy.
2. Residual FDG uptake in a mass is typically but not invariably indicative of residual cancer.

Case 4.6.13 TUMOR–METACHRONOUS LUNG CANCER (FIG. 4.6.13)

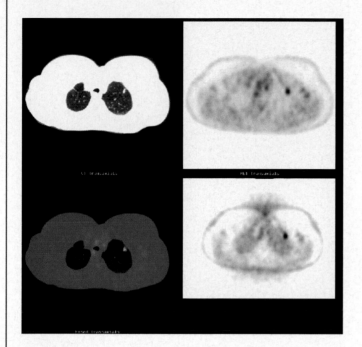

Brief History

A 67-year-old patient with a history of squamous cell lung carcinoma, status post–right upper lobectomy 2 years before this study, presented with a left upper lobe nodule on CT, increasing in size from previous studies. PET/CT was obtained to characterize this lesion.

Findings

PET/CT images demonstrate intense FDG activity in a 9-mm left upper lobe nodule seen on both attenuation-corrected (upper right) and noncorrected (lower right) images. These findings are consistent with a malignant lesion, in a contralateral location to the previous tumor.

A second primary large cell lung cancer was diagnosed at surgery.

Main Teaching Point and Summary

1. Patients with lung cancer are at risk for recurrence of that tumor or a second, new primary lung cancer.

Case 4.6.14 TUMOR–RECURRENT MESOTHELIOMA AND POSTSURGICAL CHANGES (FIG. 4.6.14)

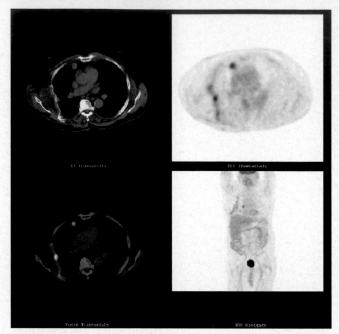

A

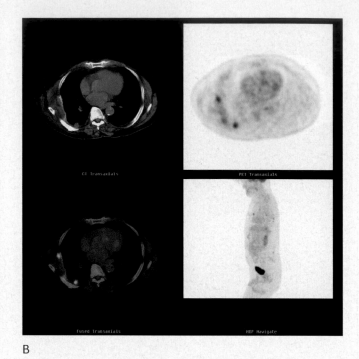

B

Brief History

A 73-year-old patient with a history of right thoracic mesothelioma, status post–resection and chest wall reconstruction 6 months pre-PET/CT, was referred for further assessment of new pleural based nodules seen on CT.

Findings

A and B. PET/CT images at the level of the midthorax demonstrate several pleural-based nodules with intense FDG uptake, consistent with recurrent cancer. In addition, there is linear FDG uptake of mild to moderate intensity in the surgical site in the right chest wall.

Main Teaching Point and Summary

1. FDG uptake in recurrent tumor is typically considerably of greater extent, intensity and focality than postsurgical changes, which are usually linear in shape.

Case 4.6.15 MULTIPLE LESIONS, MULTIFOCAL PRIMARY LUNG CANCER (FIG. 4.6.15)

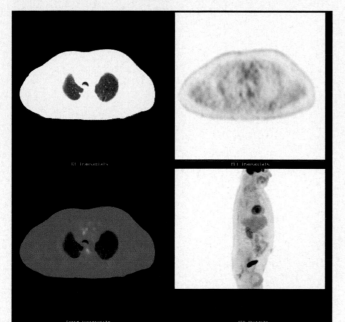

A

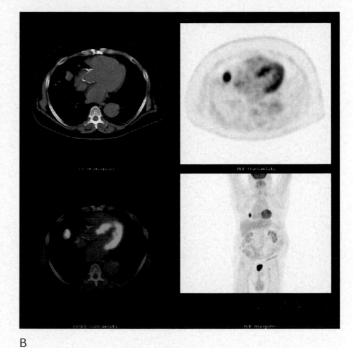

B

Brief History

A 68-year-old patient with history of thoracic aortic aneurysm, showed two new lung nodules on follow-up CT. PET/CT was obtained to assess for possible malignancy.

Findings

A and B. PET/CT images at upper and midthoracic levels demonstrate two pulmonary nodules, one 0.5-cm in diameter in the posterior paramediastinal aspect of the right upper lobe showing moderately intense FDG uptake (A) and another 2.5 cm in diameter in the right middle lobe with intense FDG uptake (B).

Biopsy of both lesions revealed non–small cell lung carcinoma.

Main Teaching Points and Summary

1. Lung cancer may be multifocal at presentation.
2. Even moderately increased FDG uptake in a 5-mm nodule must be viewed as suspicious for lung cancer, even though the absolute SUV is not very high due to partial volume effects.

Case 4.6.16 TUMOR—MULTIPLE LESIONS, LYMPHOMA (FIG. 4.6.16)

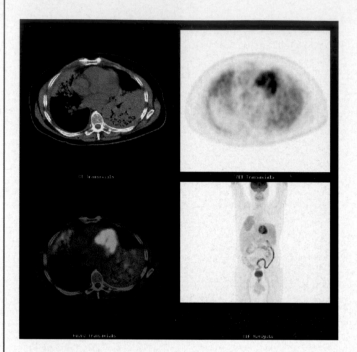

Brief History

A 63-year-old patient with history of biopsy-proved MALT lymphoma involving the lungs and stomach was evaluated for activity of disease. The patient did not have any clinical evidence of active infection.

Findings

PET/CT images show volume loss and air bronchograms in pulmonary lesions involving the right middle and left lower lobe, which have associated mild to moderate FDG uptake (SUV of 1.9 and 3.8), consistent with active lymphoma.

Main Teaching Points and Summary

1. Pulmonary MALT can have relatively modest FDG uptake on PET and air bronchograms on CT.
2. In some cases, it may be difficult to differentiate pneumonia from pulmonary lymphoma.

Case 4.6.17 TUMOR–MULTIPLE LESIONS AND INHOMOGENEOUS PATTERN, LYMPHOMA (FIG. 4.6.17)

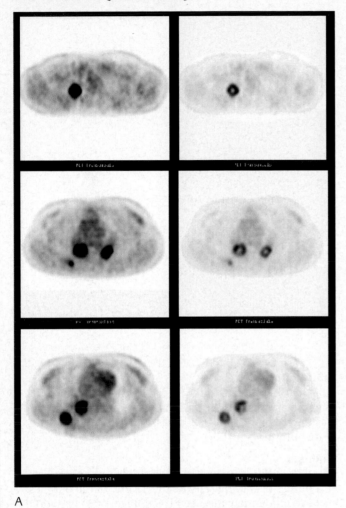

A

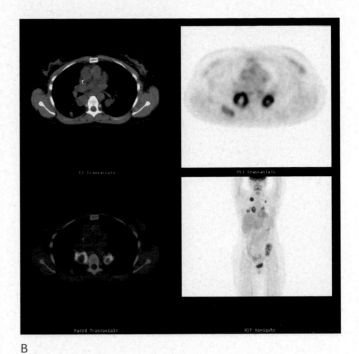

B

Brief History

A 39-year-old patient with a history of renal transplant on immunosuppression showed new pulmonary nodules on chest x-rays. Whole body FDG-PET/CT was obtained because of a suspicion of posttransplant lymphoproliferative disease.

Findings

A. Selected transaxial PET images show multiple FDG-avid lesions in both lungs. When windowed incorrectly (left column), they appear solid, whereas when displayed with appropriate intensity (right column), they appear to be centrally hypometabolic.

B. PET/CT images show multiple cavitary lesions in both lungs, with a highly intense peripheric rim of FDG uptake but cold in the center.

The final diagnosis was aggressive lymphoma.

Note on MIP: The renal transplant is evident in the left pelvis.

Main Teaching Points and Summary

1. Posttransplant lymphoma demonstrates intense FDG uptake, is aggressive, and grows very rapidly.
2. Proper windowing of PET images is essential to identify correctly the necrotic center of pulmonary nodules and other masses.

Case 4.6.18 TUMOR–MULTIPLE LESIONS, METASTASES (FIG. 4.6.18)

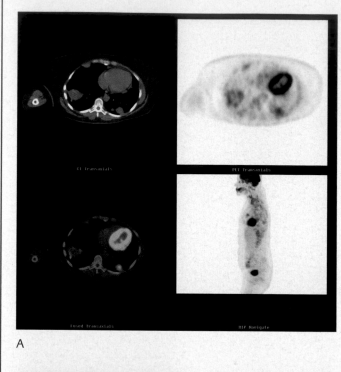

A

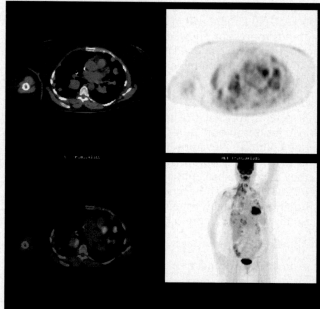

B

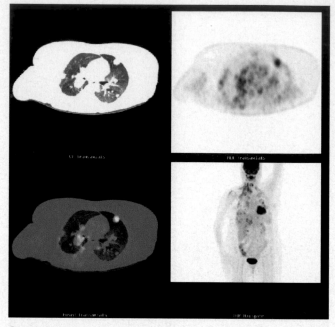

C

Brief History

A 55-year-old patient with history of osteosarcoma and lung metastases, had new pulmonary nodules on CT and was referred for PET/CT to assess the extent and activity of the tumor.

Findings

A and B. PET/CT images show multiple pulmonary nodules of varying size on CT. Several of the nodules have moderately intense FDG uptake. A small nodule just medial to the left lower lobe nodule (B) appears as FDG-negative, likely because of its small size.

C. CT images displayed with lung window show more nodules than are seen with mediastinal windows.

Main Teaching Points and Summary

1. Multiple pulmonary nodules are typical of lung metastases.
2. Lung metastases of sarcoma often demonstrate lower intensity FDG uptake than lung cancer.
3. Small, subcentimeter lung metastases can be more evident on CT, especially when assessed with lung windows, as compared to PET.

Case 4.6.19 TUMOR—MULTIPLE FDG-NEGATIVE LESIONS, METASTASES (FIG. 4.6.19)

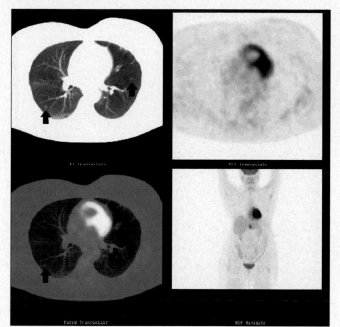

Brief History
A 62-year-old patient with history of breast cancer and suspected recurrence in the liver was assessed for the presence and extent of active tumor.

Findings
PET/CT images show several subcentimeter pulmonary nodules (arrows) that do not accumulate FDG.

The pulmonary nodules were new and considered to indicate metastatic breast cancer despite being FDG negative. All lesions responded to chemotherapy.

Note on MIP: Metastasis is seen in the left lobe of the liver.

Main Teaching Points and Summary
1. New small lung nodules in a cancer patient often indicate tumor progression, even if FDG negative.
2. Small pulmonary metastases are, as a rule, better seen on CT than PET, and therefore CT must be closely examined in the appropriate lung windows, in addition to PET, to arrive at the correct diagnosis.

Case 4.6.20 TUMOR—MULTIPLE LESIONS, TREATED AND NEW METASTASES (FIG. 4.6.20)

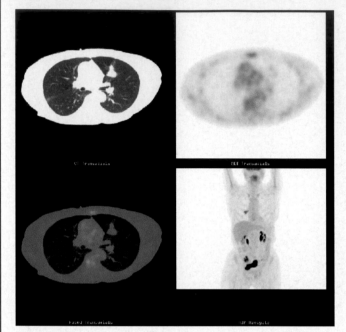

A

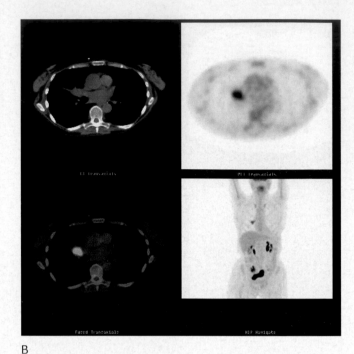

B

Brief History

A 59-year-old patient with a history of carcinoma of the cervix, metastatic to the thorax, had been treated with radiofrequency ablation to the lesion in the left lung. PET/CT was obtained to determine whether there is evidence of residual active cancer.

Findings

A. PET/CT images show a focal abnormality, about 2.5 cm in diameter, in the left lung on CT, at the site of prior radiofrequency ablation, with no corresponding FDG uptake, consistent with metabolically inactive residual scar tissue.

B. PET/CT images at a lower level show a focus of intense FDG uptake in a lesion located in the right pulmonary hilum, consistent with a new, previously untreated, metabolically active metastasis.

Main Teaching Points and Summary

1. Radiofrequency ablation is increasingly applied in the treatment of inoperable lung tumors.
2. Disparity between CT and PET findings after treatment is common, with PET more predictive of outcome than CT.

4.7 THORACIC LYMPH NODES

Case 4.7.1 SUPRACLAVICULAR LYMPH NODES (FIG. 4.7.1)

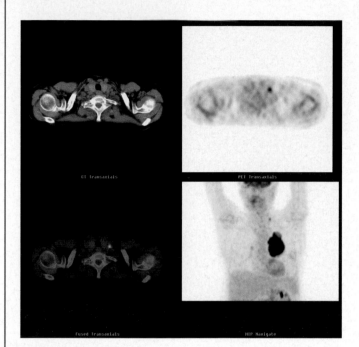

Brief History
A 67-year-old patient with history of weight loss and an abnormal chest radiograph was assessed in search of malignancy.

Findings
PET/CT images show a focal area of intense FDG uptake in a normal sized, 8 mm diameter, left supraclavicular lymph node.

Note on MIP: A left primary lung cancer is evident.

Main Teaching Point and Summary
1. The ability to detect normal-sized metastatic lymph nodes is a key advantage of PET.
2. PET/CT provides the precise localization required to perform biopsy to confirm malignancy located outside of the thorax.

Case 4.7.2 RETROCLAVICULAR AND PECTORALIS LYMPH NODES (FIG. 4.7.2)

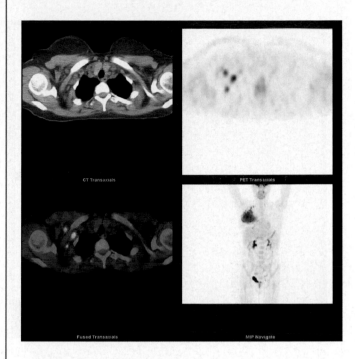

Brief History
A 28-year-old patient with a recently diagnosed large invasive ductal right breast cancer underwent PET/CT for systemic staging following the detection of a small nodule in the right upper lung lobe on CT.

Findings
PET/CT images show foci of abnormally increased FDG uptake in right retroclavicular and pectoralis lymph nodes, consistent with metastatic lymphadenopathy.

Note on MIP: Intense tracer activity is seen in the right primary breast tumor and additional multiple nodal metastases. No increased FDG uptake is seen in the lungs.

Main Teaching Points and Summary
1. The chest wall is a region characterized by multiple anatomic structures located in close proximity.
2. Confirmation and localization of metastatic lymphadenopathy seen on FDG-PET to a specific nodal station, as well as separation of bone or lung lesions from nodes is facilitated by fused PET/CT images.

Case 4.7.3 AXILLARY AND PECTORALIS LYMPH NODES (FIG. 4.7.3)

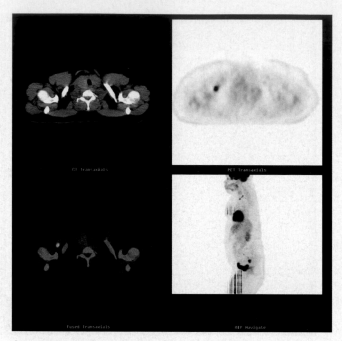

A

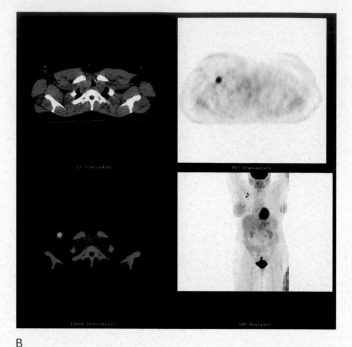

B

Brief History
A 49-year-old patient with recently diagnosed breast cancer with negative surgical margins was referred to stage for systemic disease.

Findings
A. PET/CT images show a focal area of abnormal FDG uptake in a slightly enlarged lymph node in the right axilla.
B. PET/CT images at a more proximal level show an additional node with focally increased FDG uptake in a somewhat atypical location, between the pectoralis major and minor.

Main Teaching Points and Summary
1. Focal intense nodal activity as in this case is nearly always indicative of metastatic cancer if injection technique is contralateral and correct.
2. Not all nodes draining the breast are in the typical axillary location.
3. The specificity of PET/CT findings in the axilla is lower in the postoperative patient.

Case 4.7.4 AXILLARY LYMPH NODES (FIG. 4.7.4)

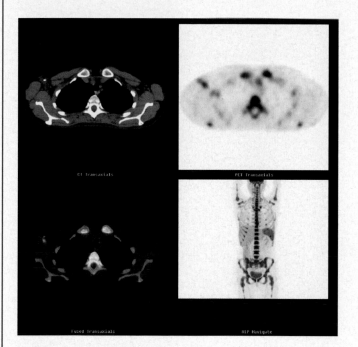

Brief History
A 41-year-old patient with newly diagnosed breast cancer had a positive sentinel node biopsy for malignancy and had recently received one dose of chemotherapy. The patient was being assessed for residual active tumor.

Findings
PET/CT images demonstrate a deep focus of intense FDG uptake in the right axilla close to the surgical clips, in metastatic lymph nodes. There is also mild tracer uptake in the skin at the biopsy site in the axilla.

Note on MIP: Intense bone marrow tracer activity, due to recent administration of pegfilgrastim, is evident.

Main Teaching Point and Summary
1. Axillary lymph nodes involved with malignancy usually have a pattern of focal and distinct activity.
2. Confounding factors for interpretation of these studies may include recent surgery and drug effects such as colony-stimulating factors. PET sensitivity is reduced by recent effective chemotherapy.

Case 4.7.5 INTERNAL MAMMARY LYMPH NODE VERSUS STERNAL LESION (FIG. 4.7.5)

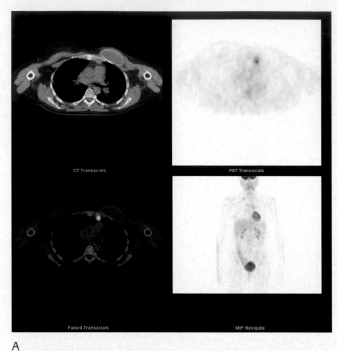

A

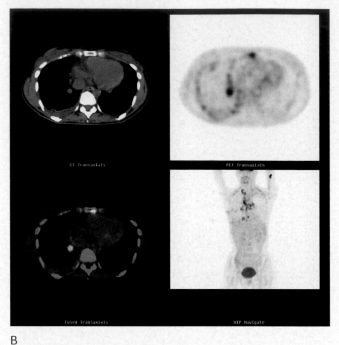

B

Brief History

A 49-year-old patient with history of medial left breast cancer, status postmastectomy, followed by left axillary dissection received chemotherapy and radiotherapy for a local recurrence. PET/CT was performed to monitor response to treatment

Findings

A. PET/CT images demonstrate moderate focal FDG uptake in a slightly enlarged left internal mammary lymph node, consistent with metastatic lymphadenopathy.

Note on MIP: Additional foci of abnormal tracer activity in multiple mediastinal and right supraclavicular lymph node metastases is seen.

B. For comparison: PET/CT images in another patient demonstrate an intense focus of increased FDG uptake similar in appearance on PET, located by PET/CT in the sternum, anterior to and adjacent to the left internal mammary chain, representing a bone metastasis. There is an additional focus in a right lower mediastinal node.

Note on MIP: Multiple foci of increased FDG uptake throughout the right mediastinum are seen.

Main Teaching Points and Summary

1. This intensity of uptake in a relatively small node is particularly concerning because the primary tumor was medially located.
2. Medial breast cancers are more likely to drain to the internal mammary lymphatic chain.
3. Diagnosis and precise localization of these nodes is important when histologic confirmation is sought (which is only rarely the case) and mainly for inclusion in radiation fields.
4. Sternal lesions can originate from direct invasion from internal mammary nodes tissue or can be related to hematogenous spread.
5. The close anatomic proximity makes it difficult with PET alone to separate between sternal metastases and internal mammary nodes. They have, however, a different prognostic significance. Nodal lesions represent only locoregional disease while a bone lesion indicates stage IV disease.

Case 4.7.6 SUPRADIAPHRAGMATIC LYMPH NODES (FIG. 4.7.6)

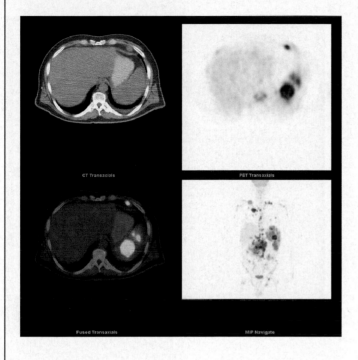

Case 4.8.1 ANTERIOR MEDIASTINAL AND PARATRACHEAL LYMPH NODES (FIG. 4.8.1)

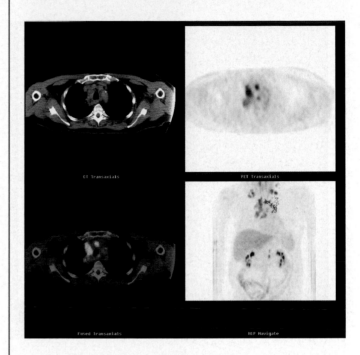

Brief History
A 46-year-old patient with newly diagnosed diffuse large cell non-Hodgkin's lymphoma was referred for initial staging before treatment.

Findings
PET/CT images demonstrate a focal site of abnormally increased FDG uptake in a left supradiaphragmatic lymph node. There are also foci of intense tracer activity in the spleen.

Note on MIP: Highly intense FDG uptake in multiple sites of nodal, splenic, and bone lymphoma is seen.

Main Teaching Point and Summary
1. Focal lesions in the periphery of the thoracic base can be located in various anatomic structures such as ribs, muscles, pleura, and supradiaphragmatic lymph nodes.
2. When presenting as single sites, precise localization of a hypermetabolic focus in lymphoma patients is of prognostic significance and also of value for diagnostic biopsy and further treatment planning.

Brief History
A 57-year-old patient with a history of melanoma presented with a loss of consciousness. Brain lesions were detected on CT. The patient also had a 1.7 × 3.4–cm right upper lobe lung density. PET/CT was ordered to determine whether active tumor was present in the thorax.

Findings
PET/CT images at the level of the thoracic inlet demonstrate the presence of an anterior mediastinal lymph node (ATS region 6) and a right paratracheal node (ATS 2R).

Note on MIP: Multiple FDG-avid lesions in supraclavicular and mediastinal metastatic lymphadenopathy, more on the right, are seen.

Metastatic lung cancer was diagnosed.

Main Teaching Points and Summary
1. This distribution of nodes is typical of advanced non–small cell lung cancer.
2. PET/CT can provide important data for guiding biopsy to the site with highest probability to confirm suspected advanced tumor.

Case 4.8.2 PREVASCULAR LYMPH NODES, NORMAL SIZE (FIG. 4.8.2)

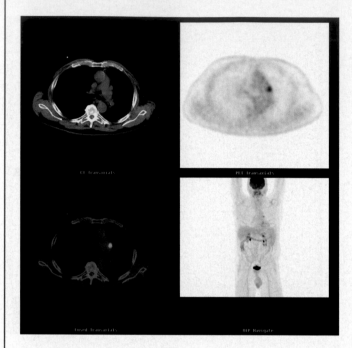

Brief History

A 76-year-old patient with non–small cell lung cancer, status post–left upper lobectomy 3 years before PET/CT, was assessed during follow-up.

Findings

PET/CT images demonstrate a 1-cm prevascular lymph node showing intense FDG uptake, consistent with nodal metastases. A previous contrast-enhanced CT was deemed normal.

Main Teaching Point and Summary

1. PET/CT is a valuable tool in assessing the postoperative thorax because it can distinguish between treatment-induced changes and recurrent cancer.
2. Normal-sized nodal metastases can fail to be detected on conventional imaging modalities; FDG-PET is more sensitive than CT for lung cancer nodal metastases.

Case 4.8.3 AORTOPULMONARY WINDOW LYMPH NODES (FIG. 4.8.3)

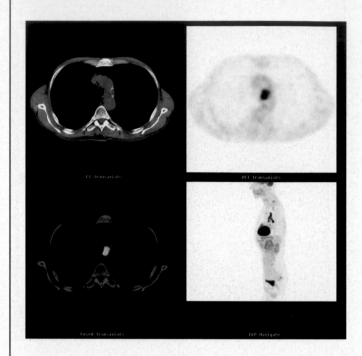

Brief History

A 71-year-old patient with history of lung cancer showed an incidental pulmonary nodule on follow-up CT, suspected to represent a recurrent tumor. PET/CT was performed to characterize the nodule and to restage the patient.

Findings

PET/CT images demonstrate a large FDG-avid lymph node in the region of the aortopulmonary window (APW).

Note on lateral MIP: Multiple mediastinal nodal metastases are seen.

Main Teaching Points and Summary

1. Centrally located nodal involvement in the region of the APW typically indicates inoperable lung cancer.
2. PET/CT clearly defines the localization of this lymph node, in immediate contiguity with the trachea, the upper aspect of the pulmonary artery, and the aorta.

Case 4.8.4 PRE- AND SUBCARINAL LYMPH NODES (FIG. 4.8.4)

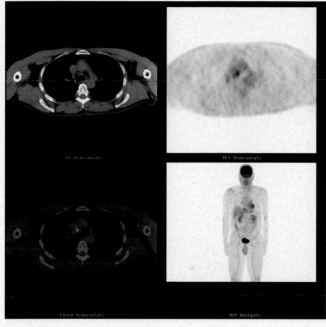

A

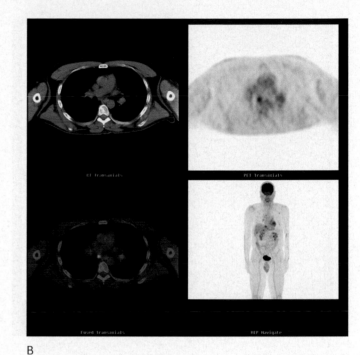

B

Brief History

A 50-year-old patient with malignant melanoma had biopsy-proved tumor involvement in lymph nodes of the left neck following sentinel node assessment. The patient was assessed for the extent of tumor involvement before therapy.

Findings

A and B. PET/CT images show increased FDG uptake in several lymph nodes including a precarinal (A) and subcarinal node, at the American Thoracic Surgery (ATS) Nodal Station VII (B).

Main Teaching Points and Summary

1. PET/CT can identify metastatic lymph nodes that are not enlarged. Histologic proof is required, however, to separate malignant from inflammatory lymphadenopathy.
2. CT can allow precise definition of the involved nodal group.
3. In this patient, the first PET/CT study provided a precise baseline from which treatment effects could be assessed in future.

Case 4.8.5 PARAESOPHAGEAL LYMPH NODES (FIG. 4.8.5)

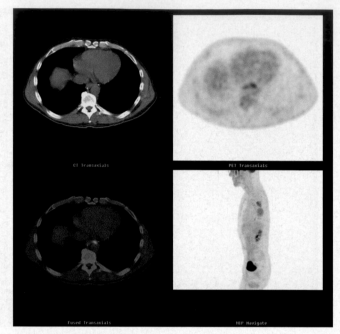

A

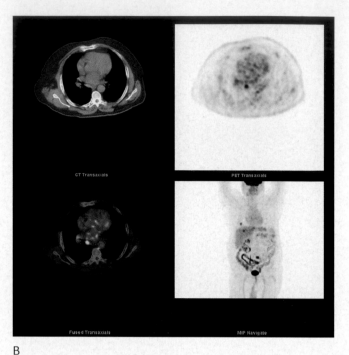

B

Brief History

A 63-year-old patient with known sarcoidosis involving lungs and lymph nodes was referred to assess the extent of nodal involvement.

Findings

A. PET/CT images show increased FDG uptake in pre-esophageal lymph nodes of borderline size, consistent with sarcoid involvement.

Note on lateral MIP: A pulmonary infiltrate proved to be active sarcoid.

B. For comparison: PET/CT images in another patient with a history of renal cell carcinoma show increased FDG uptake in a 22-mm lymph node located in the azygoesophageal recess, consistent with metastatic lymphadenopathy.

Note on MIP: Additional metastatic foci in liver and the right lung are seen.

Main Teaching Points and Summary

1. PET/CT can differentiate abnormal FDG uptake in lymph node metastases from increased tracer activity in adjacent normal or diseased organs the posterior mediastinum, such as the esophagus or large vessels.
2. Although tumor is a common cause for nodal FDG uptake, sarcoidosis and other granulomatous or inflammatory processes can also show intense tracer activity and be indistinguishable from malignancy based on visual and SUV characteristics alone.
3. Biopsy is not uncommonly needed to characterize histologically mediastinal FDG avid nodal lesions.

Case 4.8.6 PRETRACHEAL, PARATRACHEAL, TRACHEOBRONCHIAL, AND HILAR LYMPH NODES (FIG. 4.8.6)

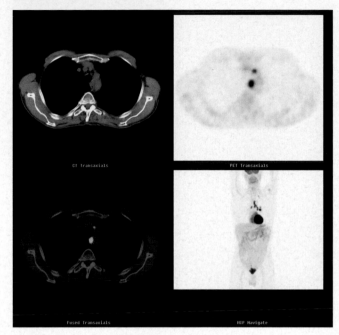

A

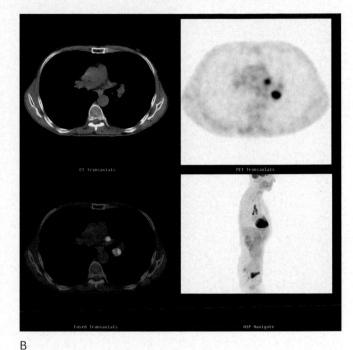

B

Brief History

A 71-year-old patient with a new left apical lung nodule suspicious for malignancy was referred for further PET/CT evaluation.

Findings

A. PET/CT images at the level of the upper thorax demonstrate two FDG-avid lymph nodes, including a pretracheal (2L) and a left paratracheal node (2L).
B. PET/CT images at a lower thoracic level demonstrate a left tracheobronchial (10L) and left hilar (ll L) node with abnormally increased FDG uptake.

Note on anterior and lateral MIPs: Focal FDG uptake in the primary left apical lung cancer and in multiple additional mediastinal lymph node metastases including 4L, paratracheal, are seen.

Main Teaching Points and Summary

1. Delineating nodal metastases by ATS stage can be helpful for consistency in nomenclature within a department.
2. The extensive adenopathy in this patient is somewhat unexpected given the small size of the primary tumor but was confirmed histologically as malignant, with the patient defined as inoperable after staging.
3. Tissue validation of nodal metastases, mainly in the presence of an unusual pattern as in the present case, is strongly recommended because false-positive results from other nonmalignant causes can occur.

Case 4.8.7 RETROCAVAL-PARATRACHEAL, PARASPINAL LYMPH NODES AND RESPONSE TO TREATMENT (FIG. 4.8.7)

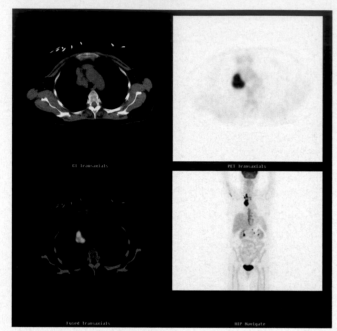

A

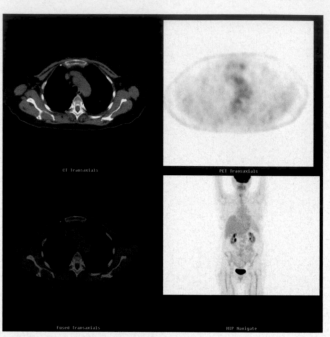

C

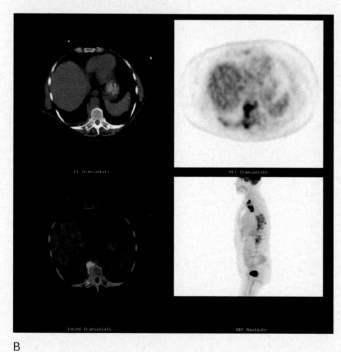

B

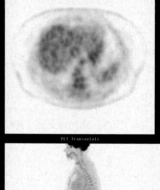

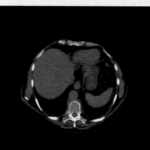

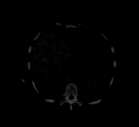

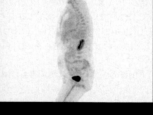

D

Brief History

A 64-year-old patient with Stage IIb diffuse large cell non-Hodgkin's lymphoma was monitored for treatment response. The initial PET/CT study was performed for staging, the follow-up study during chemotherapy.

Findings

A. PET/CT images at presentation demonstrate a bulky mass of retrocaval-paratracheal lymph nodes with intense, abnormally increased FDG uptake (2R and 4R) that are aggregated into a bulky mass.

B. PET/CT images at a lower level demonstrate a right thoracic paraaortic mass likely originating from posterior mediastinal nodes in the paraspinal region.

C and D. PET/CT images after three cycles of R-CHOP (rituximab + cyclophosphamide + doxorubicin + vincristine + prednisone) chemotherapy demonstrate complete resolution of the metabolic abnormalities and a significant decrease in the size of the anatomic findings, which have not reached complete resolution, however.

Main Teaching Points and Summary

1. Lymphoma and lung cancer are two of the more common causes of mediastinal adenopathy.
2. This case illustrates that the metabolic response assessed with FDG occurs more rapidly than change in tumor size seen on CT.

4.9 MEDIASTINUM

Case 4.9.1 PITFALL—BROWN FAT (FIG. 4.9.1)

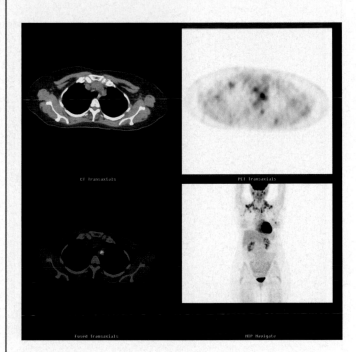

Brief History

A 56-year-old patient with recently diagnosed left breast cancer was evaluated for the suspicion of metastases because of equivocal findings on CT.

Findings

PET/CT images show a focus of increased FDG uptake in the mediastinum, just left of the trachea, localized to tissues with fatty density on CT.

Note on MIP: Extensive brown fat activity in the neck extending caudally and increased FDG uptake in the left primary breast cancer are seen.

Main Teaching Points and Summary

1. Most focal areas of increased mediastinal FDG uptake are pathologic, mainly metastatic.
2. Brown fat, in particular in locations other than the neck and shoulder girdle, should not be confused with tumor.
3. Accurate differential diagnosis can be achieved through careful examination of PET/CT images for the precise location of the focal area of tracer uptake.

Case 4.9.2 PITFALL—BLOOD CLOT (FIG. 4.9.2)

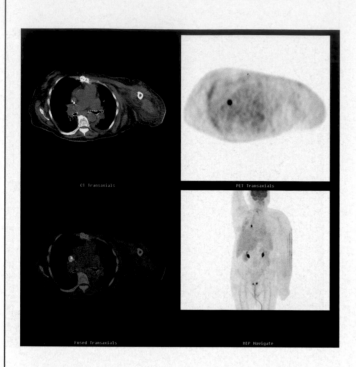

Brief History
A 68-year-old patient with history of left breast cancer 20 years pre-PET/CT was diagnosed with recurrence. The patient is status post–left mastectomy, has an enlarged left arm secondary to lymphedema following axillary dissection and radiation of the axilla, and had received chemotherapy via a right subclavian catheter. The patient was referred for whole body restaging and was injected through her central line.

Findings
PET/CT images show a focus of intense FDG activity at the tip of the catheter in the right paramediastinal region, likely in a small catheter-related "hot clot."

Note on MIP: Mild tracer activity in the right chest wall musculature, possibly due to muscle strain following the positioning of her right arm upward, is seen.

Main Teaching Point and Summary
1. Intense focal tracer uptake in or near a blood vessel should raise the question of the tracer injection route and technique.
2. Focal FDG uptake can be seen especially at the tip of a central line, more often if the flush is less than thorough. This pattern is often worrisome in appearance but usually not pathologic.

Case 4.9.3 BENIGN—THYMUS (FIG. 4.9.3)

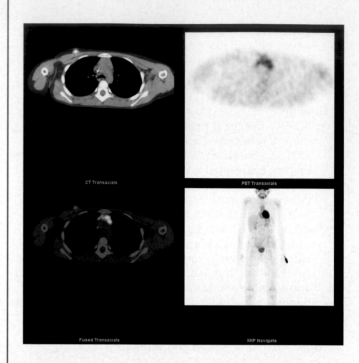

Brief History
A 10-year-old patient with Hodgkin's lymphoma was assessed for monitoring response at the end of chemotherapy.

Findings
PET/CT images show an anterior area of increased FDG uptake localized to the thymus that is reconstituting after chemotherapy, consistent with physiologic hyperplasia.

Main Teaching Points and Summary
1. The normal thymus can be visualized on FDG-PET mainly in young children and some young adults.
2. In older children and young adults, hyperplasia of the thymus can occur, especially after chemotherapy, and should not be confused with disease.

Case 4.9.4 TUMOR—BULKY DISEASE (FIG. 4.9.4)

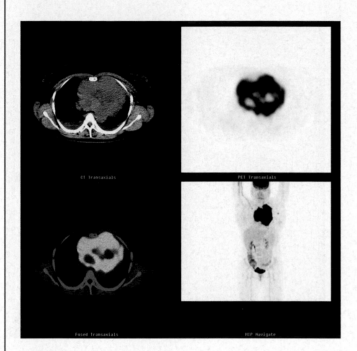

Brief History
A 51-year-old, previously healthy patient developed shortness of breath. A biopsy from a mediastinal mass seen on CT revealed lymphoma, and PET/CT was performed for staging.

Findings
PET/CT images show a huge, metabolically heterogeneous mass filling most of the anterior mediastinum and displacing the carina posteriorly and to the right. There are also bilateral FDG-negative pleural effusions.

Note on MIP: Left axillary and supraclavicular adenopathy is seen.

Main Teaching Points and Summary
1. A large anterior mediastinal mass in adults most commonly represents lymphoma.
2. On occasion teratoma, thymoma, and, rarely, thyroid cancer can have a similar appearance.
3. The heterogeneity in the mass can be seen best with proper adjustment of the contrast windows on PET.
4. FDG-negative pleural effusions are likely due to obstruction of the mediastinal lymphatic drainage and not necessarily to the presence of malignant cells in the pleural fluid

Case 4.9.5 TUMOR—ENDOTRACHEAL RECURRENT LUNG CANCER (FIG. 4.9.5)

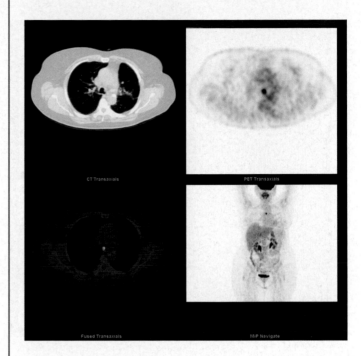

Brief History
A 64-year-old patient with a history of lung cancer, status post–left lower lobectomy 1 year pre-PET/CT, was assessed for the clinical suspicion of recurrent disease.

Findings
PET/CT images show a focus of increased FDG activity in the midmediastinum, localized to an endobronchial space-occupying lesion, further confirmed by biopsy as a recurrent lung cancer.

Note on MIP: A left adrenal metastasis is seen.

Main Teaching Points and Summary
1. Mediastinal lesions may be difficult to locate by stand-alone PET.
2. In this case, the hypermetabolic focus fuses to a previously unknown endobronchial anatomic lesion.

4.10 ESOPHAGUS

Case 4.10.1 PITFALL—HIATAL HERNIA (FIG. 4.10.1)

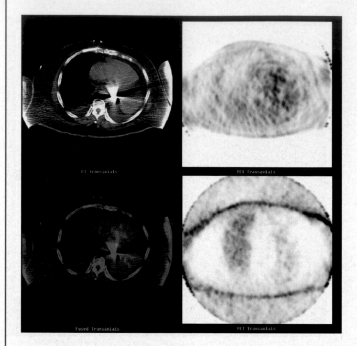

Case 4.10.2 PITFALL—GASTRIC PULL UP (FIG. 4.10.2)

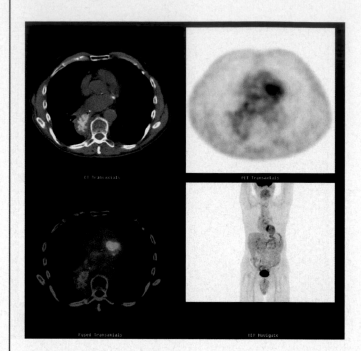

Brief History

A 71-year-old patient with recent difficulty in swallowing and a new diagnosis of carcinoma in the proximal third of the esophagus was referred for whole body PET/CT staging.

Findings

PET/CT images at the level of the lower thorax demonstrate apparently increased tracer uptake in the distal esophagus in an area of radiodense CT contrast. This is, however, artifactual, because of residual dense barium in a hiatal hernia and is not apparent on the non–attenuation-corrected image (lower right panel).

Note on MIP: Artifacts at the edge of the field of view due to image truncation in a large patient are seen.

Main Teaching Point and Summary

1. Dense barium and large patients can cause image reconstruction artifacts on PET that have propagated from the CT.

Brief History

A 73-year-old patient with esophageal carcinoma was treated with chemotherapy and radiotherapy, followed by surgery. A gastric pull-up procedure was performed in which much of the esophagus was removed and replaced with an intrathoracic location of the stomach. The patient was referred to PET/CT for follow-up restaging 1 year after surgery.

Findings

PET/CT images demonstrate curvilinear FDG activity of mild intensity in the right paraspinal region, corresponding to the wall of the partly contrast-filled stomach, which is now located in the thorax.

Main Teaching Points and Summary

1. The postoperative anatomy in patients with esophageal cancer can be complex, and it is essential to know the type of surgical procedure performed.
2. Postsurgical changes, such as an intrathoracic stomach, could be inadvertently interpreted as tumor recurrence on PET alone, but PET/CT and the clinical history clarify the diagnosis.

Case 4.10.3 BENIGN—ESOPHAGITIS, RADIATION-INDUCED (FIG. 4.10.3)

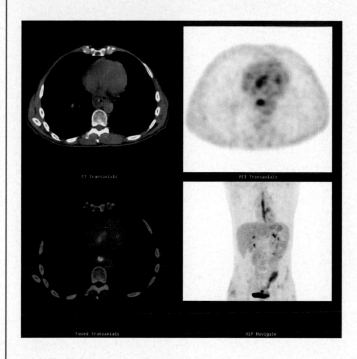

Case 4.10.4 TUMOR—CANCER OF PROXIMAL ESOPHAGUS (FIG. 4.10.4)

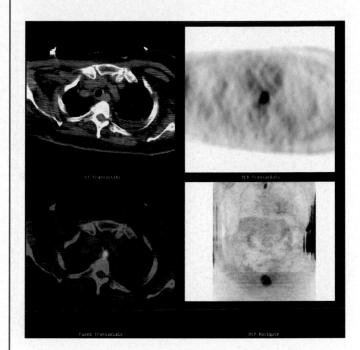

Brief History

A 50-year-old patient with adenocarcinoma of the distal esophagus was reassessed at 2 weeks following the conclusion of chemotherapy and radiotherapy.

Findings

PET/CT images after treatment demonstrate increased FDG uptake showing a linear pattern throughout the esophagus, extending cephalad to the location of the tumor at presentation, consistent with radiation esophagitis.

Results of the current study indicate that the patient had an excellent response to therapy.

Main Teaching Points and Summary

1. Effects of chemotherapy and radiotherapy of esophageal carcinomas can be monitored by PET/CT.
2. Mild linear uptake in the radiation port is common in the weeks and months immediately following treatment and should not be confused with tumor.

Brief History

A 71-year-old patient with recent difficulty swallowing and a new diagnosis of carcinoma in the proximal third of the esophagus was referred for whole body PET/CT staging.

Findings

PET/CT images clearly define abnormal FDG uptake in the primary tumor in the lower neck and upper thorax. A left pleural effusion on CT shows no increased FDG uptake.

Note on MIP: No metastases are identified. Artifacts at the edge of the field of view due to image truncation in this large patient are seen.

Main Teaching Points and Summary

1. Esophageal carcinomas are increasing in frequency and can occur anywhere along the course of the esophagus.
2. Early diagnosis improves the chances for cure by surgery and radiation/chemotherapy.

Case 4.10.5 TUMOR—CANCER OF DISTAL ESOPHAGUS (FIG. 4.10.5)

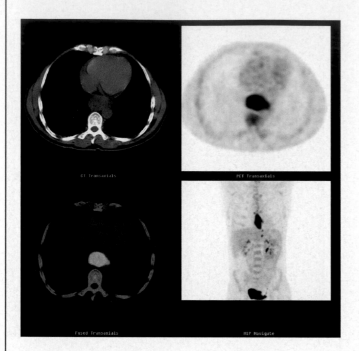

Brief History

A 50-year-old patient with swallowing difficulties diagnosed with adenocarcinoma of the distal esophagus was referred for whole body staging.

Findings

PET/CT images show a large distal esophageal mass with intense FDG avidity, consistent with the primary tumor.

Note on MIP: Nodal metastases in the region of the gastrohepatic ligament are seen.

Main Teaching Point and Summary

1. FDG-PET/CT is an excellent clinical tool for staging and treatment tailoring in patients with newly diagnosed esophageal cancer.

Case 4.10.6 TUMOR–RESPONSE TO TREATMENT, CANCER OF DISTAL ESOPHAGUS (FIG. 4.10.6)

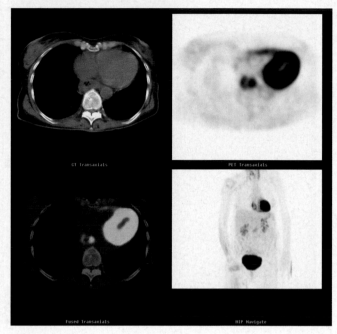

A

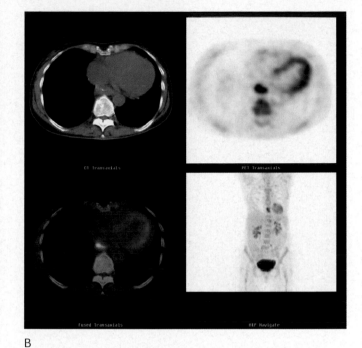

B

Brief History

A 65-year-old patient with esophageal carcinoma was assessed at presentation and after neoadjuvant chemotherapy before planning of possible surgery.

Findings

A. PET/CT images at presentation show focal intense FDG uptake in the thickened wall of the distal esophagus with no obvious distant metastases.

B. PET/CT images after chemotherapy show only mild decrease in the intensity of the tracer uptake and in the size of the anatomic esophageal lesion, representing a lack of response to therapy.

Note on MIP (B): Increased FDG marrow uptake after treatment, suggestive of reactive marrow rather than recurrent tumor, is evident.

Main Teaching Points and Summary

1. A decline in tumor FDG uptake is expected to occur by the conclusion of effective chemotherapy.
2. In this patient, treatment was not effective and disseminated metastatic disease was soon diagnosed.

4.11 CARDIOVASCULAR

Case 4.11.1 BENIGN—TAKAYASU'S AORTITIS (FIG. 4.11.1)

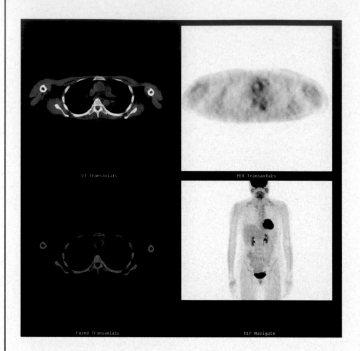

Brief History
A 25-year-old patient with Takayasu's aortitis had PET/CT to assess the activity of disease.

Findings
PET/CT images demonstrate moderately intense FDG uptake in the wall of the ascending aorta, which is somewhat dilated on CT.

Main Teaching Point and Summary
1. Active aortitis can show intense FDG uptake located to the vascular wall and not to the vascular lumen.
2. It is likely that FDG PET-CT will play a growing role in diagnosis and therapeutic monitoring of vasculitis.

Case 4.11.2 BENIGN—CORONARY CALCIFICATIONS AND PERICARDIAL EFFUSION (FIG. 4.11.2)

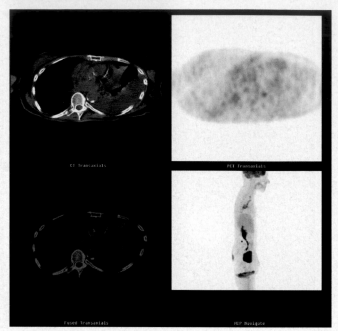

Brief History
A 70-year-old patient with fever and history of smoking was referred for further assessment of a pleural effusion and pulmonary nodule on CT.

Findings
PET/CT images show extensive coronary artery calcifications, which are FDG negative, and a large pericardial effusion with only modest FDG accumulation. On other images an FDG-avid pulmonary mass was seen.

Main Teaching Point and Summary
1. Although most PET/CT studies are performed to assess known or suspected cancer, there are additional findings that may be apparent only on the CT portion of the study although FDG-negative.
2. The presence of pericardial effusion and coronary calcifications raise concern for the presence of cardiac pathology in addition to the pulmonary lesions.

Case 4.11.3 ASSESSMENT OF MYOCARDIUM—SCAR (FIG. 4.11.3)

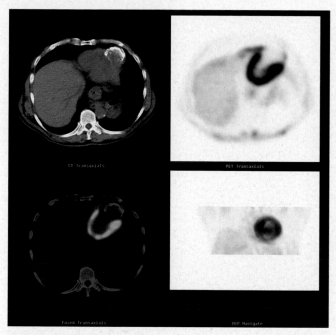

A

Brief History

A 66-year-old patient with a history of coronary artery disease and typical angina, status post–myocardial infarction 20 years before PET/CT, was evaluated to determine whether there was viable myocardium.

Findings

A and B. PET/CT images demonstrate the presence of calcification in the region of the myocardial apex on CT. On the FDG-PET study, there is a large focal defect at the left ventricular apex and splaying of the myocardial walls as they approach the apex. These findings are consistent with an apical aneurysm surrounded by nonviable myocardium.

Main Teaching Point and Summary

1. In contrast to cancer imaging, the patient preparation protocol for cardiac FDG-PET studies for myocardial viability includes administration of 50 g of glucose orally about 2 hours before the test. The patient may also be given insulin. FDG is typically injected when the glucose levels have declined to less than 150 mg/dl.
2. Myocardial viability studies with FDG are a sensitive method to detect biologically relevant residual viable tissue and separate hypoperfused viable from nonviable myocardium.
3. For PET/CT of the heart to work properly, it is critical that the CT and PET components be correctly aligned, as seen in this case, which is thus suitable for interpretation.

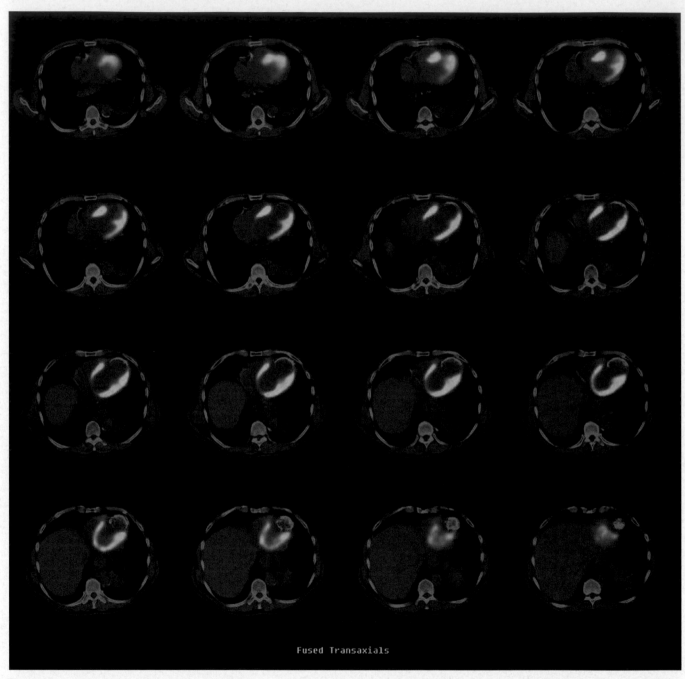

Fused Transaxials

B

Case 4.11.4 ASSESSMENT OF MYOCARDIUM—VIABILITY AND APICAL SCAR (FIG. 4.11.4)

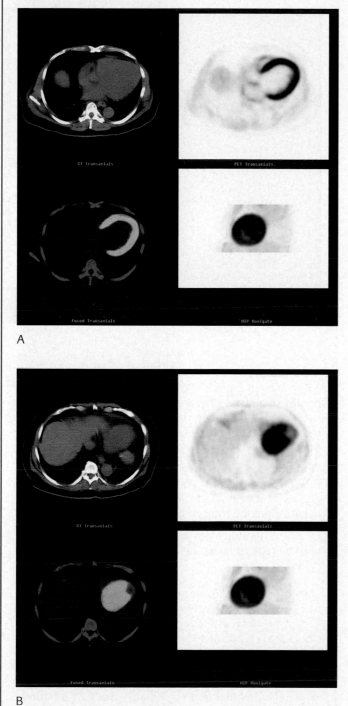

A

B

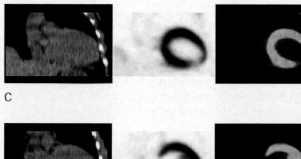

C

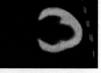
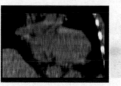
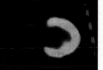

D

E

Brief History

A 63-year-old patient with an idiopathic dilated cardio-myopathy for nearly 10 years (ejection fraction by echo 25%) had a recent myocardial perfusion stress study with Tc99m methoxyisobutyl isonitrile (MIBI) showing reduced flow in the proximal midinferior wall suggesting an infarct in the distal inferior and inferoapical walls. The patient was assessed for the presence of myocardial viability.

Findings

A–E. PET/CT images show that nearly all of the myocar-dium has preserved glucose metabolism except for the distal inferoapical wall and the apex, with the infarct best seen on (B) and (C). The left ventricle is substan-tially dilated, but the atria and right ventricle are not enlarged (A). The anterior and posterior papillary muscles are both well seen (D and E).

Main Teaching Point and Summary

1. Assessment of myocardial viability includes evalua-tion of perfusion followed by that of glycolysis using PET.
2. In this patient, only a small area of infarction was identified compared with the large perfusion defects reported on Tc-MIBI perfusion imaging.
3. This patient appears to be a suitable candidate for revascularization.

Case 4.11.5 ASSESSMENT OF MYOCARDIUM–CARDIOMYOPATHY (FIG. 4.11.5)

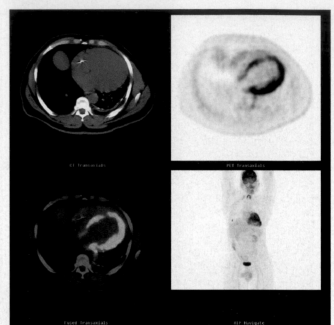

Brief History

A 46-year-old patient with history of familial cardiomy-opathy of at least 12 years had a ventricular defibrillator in place and was being considered for a heart transplant. He was referred for assessment of a new pulmonary nodule by PET/CT.

Findings

PET/CT images show a dilated left ventricle and reduced glycolytic activity in the septum. There is also FDG-negative pleural thickening and calcification.

Of note: This study was performed for cancer imaging, and the patient fasted for 4 hours before the FDG injection.

Main Teaching Point and Summary

1. The reduced glycolysis in the septum is suspicious for previous infarction and scar.
2. However, because the patient was imaged in the fasting setting, as opposed to conditions of high insulin levels following a glucose load that are required for a myocardial viability study, it cannot be concluded that there is reduced septal myocardial viability.

Case 4.11.6 CARDIAC PET/CT—NORMAL MYOCARDIAL PERFUSION AND CORONARY ANATOMY (FIG. 4.11.6)

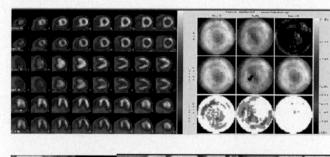

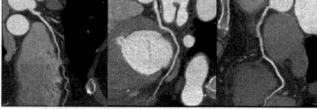

LAD   LCX   RCA

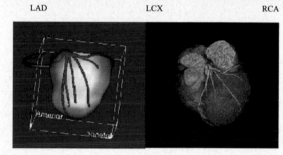

Brief History

A 46-year-old patient with hypercholesterolemia as a major risk factor for coronary artery disease underwent a Ru-82 perfusion study at rest and stress using adenosine. In addition, the patient had a 64-slice CT angiography (CTA) and a cardiac catheterization.

Findings

The myocardial perfusion is normal, as is the cardiac CTA and catheterization.

Main Teaching Point and Summary

1. This is a normal study by PET and anatomic imaging.

(Images courtesy of Dr. Tracy Faber, Emory University, Atlanta, Georgia).

Case 4.11.7 CARDIAC PET/CT—ISCHEMIA AND CORONARY CALCIFICATIONS AND NARROWING (FIG. 4.11.7)

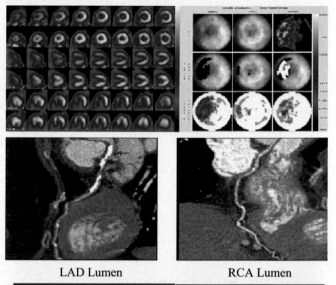

LAD Lumen   RCA Lumen

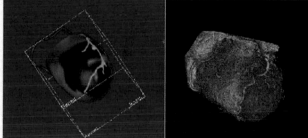

Brief History

A 52-year-old patient with chest pain and suspected coronary artery disease underwent adenosine stress and rest Ru-82 PET studies followed by CTA and cardiac catheterization.

Findings

A large reversible defect in the anteroseptal myocardium is seen on the Ru-82 perfusion stress/rest studies (upper row, left), quantitatively significant by polar map (upper row, right). CTA shows substantial calcification and narrowing of the left anterior descending artery (LAD; middle row, left) and a thinned right coronary artery (RCA; middle row, right). Fused images (lower row) indicate that the myocardial ischemia is related to the territory of the LAD perfusion.

Main Teaching Point and Summary

1. Hybrid PET/CT imaging can provide the anatomic and functional information needed to manage coronary artery disease in many instances.
2. Dense calcifications can degrade the quality of CTA studies.

(Images courtesy of Dr. Tracy Faber).

PET/CT of the Abdomen

Ora Israel • Ahuva Engel

5.1 NORMAL PATTERN

Case 5.1.1 NORMAL PATTERN PET/CT OF THE ABDOMEN (FIG. 5.1)

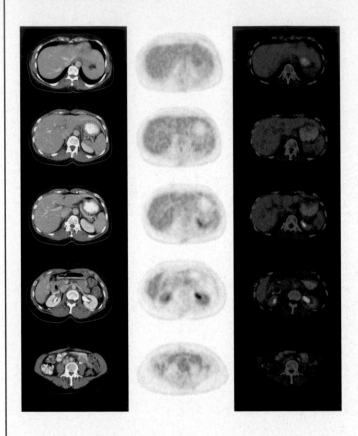

This is an example of a normal PET/CT of the abdomen. The study was performed following administration of diluted oral and standard intravenous (IV) contrast, which facilitates location of bowel and blood vessels and thus better distinguishes them from nodal or other pathologic findings. This protocol may also be of value for assessment of hepatic lesions. Care must be taken to ensure that no PET imaging or quantitative artifacts are induced by highly concentrated oral contrast or very high levels of IV contrast, which should not be used.

Normal FDG uptake is identified in the liver, spleen, stomach, kidneys, renal collecting system, and bowel loops.

5.2 ABDOMINAL WALL

Case 5.2.1 PITFALL—COLOSTOMY (FIG. 5.2.1)

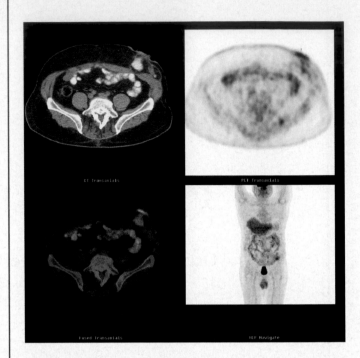

Brief History

A 60-year-old patient with a history of colon cancer, status post–left hemicolectomy and wedge resection of liver metastases, was assessed by PET/CT for the new onset of abdominal pain.

Findings

PET/CT images show a superficial area of increased 2-[18F] fluoro-2-deoxy-D-glucose (FDG) uptake in the left lower abdomen at the site of colostomy. CT also demonstrates the presence of an FDG-negative pericolostomy hernia containing small bowel.

Main Teaching Points and Summary
1. Increased FDG uptake in colostomies is common and should not be confused with tumor.
2. Not all pericolostomy hernias are FDG avid.

Case 5.2.2 PITFALL—PARARENAL BROWN FAT (FIG. 5.2.2)

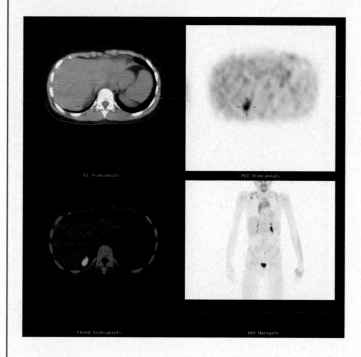

Case 5.2.3 PITFALL—ANTERIOR ABDOMINAL BROWN FAT (FIG. 5.2.3)

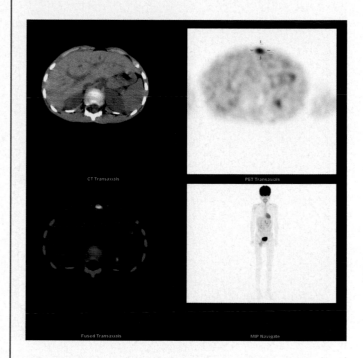

Brief History

A 9-year-old patient with abdominal Burkitt's lymphoma was assessed for monitoring response to treatment following four cycles of chemotherapy.

Findings

A. PET/CT images show a focal area of increased FDG uptake in the right lower flank region, localized to suprarenal fatty tissue, considered to represent physiologic tracer uptake in activated infradiaphragmatic brown fat, unrelated to malignancy.

Note on MIP: Foci of supradiaphragmatic adipose tissue uptake ("USA fat") in shoulder girdle as well as increased tracer activity in thymic rebound after treatment.

The patient had no evidence of active lymphoma on a follow-up of 8 months.

Main Teaching Points and Summary
1. Physiologic increased FDG uptake has been reported in supra- and infradiaphragmatic brown fat.
2. Brown fat uptake of FDG is more common in young patients and if the patient is in a low-temperature environment during tracer uptake.
3. An asymmetric pattern of FDG uptake, mainly below the diaphragm, may pose a diagnostic challenge. Abdominal brown fat is, however, usually associated with increased FDG uptake in USA fat.
4. PET/CT localization of these foci of tracer uptake to adipose tissue indicates their benign nature.

Brief History

A 7-year-old patient with newly diagnosed Ewing's sarcoma of the right pelvis was referred for staging.

Findings

PET/CT images show a focal area of abnormally increased FDG uptake in prehepatic fatty tissue in the anterior upper midabdomen just below the skin.

Note on MIP: The known primary tumor in the right inguinal region and physiologic excretion of FDG in the left renal collecting system are evident.

Main Teaching Point and Summary
1. Physiologic increased FDG uptake in infradiaphragmatic adipose tissue is less frequent as compared to foci of a similar etiology above the diaphragm.

Case 5.2.4 PITFALL—PARACOLIC BROWN FAT (FIG. 5.2.4)

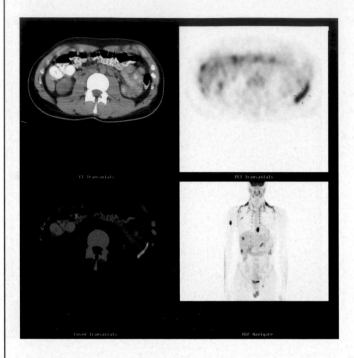

Case 5.2.5 BENIGN—SURGICAL SCAR (FIG. 5.2.5)

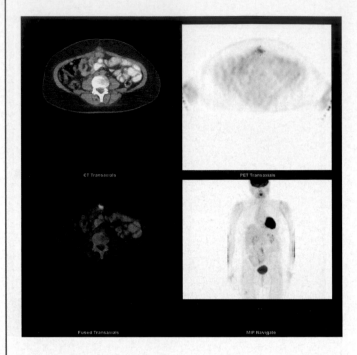

Brief History
An 18-year-old patient with newly diagnosed metastatic melanoma was referred for total body assessment before treatment planning.

Findings
PET/CT images show a focal area of abnormally increased FDG uptake in the lateral aspect of the left lower abdomen, located in paracolic fatty tissue. Additional foci of FDG uptake at this level are related to physiologic bowel excretion.

Note on MIP: Multiple metastatic sites in the liver, mediastinum, axillary, retroperitoneal, and inguinal lymph nodes, as well as the right humerus; physiologic foci of supradiaphragmatic brown fat in the cervical, shoulder girdle, and medial intercostal regions bilaterally; and normal testicular tracer activity are evident.

Main Teaching Points and Summary
1. Physiologic increased FDG uptake in brown fat below the diaphragm may be located in the parahepatic, paracolic, and perirenal spaces and may be symmetrical or unilateral.
2. As a rule, infradiaphragmatic FDG uptake in fatty tissues is associated with similar findings in sites above the diaphragm.
3. PET/CT is of major clinical value when asymmetric physiologic FDG uptake has to be differentiated from uptake in coexistent malignant lesions.

Brief History
A 56-year-old patient with history of carcinoma of the distal esophagus, status post-surgery 18 months pre-PET/CT, was assessed for new onset of swallowing difficulties. Recent CT had been reported as negative.

Findings
PET/CT images show an area of increased FDG uptake in the anterior midabdomen, corresponding to the surgical scar in the abdominal wall.

Main Teaching Points and Summary
1. FDG uptake in a recent surgical incision is generally related to an inflammatory or healing process.
2. In most patients, there is a gradual decrease in the intensity of FDG uptake over time in scars.

Case 5.2.6 BENIGN—RIB FRACTURE (FIG. 5.2.6)

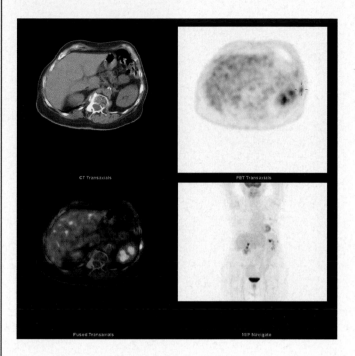

Brief History

A 72-year-old patient, 5 years after left lumpectomy for breast cancer, was assessed for suspected bone metastases due to equivocal bone scintigraphy results.

Findings

PET/CT images show a focus of increased FDG uptake in the lateral aspect of the abdominal wall, adjacent to the left kidney, localized to a healing fracture of a left lower rib.

Note on MIP: Foci of faint FDG uptake in the left anterior hemithorax, localized by PET/CT (not shown) to additional left rib fractures, are seen.

Main Teaching Points and Summary

1. Foci of increased FDG uptake in the abdominal wall may be located in different structures, including the skin, subcutaneous tissues, muscles, bones, bowel, and adjacent lymph nodes.
2. Recent healing fractures can show increased FDG uptake.
3. Older fractures often show no or less intense FDG uptake.

Case 5.2.7 TUMOR–METASTASIS (FIG 5.2.7)

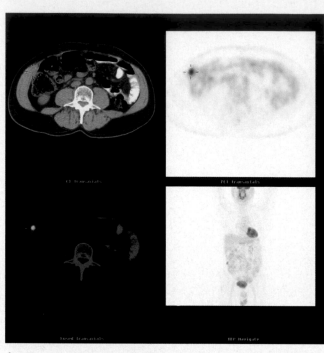

A

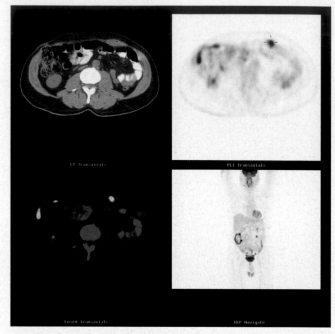

B

Brief History

A 49-year-old patient with a history of carcinoma of the pancreas, status post–distal pancreatectomy and wedge resection of the stomach 14 months pre-PET/CT, was assessed for suspected recurrence due to rising CA 19-9 serum levels in the presence of a whole body CT reported as normal.

Findings

A. PET/CT images show a focal area of abnormally increased FDG uptake in the anterolateral aspect of the abdomen corresponding to a hypodense area in the right external abdominal oblique muscle, adjacent to the surgical incision.

The patient underwent PET/CT guided fine-needle biopsy followed by surgical excision of a recurrent tumor of pancreatic origin in the abdominal wall. After an initial transient decrease, CA 19-9 serum levels increased again.

B. PET/CT performed 2 months later shows a new focus of abnormally increased FDG uptake in the left anterior midabdominal wall representing a new site of metastatic disease.

Note on MIP (B): A circular linear area of increased FDG uptake in the right midabdomen located by PET/CT (not shown) to inflammatory reactive changes in the abdominal wall following recent surgery and herniated bowel loops is seen.

Main Teaching Points and Summary

1. Recurrent disease in the abdominal wall may be difficult to detect by conventional imaging modalities, mainly if located adjacent to sites of previous surgery.
2. Increased FDG uptake in the sites of previous surgery for a malignant tumor may be related to a local inflammatory reaction or recurrent cancer.
3. PET/CT allows for precise guidance of confirmatory invasive diagnostic procedures and therefore early detection of recurrence.

5.3 LIVER AND SPLEEN

Case 5.3.1 PITFALL—INTRACHOLEDOCAL STENT (FIG. 5.3.1)

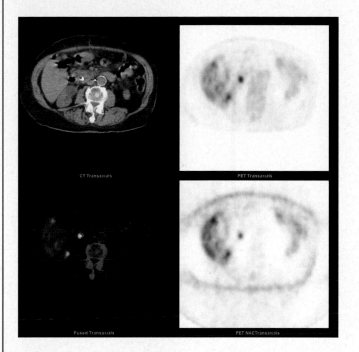

Brief History
An 80-year-old patient with a history of endometrial cancer and recently diagnosed carcinoma of the cecum was referred for further assessment of elevated serum CA 19-9 levels. The patient had previously undergone endoscopic papillotomy with intracholedochal stent insertion due to a malignant lesion diagnosed by endoscopic retrograde cholangiopancreatography at the level of the papilla.

Findings
PET/CT images show an area of abnormally increased FDG uptake at the level of the intracholedochal stent in the right upper abdomen. This focus is seen on both attenuation corrected (right upper) and uncorrected (right bottom) PET images.

PET/CT was reported as negative for malignancy, and the patient had no evidence of active disease on further clinical follow-up.

Main Teaching Points and Summary
1. Focal increased FDG uptake has been reported in areas of implants and stents. This may be due to a regional inflammatory reaction or to artifacts related to CT attenuation correction.
2. The similar findings seen in present case on corrected and uncorrected PET images substantially exclude an attenuation correction related artifactual etiology of this focus.
3. PET/CT can precisely localize a focus of abnormal FDG uptake to a device seen on the CT component and therefore reduce the rate of false-positive results and increase the specificity of the PET examination.

Case 5.3.2 PITFALL—LESIONS AT LIVER—LUNG INTERFACE (FIG. 5.3.2)

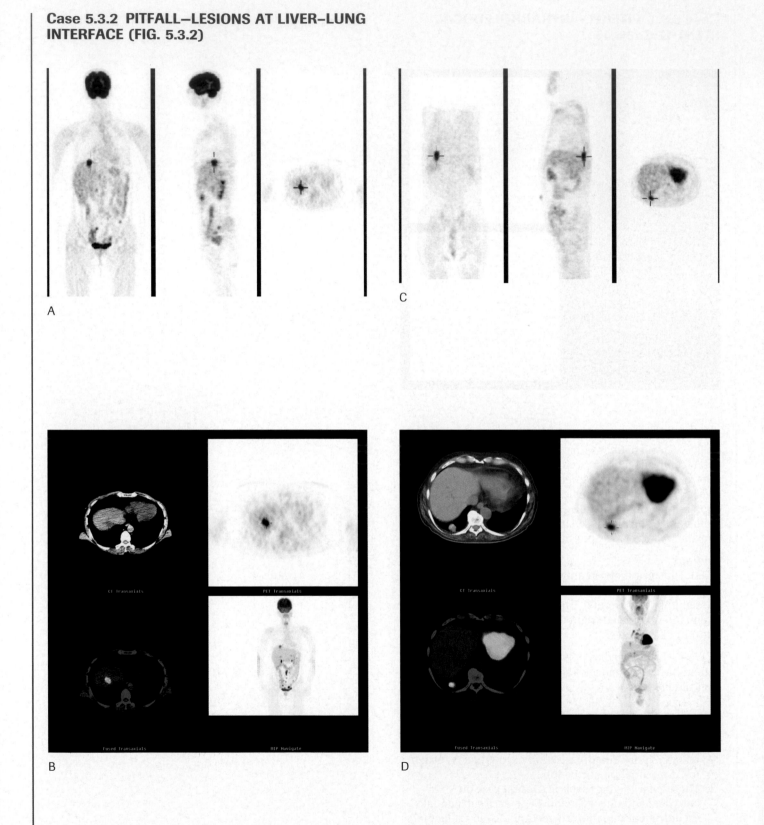

Brief History

A 55-year-old patient with history of carcinoma of the ovary, 2 years after surgery and chemotherapy, was referred because of rising serum tumor markers for a clinical suspicion of recurrence in the presence of a CT study reported as negative.

Findings

A. PET images show a focus of abnormally increased FDG uptake in the posterior aspect of the right liver–lung interface, consistent with a malignant lesion of unclear location, either in the lower lobe of the right lung or the upper pole of the liver.

B. PET/CT localizes this suspicious focus to a hypodense lesion in segment 8 in the hepatic dome. This liver metastasis was initially missed and only retrospectively detected on the high-resolution, contrast-enhanced CT study that had been previously performed.

Note on MIP: There are multiple additional foci of abnormal FDG uptake in the abdomen and pelvis, defined by PET/CT as peritoneal seeding, as well as retroperitoneal and pelvic metastatic lymphadenopathy.

C. For comparison purposes, PET images in another patient show a focal area of abnormal FDG uptake in the posterior aspect of the right liver–lung interface, consistent with a malignant lesion of unclear location.

D. PET/CT localizes the suspicious focus in this patient to a pulmonary nodule, 20 mm in diameter, in the right costophrenic region. The diagnosis of a second primary lung cancer was confirmed at surgery.

Note on MIP: Moderately intense FDG uptake in multiple mediastinal lymph nodes is seen.

Main Teaching Points and Summary

1. The posterior lower aspect of the lungs, costophrenic angles, retroperitoneum, and posterior liver interface are challenging areas to assess.

2. Abnormally increased FDG foci at the liver–lung interface can be difficult to localize to either lung or liver even on PET/CT because of potential breathing-related misregistration artifacts.

3. Close examination of the CT images of the area in question is necessary.

4. The presence of a congruent lesion on the CT component of the PET/CT study helps in the precise characterization of these findings.

Case 5.3.3 BENIGN—CHRONIC CHOLECYSTITIS (FIG. 5.3.3)

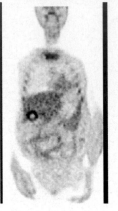
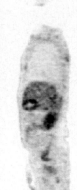
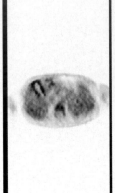

A

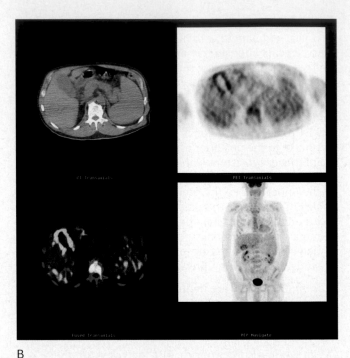

B

Brief History

A 74-year-old patient with aggressive non-Hodgkin's lymphoma was assessed for monitoring response to treatment at the completion of chemotherapy.

Findings

A. PET images show a large area with a rim of intense abnormal FDG uptake and a photopenic central region, adjacent to the anterior aspect of the liver.

B. PET/CT localizes this lesion to the wall of the gallbladder. The findings were considered to be unrelated to malignancy and represent an inflammatory process of the gallbladder.

Diagnosis of cholecystitis was confirmed by ultrasound and further surgery.

Main Teaching Point and Summary

1. Increased FDG uptake along the entire wall of the gallbladder is clearly abnormal but is much more suggestive of inflammatory changes than of malignancy although gallbladder cancer can have a similar appearance.

Case 5.3.4 TUMOR—PRIMARY HEPATOCELLULAR CARCINOMA (FIG. 5.3.4)

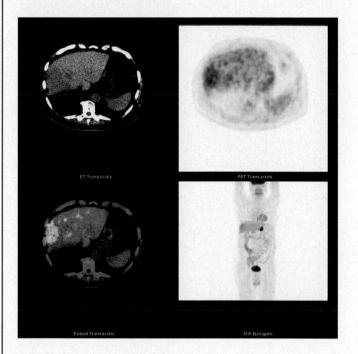

Brief History

An 82-year-old patient with recently diagnosed hepatocellular carcinoma in segment 6 of the liver was referred for staging in the presence of several additional hepatic lesions and an extraluminal gastric mass, 30 mm in diameter, seen on CT. The gastric lesion had been known for 7 years; endoscopic biopsy had been negative for malignancy and indicated only the presence of a chronic inflammatory process.

Findings

PET/CT shows a low-intensity, ill-defined focus of abnormal FDG uptake in the lateral aspect of the right lobe of the liver, corresponding to the known primary liver tumor.

Note on MIP: Increased FDG uptake in the known gastric inflammatory process is seen.

Main Teaching Points and Summary

1. FDG uptake in hepatocellular carcinoma is, not uncommonly, of lower intensity compared with other malignant liver lesions.
2. Hepatocellular carcinoma often shows an infiltrative pattern on CT.
3. Superimposition of ill-defined and at times equivocal metabolic and structural changes on fused PET/CT images can improve the diagnostic accuracy and detectability rate of hepatocellular carcinoma.

Case 5.3.5 TUMOR–SINGLE METASTASIS, LOWER POLE OF RIGHT LIVER LOBE (FIG. 5.3.5)

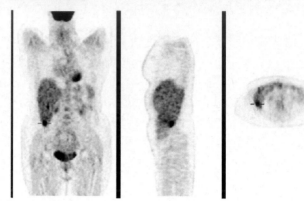

A

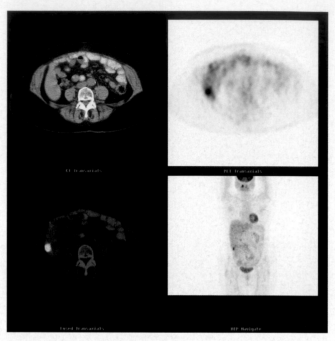

B

Brief History

A 65-year-old patient with colon cancer metastatic to the liver was assessed for the presence of residual active disease following neoadjuvant chemotherapy.

Findings

A. PET images show an area of increased FDG uptake in the right midlateral abdomen, which could represent a focal site of physiologic tracer activity in the ascending colon or residual active liver malignancy.

B. PET/CT demonstrates the localization of this hypermetabolic focus to the lower pole of a hepatic Riedel's lobe, consistent with residual viable tumor.

Main Teaching Points and Summary

1. PET/CT can precisely localize the foci of increased FDG uptake to a specific structure in regions with "crowded" and complex anatomy.

2. The ability of PET/CT to differentiate between physiologic bowel activity and a liver metastasis nearby is of critical importance for further treatment planning.

Case 5.3.6 TUMOR—MULTIPLE LIVER METASTASES (FIG. 5.3.6)

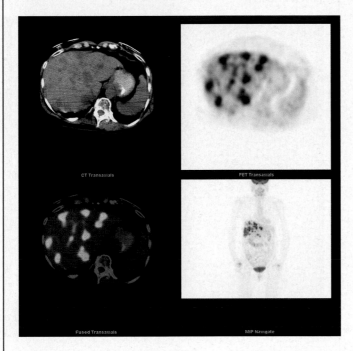

Brief History
A 67-year-old patient with ovarian cancer, metastatic to the liver, was referred to assess the extent of disease prior to chemotherapy.

Findings
PET/CT images show multiple hypodense lesions on CT with corresponding high FDG uptake in both lobes of the liver, consistent with disseminated hepatic metastases.

Main Teaching Points and Summary
1. Multiple foci of abnormally increased FDG uptake in the liver identified on PET indicate the presence of disseminated hepatic metastases.
2. PET/CT can be of additional value when surgical resectability is considered as a therapeutic option; in the presence of associated hepatic pathology such as fatty infiltration; or in the differential diagnosis of liver versus extrahepatic metastatic foci.

Case 5.3.7 TUMOR—LIVER METASTASIS, RECURRENCE AT SITE OF SURGERY (FIG. 5.3.7)

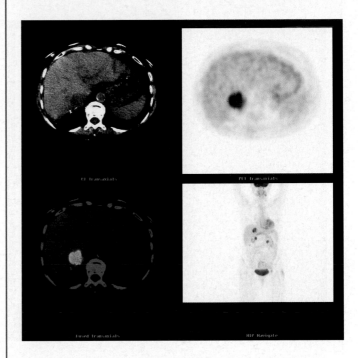

Brief History
A 67-year-old patient with history of sigmoid colon cancer, status post–resection of the primary tumor and of a liver metastasis, was assessed following elevated serum CEA levels and equivocal findings on CT for a suspected recurrence at the site of previous liver surgery.

Findings
PET/CT demonstrates an area of intense abnormally increased FDG uptake located in a hypodense lesion, 30 mm in diameter, in the posterior aspect of the right lobe of the liver, in the region of surgical clips related to previous hepatic metastasis resection.

The diagnosis of a new liver metastasis in this location was confirmed at surgical re-exploration.

Main Teaching Points and Summary
1. PET/CT matches hypermetabolic lesions and equivocal CT findings, defining them as malignant when appropriate.
2. Contrast enhanced CT remains important especially to define the vascular supply of the lesion in cases where surgery is planned.

Case 5.3.8 TUMOR—SINGLE METASTASIS IN SPLEEN (FIG. 5.3.8)

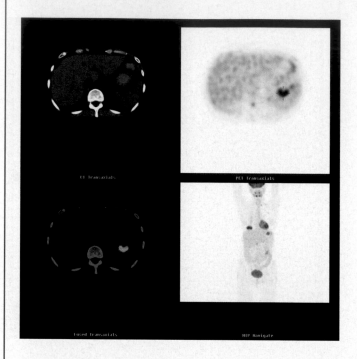

Brief History

A 45-year-old patient with cancer of the colon metastatic to the liver, status post–right hemicolectomy, was assessed to monitor response to chemotherapy.

Findings

PET/CT images show an area of abnormally increased FDG uptake in a hypodense lesion in the midportion of the spleen, consistent with a metastatic lesion.

Note on MIP: Additional foci of abnormal FDG uptake in a right lower lobe lung metastasis and in para-aortic lymphadenopathy in the upper retroperitoneum are seen.

Main Teaching Point and Summary

1. Splenic metastases are difficult to diagnose with certainty on CT alone. PET adds sensitivity and specificity to this region.

Case 5.3.9 TUMOR—MULTIPLE LESIONS IN SPLEEN AND NODAL INVOLVEMENT (FIG. 5.3.9)

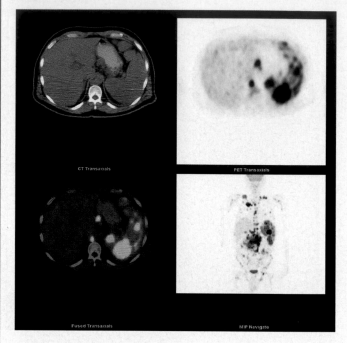

Brief History

A 45-year-old patient with newly diagnosed diffuse large cell non-Hodgkin's lymphoma was referred for staging before chemotherapy.

Findings

PET/CT images show multiple foci of abnormally increased FDG uptake in an enlarged spleen. There is also increased tracer uptake in enlarged para-aortic and gastrohepatic ligament lymph nodes.

Note on MIP: Multiple sites of lymphoma involving lymph nodes above and below the diaphragm, the spleen, and skeleton are seen.

Main Teaching Points and Summary

1. Lymphoma involving the spleen is common and can show variable patterns on PET of single or multifocal disease.
2. CT may fail to show tumor foci in the spleen.

Case 5.3.10 TUMOR—SPLENOMEGALY AND DIFFUSE INVOLVEMENT BY LYMPHOMA (FIG. 5.3.10)

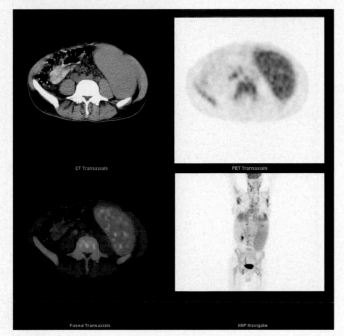

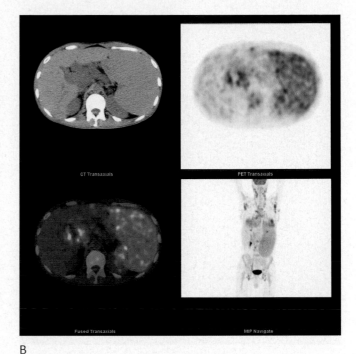

A

B

Brief History

A 41-year-old patient was referred for baseline evaluation of a newly diagnosed low-grade, follicular-cell non-Hodgkin's lymphoma.

Findings

A and B. PET/CT images show increased FDG uptake in a very large spleen, with its lower pole reaching the level of the left iliac crest. On the transaxial PET/CT slices at a more cephalad level (A), involvement of lymph nodes located at the hepatic hilum is also demonstrated.

Note on MIP images: There is evidence for extensive disease in supra- and infradiaphragmatic locations, involving multiple nodal sites, the spleen, and lungs.

Main Teaching Points and Summary

1. The normal FDG biodistribution patterns include liver and spleen activity of variable intensity.
2. Splenic FDG activity is, in normals, typically lower or equivalent as compared with uptake in the liver.
3. Lymphoma involving the spleen can display a focal or diffuse pattern, with or without splenic enlargement.
4. Increased FDG uptake associated with splenomegaly can represent active lymphoma but may also be related to recent administration of granulocyte colony stimulation factor. Detailed patient history is therefore important.

5.4 PANCREAS

Case 5.4.1 TUMOR—CANCER IN HEAD OF PANCREAS (FIG. 5.4.1)

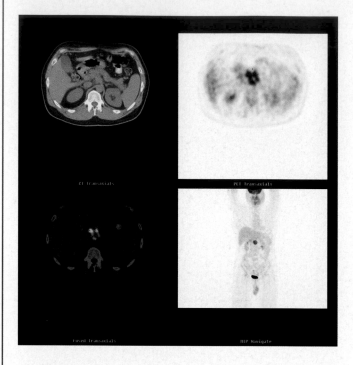

Case 5.4.2 TUMOR—CANCER IN TAIL OF PANCREAS (FIGURE 5.4.2)

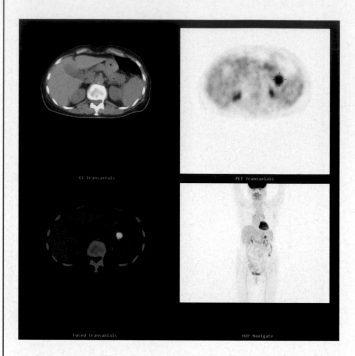

Brief History

A 44-year-old patient with newly diagnosed cancer of the pancreas was referred because of a suspicious splenic lesion on CT for staging before surgery.

Findings

PET/CT images show a focus of abnormally increased FDG uptake in the upper midabdomen, localized to a space-occupying lesion, 33 mm in diameter, involving the head of the pancreas, the uncinate process, and peripancreatic celiac axis lymph nodes. These findings are consistent with the known primary malignant tumor and metastatic lymphadenopathy.

Note that no abnormal FDG uptake was seen in the spleen.

Main Teaching Point and Summary

1. PET/CT can detect many primary pancreatic cancers as well as locoregional lymph node and systemic metastases.

Brief History

A 78-year-old patient with a history of rectal and bronchioloalveolar lung cancer was referred for further assessment of weight loss, abdominal pain, rising serum tumor markers, and equivocal findings on abdominopelvic CT.

Findings

PET/CT images show a focal area of abnormally increased FDG uptake in the upper left abdomen, medial to the spleen, located in a mildly enlarged pancreatic tail.

This lesion had been previously undiagnosed and only retrospectively detected on contrast-enhanced, high-resolution CT. A third primary tumor, ductal adenocarcinoma of the pancreas, was diagnosed at surgery.

Main Teaching Points and Summary

1. PET/CT can match metabolic PET and structural CT findings, facilitating diagnosis of lesions that may be missed at independent reading of the two diagnostic modalities.
2. Subtle CT findings are often detected only after the PET study is abnormal in a specific location.

Case 5.4.3 TUMOR AND INFLAMMATION—MULTIPLE PANCREATIC LESIONS (FIG. 5.4.3)

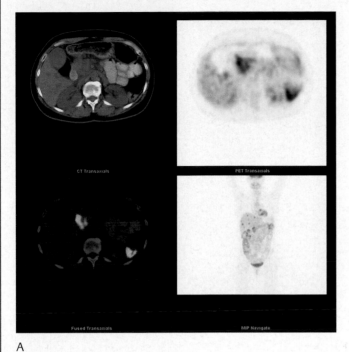

A

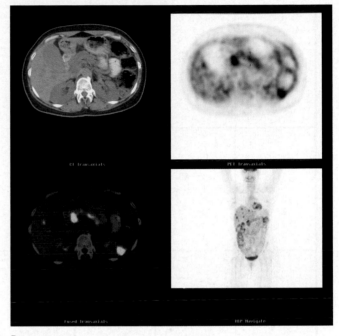

B

Brief History

A 54-year-old patient with newly diagnosed pancreatic cancer and suspicious CT findings in the liver was referred for staging before surgery.

Findings

A. PET/CT images show an area of abnormally increased FDG uptake in the right paramedian midabdomen, localized to a heterogeneous mass in the head of the pancreas, 40 mm in diameter, consistent with the known primary tumor.

B. PET/CT images at a cephalad level show an additional area of abnormally increased FDG uptake of moderate intensity in the left paramedian, midabdominal region, localized to a slightly edematous body of the pancreas, most probably consistent with an inflammatory postobstructive process.

Note on MIP: Multiple areas of abnormal FDG uptake in both lobes of the liver, consistent with hepatic metastases, and physiologic tracer activity in the bowel are seen.

Main Teaching Points and Summary

1. Increased FDG uptake may be related to either a malignant tumor or an inflammatory process, which is a common postobstructive reaction.
2. PET/CT may localize hypermetabolic areas to focal or diffuse anatomic abnormalities and thus differentiate between the two potential causes of increased tracer uptake.

5.5 STOMACH

Case 5.5.1 PHYSIOLOGIC–GASTRIC UPTAKE (FIG. 5.5.1)

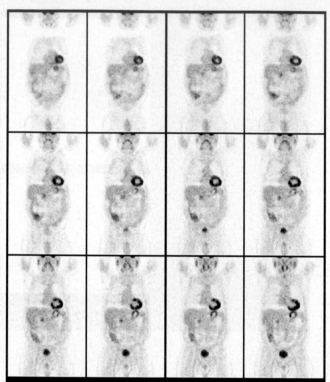

A

B

Brief History

A 71-year-old patient, 7 years after left upper lobectomy for lung cancer, was referred to assess a new right upper lobe cavitary lung lesion, 22 mm in diameter, seen on a follow up CT study.

Findings

A and B. Selected coronal PET and transaxial PET/CT images show diffuse increased FDG uptake of moderate intensity in the gastric wall.

There was abnormally increased FDG uptake in the new pulmonary nodule in the right upper lobe (not shown) histologically proved to represent a second primary lung cancer.

Main Teaching Points and Summary

1. Nonmalignant gastric FDG uptake representing physiologic tracer accumulation or less commonly, gastritis, is frequently encountered.
2. Differential diagnosis versus diffuse tumor involvement may be difficult but tumor uptake is typically more focal.

Case 5.5.2 TUMOR–LYMPHOMA IN DISTAL ANTRUM (FIG. 5.5.2)

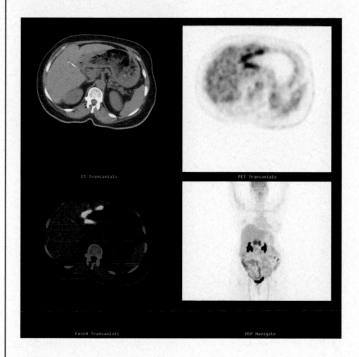

Brief History
A 59-year-old patient was referred for initial staging of large cell non-Hodgkin's lymphoma of the stomach.

Findings
PET/CT images show intense abnormal FDG uptake in the upper midabdomen, located in a severely thickened gastric wall at the level of the distal antrum, consistent with involvement of the known lymphoma.

Main Teaching Points and Summary
1. Lymphoma or other malignant gastric tumors may involve the whole organ or be localized to a small region in the stomach.
2. Focal FDG uptake is more suggestive of malignant involvement than a pattern of diffuse increased tracer activity.

Case 5.5.3 TUMOR–DIFFUSE PATTERN, GASTRIC CANCER, AND NODAL METASTASES (FIG. 5.5.3)

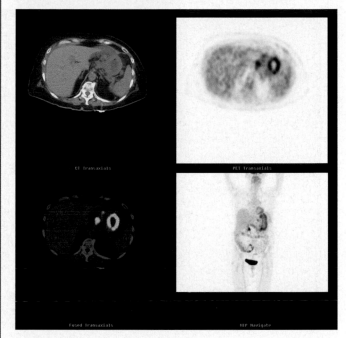

Brief History
A 68-year-old patient with newly diagnosed adenocarcinoma of the stomach was referred for staging before surgery in the presence of a suspicious pulmonary lesion seen on CT.

Findings
PET/CT images show a large area of intense abnormal FDG uptake in the left upper abdomen, localized to diffuse irregular thickening of the gastric wall, representing the known malignant tumor. There is also increased FDG uptake in gastrohepatic ligament lymph node metastases.

No increased tracer uptake was demonstrated in the pulmonary nodules, with no further evidence of pulmonary malignancy on clinical follow-up.

Main Teaching Points and Summary
1. Diffuse FDG uptake in the stomach may be related to physiologic tracer excretion, gastritis, or malignant tumors of variable histology.
2. Nodal FDG uptake near the stomach generally indicates the presence of metastatic lymph node involvement.

Case 5.5.4 TUMOR–LARGE GASTRIC MASS, GASTROINTESTINAL STROMAL TUMOR (GIST) (FIG. 5.5.4)

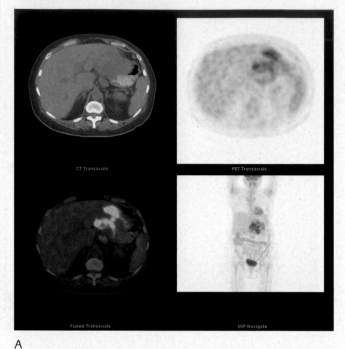

A

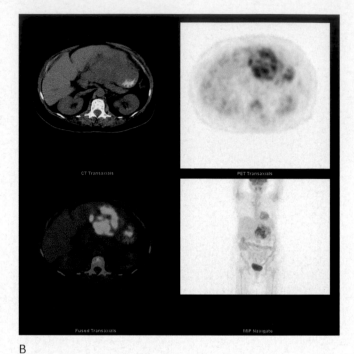

B

Brief History

A 66-year-old patient with a gastrointestinal stromal tumor (GIST) originating in the stomach, presented with recurrent episodes of gastrointestinal bleeding that continued despite chemotherapy administered over a 9-month period. He was referred to assess for possible resectability as a palliative approach.

Findings

A and B. PET/CT images at two upper abdominal levels show a huge, heterogeneous area of abnormally increased FDG uptake in the anterior midabdomen localized to a very large ulcerating mass involving most of the stomach, consistent with the known primary tumor.

Main Teaching Points and Summary

1. The majority of GISTs (approximately 70%) originate in the stomach.
2. Before the novel tyrosine kinase inhibitor therapy imatinib (Gleevec) treatment option, GIST generally had a poor prognosis.
3. Heterogeneous radiotracer uptake is common in GIST likely due to areas of necrosis.
4. PET/CT imaging is a sensitive modality for assessing response of GIST to treatment.

Case 5.5.5 TUMOR—RECURRENCE OF GASTRIC CANCER (FIG. 5.5.5)

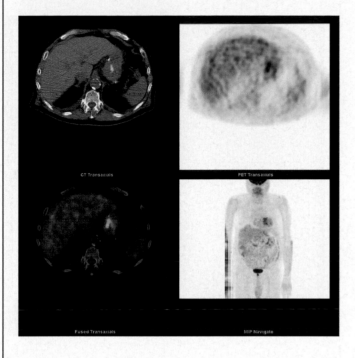

Case 5.6.1 BENIGN—ADENOMA IN COLON (FIG. 5.6.1)

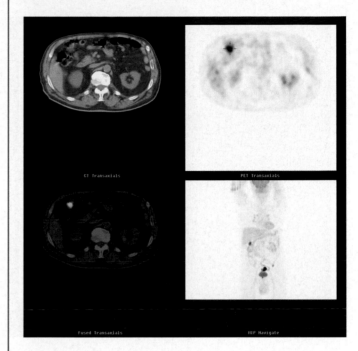

Brief History
A 73-year-old patient, 7 years after subtotal gastrectomy for an adenocarcinoma, had a new episode of gastrointestinal bleeding and was diagnosed with recurrent disease by gastroscopy. CT demonstrated the presence of mild nodal enlargement in the hepatic and splenic hilum, and PET/CT was performed for restaging before surgery.

Findings
PET/CT images show an area of mildly increased FDG uptake located to part of the thickened gastric stump, consistent with the known recurrent tumor.

Note on MIP: No additional areas of abnormal FDG uptake in the upper abdomen or other parts of the torso are seen.

Main Teaching Points and Summary
1. PET/CT can help to define the clinical significance of low-intensity FDG-avid suspicious sites when located in regions of known anatomic pathology.
2. The differential diagnosis of increased FDG uptake in the region of the stomach is difficult, mainly in the presence of distorted anatomy after surgery.

Brief History
An 83-year-old patient with newly diagnosed carcinoma of the rectum was referred for preoperative staging because of the presence of suspicious pulmonary lesions on CT.

Findings
PET/CT images show a focus of abnormally increased FDG uptake in the colon at the level of the hepatic flexure, with no corresponding abnormalities on CT.

Colonoscopy performed 2 months later indicated the presence of a large tubular adenoma corresponding to the FDG avid focus.

Note on MIP: Abnormal uptake in the primary rectal tumor and low-intensity FDG uptake in mediastinal lymph nodes, most probably granulomatous changes, are seen.

Main Teaching Points and Summary
1. Up to 70% of focally increased FDG activity localized in the colon is related to malignant or premalignant lesions.
2. Foci of intense FDG uptake located in the gastrointestinal tract require further endoscopic investigation or close follow-up PET/CT.

Case 5.6.2 TUMOR–PRIMARY COLON CANCER (FIG. 5.6.2)

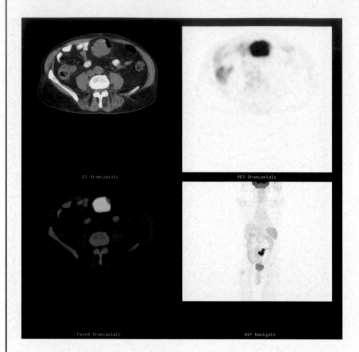

Brief History
A 79-year-old patient with newly diagnosed cancer of the colon was referred for preoperative staging because of the presence of small lung nodules on CT performed 4 weeks pre-PET/CT.

Findings
PET/CT images show an area of intense abnormal FDG uptake in the midabdomen localized to a space-occupying lesion in the transverse colon, consistent with the known primary colon cancer.

There was no increased FDG uptake in the lungs, and no pulmonary nodules were seen on the CT component of the study.

The interval changes to previously reported pulmonary findings were therefore considered to represent healing of an intercurrent respiratory tract infection. There was no evidence of pulmonary disease involvement on clinical follow-up.

Main Teaching Points and Summary
1. A pattern of highly intense focal FDG uptake located in a space-occupying colonic lesion on the CT component of the study is highly suggestive of malignancy.
2. Administration of diluted oral contrast is an important part of the imaging protocol.

Case 5.6.3 TUMOR–METASTASIS IN SMALL INTESTINE (FIG. 5.6.3)

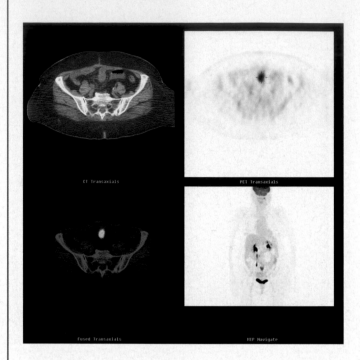

Brief History
A 73-year-old patient, status post–right hemicolectomy for adenocarcinoma, was referred with the suspicion of recurrence because of rising CEA serum levels and equivocal CT findings at the level of the surgical anastomosis.

Findings
PET/CT images show a focus of abnormally increased FDG uptake in the lower midabdomen localizing to a small intestine loop, suspicious for malignancy.

The patient was referred to surgery, and a metastasis from colon cancer was removed.

Main Teaching Points and Summary
1. A highly intense focal pattern, in the presence of an intraluminal filling defect or mass on the CT component of the study, increases the suspicion of malignant or premalignant lesions.
2. The small bowel may rarely be the site of metastases. This is relatively more common with melanoma.

5.7 PERITONEUM

Case 5.7.1 BENIGN—GRANULOMATOTIC NODULE (FIG. 5.7.1)

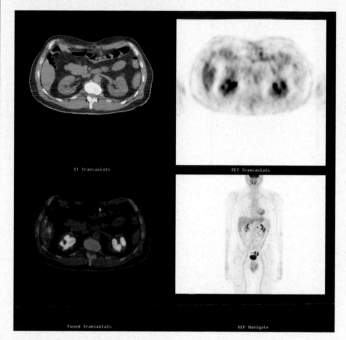

A

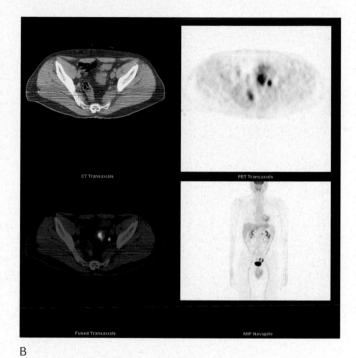

B

Brief History

A 53-year-old patient with cancer of the colon, 2 years after right hemicolectomy, was assessed before resection of a newly diagnosed second primary tumor in the sigmoid colon.

Findings

A. PET/CT images show a hypermetabolic focus in the left anterior aspect of the abdomen, located in a nodule in the peritoneal fat, behind the rectus muscle, just anterior to the transverse colon, in the vicinity of the previous surgical incision.

B. PET/CT images at the level of the midpelvis show abnormally increased FDG uptake in the primary sigmoid tumor. Additional tracer uptake is seen in the left ureter and a bowel loop.

The patient underwent surgical resection of the tumor in the sigmoid colon. Based on the precise localization provided by PET/CT, the peritoneal lesion was removed. Histologic examination revealed postsurgical granulomatous tissue, with no evidence of malignancy.

Main Teaching Points and Summary

1. Increased FDG uptake in or adjacent to sites of previous surgery may be related to a local inflammatory reaction or recurrent disease.
2. PET/CT enables precise guidance of invasive procedures that may be needed to exclude the presence of malignant lesions.

Case 5.7.2 TUMOR—SINGLE NODULE, METASTASIS (FIG. 5.7.2)

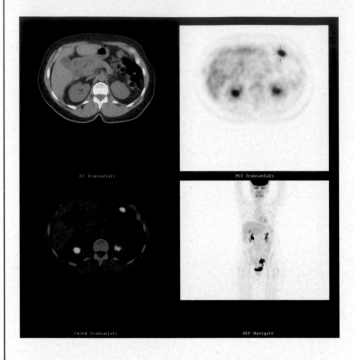

Brief History

A 65-year-old patient with carcinoma of the ovary, status post–total hysterectomy and bilateral salpingo-oophorectomy, was assessed for a clinically suspected recurrence as suggested by elevated serum levels of CA-125 and an equivocal CT in the region of previous surgery.

Findings

PET/CT images show a small focus of abnormally increased FDG uptake in a peritoneal nodule, 23 mm in diameter, at the level of the upper pole of the left kidney, consistent with a metastatic peritoneal implant.

Note on MIP: Additional foci of intense FDG uptake consistent with recurrent disease in the left anatomic pelvis and a small metastatic lesion in the liver are evident.

Main Teaching Points and Summary

1. Malignant involvement of the peritoneum may be masked or missed on PET as a stand-alone procedure because of various abdominal sites of physiologic and benign FDG uptake, most notably normal gut uptake.
2. Peritoneal seeding can be difficult to diagnose on CT in its early stages.

Case 5.7.3 TUMOR—MULTIPLE NODULES, METASTASES (FIG. 5.7.3)

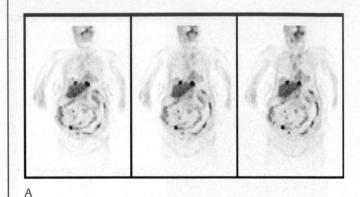

A

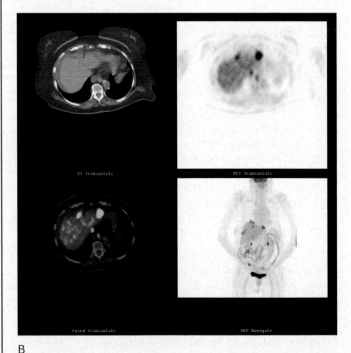

B

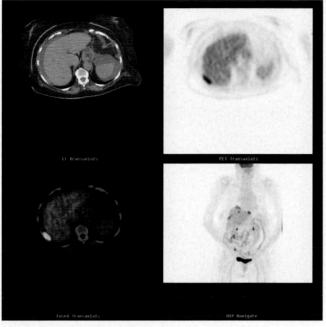

C

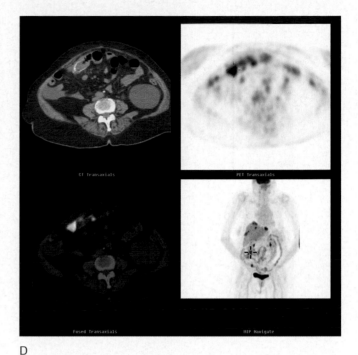

D

Brief History
A 78-year-old patient with a history of colon cancer, status post–right hemicolectomy and chemotherapy 2 years pre-PET/CT, was assessed for clinically suspected recurrence related to rising serum tumor markers and suspicious CT findings in the region of the surgical anastomosis.

Findings
A. Selected coronal PET images show multiple foci of abnormally increased FDG uptake at the margins of the liver and an additional suspicious lesion in the right lower abdomen.
B. PET/CT images at the level of the liver–lung interface localize several foci of increased FDG uptake to peritoneal nodules at the upper pole of the right lobe of the liver.
C. PET/CT images at a more caudal level localize an additional focus of increased FDG uptake to a peritoneal nodule adjacent to the posteriolateral aspect of the right lobe of the liver.
D. PET/CT images at the level of the lower abdomen show a hypermetabolic mass at the site of the surgical anastomosis, consistent with local recurrence.

Main Teaching Points and Summary
1. PET/CT improves the diagnosis of peritoneal disease over separately performed studies.
2. PET/CT often indicates the presence of corresponding subtle hypermetabolic and anatomic lesions related to peritoneal seeding.

Case 5.7.4 TUMOR–DIFFUSE PATTERN, PERITONEAL SEEDING (FIG. 5.7.4)

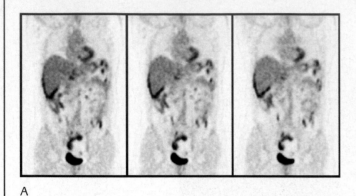

A

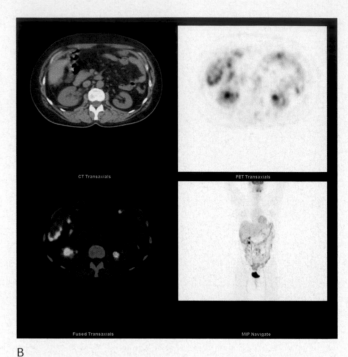

B

Brief History

A 48-year-old patient with carcinoma of the ovary, status post–total hysterectomy and bilateral salpingo-oophorectomy, was assessed for suspicion of recurrence related to elevated CA-125 levels and equivocal findings on CT of the pelvis.

Findings

A. Selected coronal PET images show a linear area of increased FDG uptake surrounding the lower part of the right lobe of the liver.

B. PET/CT images localize the increased FDG uptake to peritoneal seeding surrounding the lower pole of the right lobe of the liver, consistent with malignant peritoneal spread.

Note on MIP: Areas of linear increased FDG uptake in the vicinity of the spleen and in the right pelvis, consistent with additional sites of metastatic peritoneal involvement.

Main Teaching Points and Summary

1. Malignant involvement of the peritoneum may show a focal or diffuse pattern on PET.
2. Peritoneal seeding is difficult to diagnose on CT.
3. The "liver outline" pattern on PET is typical of disseminated peritoneal metastases, in particular from ovarian cancer.

Case 5.7.5 TUMOR–PERITONEAL MASSES, GIST, AND LIVER INVOLVEMENT (FIG. 5.7.5)

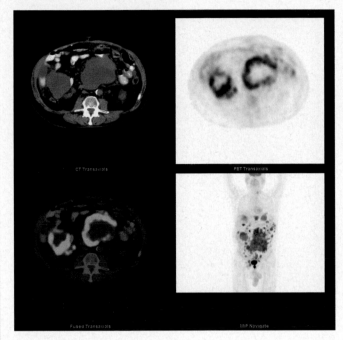

A

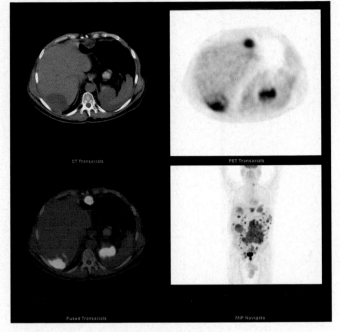

B

Brief History
A 70-year-old patient with a very large mesenteric gastrointestinal stromal tumor (GIST), status post–incomplete resection, was referred for restaging before chemotherapy.

Findings
A. PET/CT images show two large peritoneal masses with heterogeneous densities on CT and a peripheral rim of abnormally increased FDG uptake, corresponding to partially necrotic lesions.
B. PET/CT images at a more cephalad level demonstrate the presence of additional peritoneal masses, smaller in size, showing more homogeneous FDG uptake, one located in the anterior upper abdomen, adjacent to the stomach, and a second posterior lesion, close to the spleen. There is also a large hypodense, FDG-avid lesion in the posterior aspect of the right lobe of the liver. The findings are consistent with peritoneal and hepatic metastases.

Note on MIP: Multiple foci of intense FDG uptake consistent with extensive peritoneal and hepatic metastatic sites of disease involvement are seen.

Main Teaching Points and Summary
1. Sensitivity of PET and CT for staging of untreated GIST are comparable at about 90%.
2. Baseline PET/CT needs to be performed before treatment because this imaging modality appears to be the test of choice for monitoring GIST response to treatment, with FDG uptake dropping quickly with effective therapy.
3. After treatment, CT may be more sensitive than PET in detecting the presence of GIST, but if negative on FDG PET, these tumors are often functionally inactive.

5.8 KIDNEYS AND ADRENALS

Case 5.8.1 PITFALL—REGIONAL LYMPHADENOPATHY NEAR RENAL PELVIS (FIG. 5.8.1)

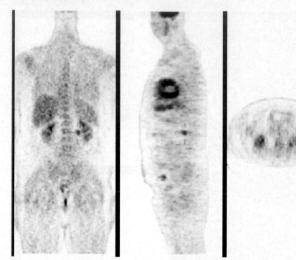

A

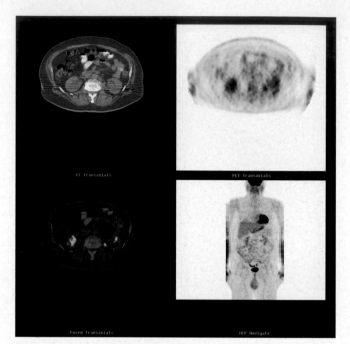

B

Brief History

A 59-year-old patient with diffuse large cell non-Hodgkin's lymphoma was referred to monitor response early during treatment.

Findings

A. PET images show a focus of increased FDG uptake near the anteriomedial aspect of the left kidney, considered on PET alone to represent physiologic tracer uptake in the urinary collecting system.

B. PET/CT images localize this focus to a slightly enlarged lymph node, 16 mm in diameter, adjacent to the medial aspect of the left renal cortex, consistent with a site of residual viable lymphoma.

Main Teaching Points and Summary

1. Physiologic excretion of FDG in the renal collecting systems has to be differentiated from pathologic uptake in regional malignant sites.

2. PET/CT may identify tumor sites masked by, or confused with, physiologic tracer activity in adjacent normal organs.

Case 5.8.2 PITFALL—SINGLE KIDNEY (FIG. 5.8.2)

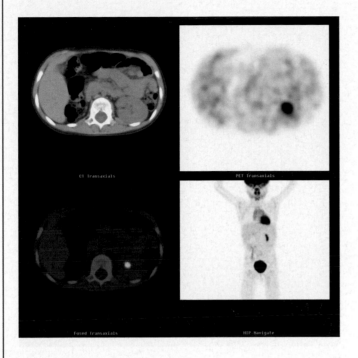

Brief History

A 10-year-old patient with Wilm's tumor, status post–surgical excision of the right kidney, was assessed for further evaluation of new small pulmonary nodules seen in the base of both lungs on CT.

Findings

PET/CT images show an area of increased FDG uptake in the left midabdomen localized to the pelvis of the single left kidney.

The presence of abdominal malignancy was excluded. Lung nodules were not seen on either the PET or CT component of the study, consistent with a resolving respiratory tract infection.

Note on MIP: There is visualization of the normal thymus in the anterior midmediastinum.

Main Teaching Points and Summary

1. Asymmetric physiologic FDG activity in the collecting system of a single kidney may present as an equivocal or suspicious site on PET.
2. PET/CT allows the differential diagnosis of physiologic FDG uptake, unrelated to cancer versus a malignant lesion.
3. Thymic visualization is normal in patients of this age.

Case 5.8.3 PITFALL—ECTOPIC KIDNEY (FIG. 5.8.3)

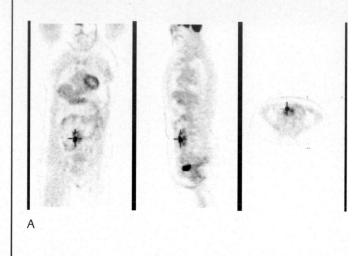

A

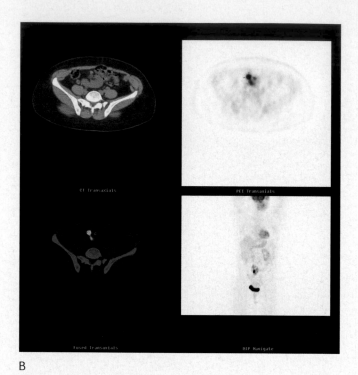

B

Brief History

A 50-year-old patient was referred for further assessment of a pulmonary nodule, 20 mm in diameter, in the lower lobe of the right lung, detected on CT.

Findings

A. PET images show a focus of increased FDG uptake in the right lower midabdomen.
B. PET/CT images localize this suspicious finding to physiologic urinary FDG excretion in the collecting system of an ectopic, rotated right pelvic kidney.

The pulmonary lesion was FDG negative, and there was no evidence of malignancy on clinical follow-up. The left kidney was visualized in its normal location (seen on anterior MIP in B).

Main Teaching Points and Summary

1. Physiologic FDG activity in the renal pelvis is common.
2. Variations in renal anatomy may lead to pitfalls and misinterpretation of FDG uptake, which can be clarified through the use of PET/CT.

Case 5.8.4 PITFALL–HORSESHOE KIDNEY (FIG. 5.8.4)

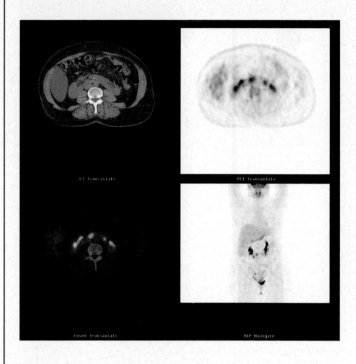

Brief History
A 49-year-old patient with low-grade non-Hodgkin's lymphoma was referred for further assessment of equivocal, slightly enlarged mesenteric lymph nodes on follow up CT.

Findings
PET/CT images show a focus of increased FDG uptake in the midabdomen, located in the central part of a horseshoe kidney, consistent with physiologic tracer uptake in an anatomic variant.

Note on MIP: Medial angulation of the lower poles of both kidneys is seen, consistent with a characteristic pattern of horseshoe kidney.

The patient had no evidence of active lymphoma for a follow-up of 8 months.

Main Teaching Points and Summary
1. Physiologic FDG activity in kidneys can be misinterpreted in cases with anatomic variants.
2. The considerable variability in the appearance of horseshoe kidneys can be clarified by PET/CT.

Case 5.8.5 PITFALL–DISTORTED RENAL PELVIS (FIG. 5.8.5)

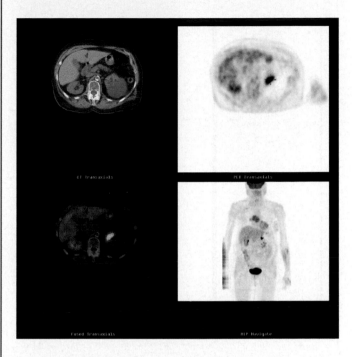

Brief History
A 79-year-old patient with a history of breast cancer was referred for initial staging of a second primary non–small cell lung cancer in the right lower lobe.

Findings
PET/CT images show a focus of increased FDG uptake in the left upper abdominal region localized to a left renal pelvis displaced by a large renal cyst, consistent with physiologic tracer uptake in an anatomic distorted kidney.

Note on MIP: A new second primary tumor in the paramediastinal superior aspect of the lower lobe of the right lung is evident.

Main Teaching Points and Summary
1. PET/CT can precisely localize increased FDG uptake to the renal pelvis, even in displaced kidneys.
2. In this patient, a suspected adrenal metastasis by assessment of PET alone was excluded by PET/CT.

Case 5.8.6 TUMOR–SINGLE RENAL METASTASIS (FIG. 5.8.6)

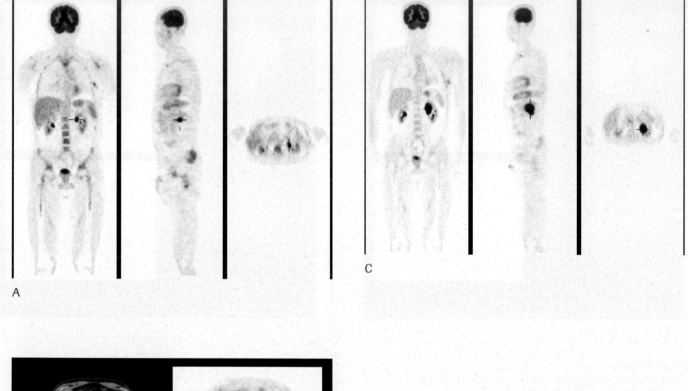

A

C

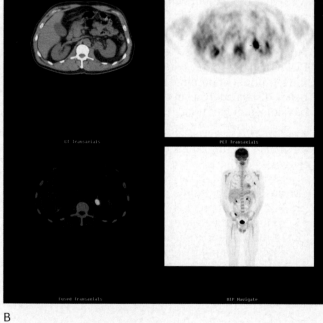

B

Brief History

A 47-year-old patient with malignant melanoma metastatic to a left axillary lymph node was assessed in search of the primary tumor.

Findings

A. PET images show a focus of increased FDG uptake at the medial aspect of the left kidney.
B. PET/CT images localize this hypermetabolic focus to a space-occupying lesion, 28 mm in diameter, in the left renal parenchyma, consistent with an additional site of metastatic melanoma.

Note on MIP: There is abnormal FDG uptake in the left axilla representing the known metastatic lymphadenopathy.

C. PET images of a study performed 4 months later for monitoring response to chemotherapy show tumor progression. The lesion in the left kidney has increased in size and intensity of uptake. There are also new sites of metastatic involvement in left supraclavicular and retroperitoneal lymph nodes (not shown).

Main Teaching Points and Summary

1. FDG activity in kidneys may be due to physiologic renal tracer excretion. Differential diagnosis with a malignant lesion is difficult using only PET.
2. A repeat delayed PET acquisition or administration of diuretics can help to evaluate lesions near or in the renal cortex.
3. PET/CT can precisely localize renal uptake of FDG to sites of normal or abnormal anatomy detected by CT.
4. It is not unusual that the primary melanoma is not localized, as in this case, although the entire torso and arms were included in the study.

Case 5.8.7 TUMOR—MULTIPLE RENAL LESIONS, LYMPHOMA (FIG. 5.8.7)

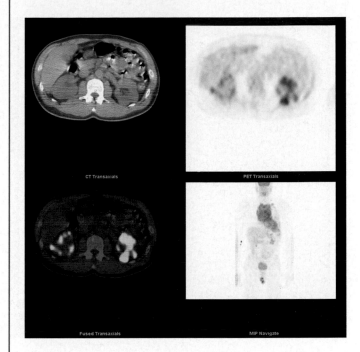

Brief History

A 32-year-old patient with newly diagnosed aggressive non-Hodgkin's lymphoma was referred for initial staging before treatment.

Findings

PET/CT images show multiple foci of abnormally increased FDG uptake localized to exophytic hyper- and isodense lesions in the cortex of both kidneys, more prominent on the left, consistent with the presence of extranodal renal lymphoma.

Note on MIP: A bulky mediastinal lesion and left cervical and supraclavicular nodal sites of disease involvement are seen.

Repeat PET/CT performed after two cycles of chemotherapy was normal, with disappearance of all nodal and renal lymphoma lesions on both the PET and CT component of the study.

Main Teaching Points and Summary

1. The differential diagnosis between malignant or physiologic FDG uptake in the renal cortex is difficult on PET alone.
2. The presence of corresponding anatomic lesions showing a mass effect or changes in tissue attenuation should lead to the correct diagnosis.

Case 5.8.8 TUMOR–SINGLE ADRENAL METASTASIS (FIG. 5.8.8)

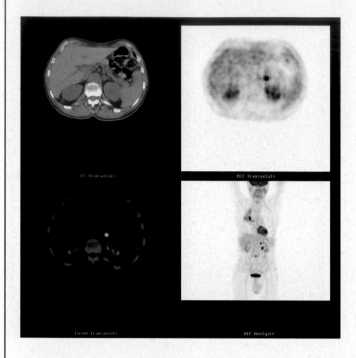

Case 5.8.9 TUMOR–BILATERAL ADRENAL INVOLVEMENT, LYMPHOMA (FIG. 5.8.9)

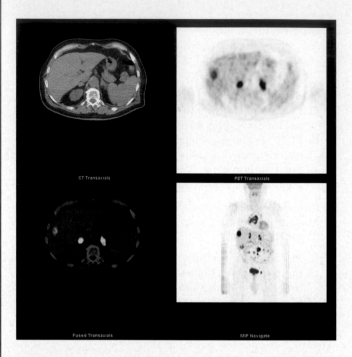

Brief History

A 71-year-old patient with locally advanced non–small cell lung cancer was referred to monitor response to neoadjuvant chemotherapy.

Findings

PET/CT images show a focus of abnormally increased FDG uptake in the left posterior abdomen, anteromedial to the upper pole of the left kidney, localized to a slightly enlarged left adrenal gland, consistent with an adrenal metastasis.

Note on MIP: Residual viable lung cancer in the right upper lobe and metastatic mediastinal lymphadenopathy are seen.

Main Teaching Points and Summary

1. Most adrenal masses seen on CT in patients with lung cancer are benign adenomas.
2. Intense FDG uptake in an adrenal mass is, however, typically diagnostic of adrenal metastasis.

Brief History

A 75-year-old patient with recurrent diffuse large cell non-Hodgkin's lymphoma was referred for restaging before second-line chemotherapy.

Findings

PET/CT images show two foci of abnormally increased FDG uptake in the left and right proximal paravertebral regions, consistent with lymphoma involving enlarged adrenal glands, bilaterally. An hepatic lymphoma lesion is also visualized in the lateral aspect of the right lobe.

Note on MIP: Additional foci of recurrent lymphoma in the mediastinum, liver, and para-aortic lymph nodes are seen.

Main Teaching Point and Summary

1. Adrenals are an uncommon site of lymphoma. When present, additional extranodal lesions are also often seen.

5.9 LYMPH NODES

Case 5.9.1 GASTROHEPATIC LIGAMENT LYMPH NODES (FIG. 5.9.1)

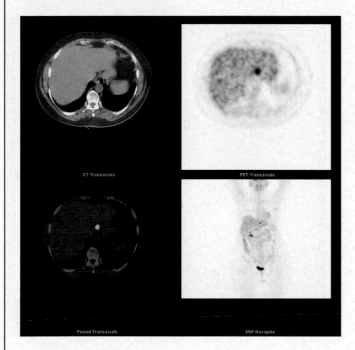

Case 5.9.2 HEPATIC HILUM LYMPH NODES AND LIVER METASTASES (FIG. 5.9.2)

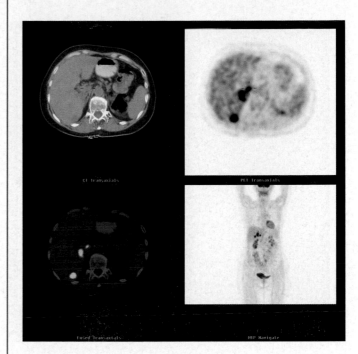

Brief History

A 65-year-old patient with history of sigmoid cancer, status postsigmoidectomy 16 months pre-PET/CT, was assessed because of rising serum tumor markers in the presence of a CT reported as negative for a clinically suspected recurrence.

Findings

PET/CT images show a focal area of abnormally increased FDG uptake in a normal sized lymph node, 9 mm in diameter, in the upper midabdomen at the level of the gastrohepatic ligament, consistent with a single nodal metastasis.

Main Teaching Points and Summary

1. FDG-PET detects hypermetabolic lesions in normal sized lymph nodes, which are often reported as normal on CT alone.
2. PET/CT provides the precise localization of hyper-metabolic lesions—in the present case in the upper midabdomen, a complex area because of the proximity of the liver to regional lymph nodes.

Brief History

A 73-year-old patient with colon cancer metastatic to the liver was referred to assess response to neoadjuvant chemotherapy prior to planning of potential surgery.

Findings

PET/CT images show multiple foci of abnormally increased FDG uptake in the right lobe of the liver. Two of these foci correspond to liver metastases in segment 7, and an additional focus is fused to a normal size, 10 mm in diameter, lymph node in the hepatic hilum, consistent with a nodal metastasis.

Main Teaching Point and Summary

1. The demonstration of extrahepatic tumor generally precludes partial hepatectomy.

Case 5.9.3 SPLENIC HILUM LYMPH NODES (FIG. 5.9.3)

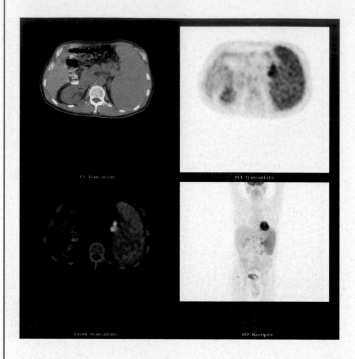

Case 5.9.4 MESENTERIC AND RETROPERITONEAL LYMPH NODES (FIG. 5.9.4)

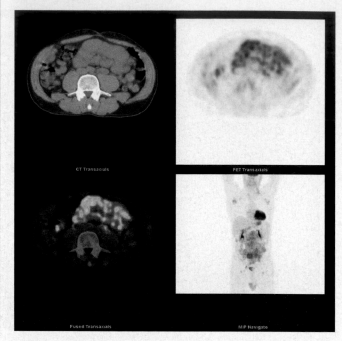

Brief History

A 71-year-old patient was referred for initial staging of follicular low-grade non-Hodgkin's lymphoma diagnosed from bone marrow biopsy.

Findings

PET/CT images show two focal areas of abnormally increased FDG activity in the left midabdomen, adjacent to the spleen. These foci correspond to enlarged lymph nodes in the splenic hilum, 15 and 18 mm in diameter, consistent with lymphomatous nodal involvement. There is also intense FDG uptake in an enlarged spleen.

Main Teaching Points and Summary

1. Nodal tumor foci near the splenic hilum can be confused with focal splenic uptake of FDG on PET alone but can be resolved on PET/CT.
2. Intense FDG uptake in an enlarged spleen in a patient with non-Hodgkin's lymphoma who is not treated with colony stimulating factor is typical of tumor involvement.

Brief History

A 46-year-old patient was assessed for initial staging of small lymphocytic low-grade non-Hodgkin's lymphoma.

Findings

PET/CT images show multiple areas of intense, inhomogeneous abdominal FDG uptake in massive mesenteric and retroperitoneal lymphadenopathy.

Note on MIP: Additional sites of lymphoma in left cervical and bilateral axillary lymph nodes are seen.

Main Teaching Points and Summary

1. Diffuse increased FDG uptake in the abdomen may be related to physiologic tracer excretion in the gastrointestinal tract, malignant lymphadenopathy, or peritoneal involvement.
2. PET/CT facilitates the differential diagnosis and defines the clinical significance of this pattern based on the presence or absence of corresponding structural lesions.
3. Small lymphocytic lymphoma may show less intense FDG uptake compared with other forms of non-Hodgkin's lymphoma.

Case 5.9.5 MESENTERIC LYMPH NODES IN REGION OF ROOT OF MESENTERY (FIG. 5.9.5)

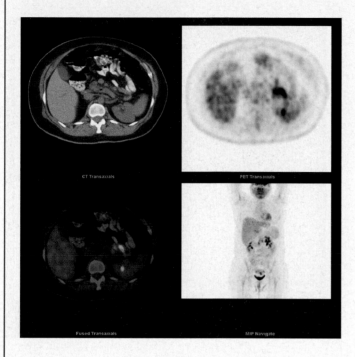

Case 5.9.6 PARA-AORTIC LYMPH NODES (FIG. 5.9.6)

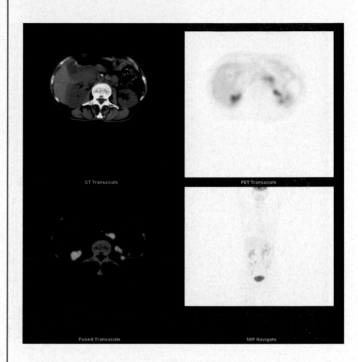

Brief History
A 45-year-old patient with a history of breast cancer was assessed following rising serum tumor markers for a clinically suspected recurrence.

Findings
PET/CT images show sites of abnormally increased FDG uptake located in enlarged inferior mesenteric lymph nodes in the region of the root of the mesentery in the left midabdomen, which is consistent with malignant lymphadenopathy.

Note on MIP: Foci of abnormally increased FDG uptake in metastatic para-aortic lymph nodes and a lesion in the midpelvis, localized by PET/CT (not shown) to an ovarian mass were seen and subsequently proved by biopsy to represent a second primary tumor.

Main Teaching Points and Summary
1. Foci of increased FDG uptake, apparently in the posterior abdomen on PET alone, can be defined as adenopathy in the root of the mesentery by PET/CT.
2. Atypical spread of nodal metastases, such as abdominal sites in this patient with known breast cancer, should raise the suspicion of a new primary malignant tumor.

Brief History
A 62-year-old patient with history of colon carcinoma, status post–low anterior resection, chemotherapy, and radiotherapy 2 years before the current study, was referred for further assessment of a presacral mass and slightly enlarged retroperitoneal lymph nodes, 15 mm in diameter, reported on a previous CT.

Findings
PET/CT images show a midabdominal focus of abnormally increased FDG uptake in an enlarged left para-aortic lymph node, 15 mm in diameter, at the level of the kidneys, consistent with metastatic involvement.

Note on MIP: Additional foci of abnormal FDG uptake in lymph nodes of the iliac chain are seen on both sides.

The presacral mass was FDG negative, thus excluding the presence of active malignancy in this location.

Main Teaching Points and Summary
1. Hypermetabolic foci representing metastatic disease may occur in borderline-sized lymph nodes.
2. PET/CT provides the matching assessment between hypermetabolic or FDG-negative findings on PET and equivocal morphologic lesions on CT.

Case 5.9.7 AORTOCAVAL LYMPH NODES (FIG. 5.9.7)

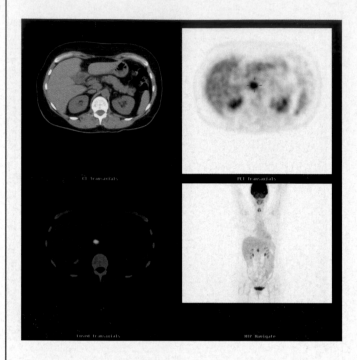

Brief History
A 55-year-old patient with history of carcinoma of the ovary, status postsurgery and postchemotherapy 4 years before the present examination, was referred for further assessment of enlarged retroperitoneal lymph nodes visualized on repeat CT examinations for a period of 8 months.

Findings
PET/CT images show a focal area of abnormally increased FDG uptake in an enlarged aorto-caval lymph node at the level of the pancreatic body, 15 mm in diameter.

The diagnosis of a single lymph node metastasis was confirmed at surgery.

Main Teaching Points and Summary
1. PET/CT may provide the matching assessment between suspicious metabolic and structural findings on PET and CT.
2. Retroperitoneal lymph node metastases are relatively common in ovarian cancer.

Case 5.9.8 ILIAC LYMPH NODES (FIG. 5.9.8)

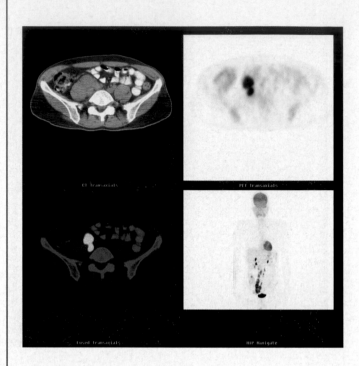

Brief History
A 41-year-old patient was referred for initial staging of Hodgkin's lymphoma.

Findings
PET/CT images show foci of abnormally increased FDG uptake in the right lower abdomen, in enlarged lymph nodes of the right iliac chain, consistent with malignant involvement.

Note on MIP: Additional sites of disease in para-aortic and both iliac chain lymph nodes, more prominent on the right.

Main Teaching Point and Summary
1. Contiguous spread of tumor is typical of Hodgkin's lymphoma.

5.10 VASCULAR

Case 5.10.1 PITFALL—AORTIC WALL CALCIFICATIONS (FIG. 5.10.1)

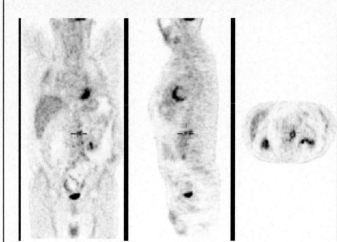

A

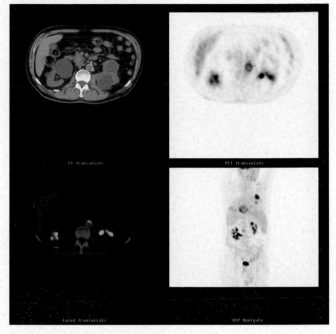

B

Brief History

A 67-year-old patient with non–small cell cancer of the right lung was referred for staging before surgery.

Findings

A. PET images show a focal area of FDG uptake in the midposterior abdomen, suspicious for left para-aortic lymph node metastasis.

B. PET/CT images localize this suspicious focus to calcifications and presumed inflammation in the wall of the abdominal aorta, unrelated to malignancy.

Note on PET and CT: Multiple FDG-negative renal cysts, increased FDG activity in a distorted renal collecting system, and increased FDG uptake in the primary right lung tumor are seen, including on the posterior MIP image in B.

On follow-up, the patient had no further evidence for abdominal metastases.

Main Teaching Point and Summary

1. Focal increased FDG uptake in the vascular wall has been reported to represent dynamic inflammatory atherosclerotic changes, associated at times, as in present case, with congruent and more commonly incongruent calcifications on CT.

Case 5.10.2 PITFALL—AORTIC ANEURYSM (FIG. 5.10.2)

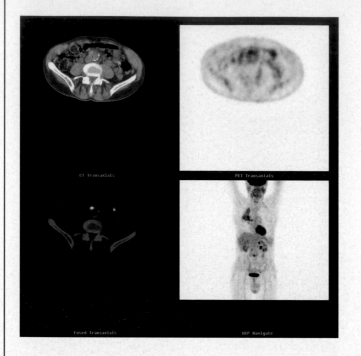

Brief History
A 71-year-old patient with locally advanced non–small cell lung cancer, was assessed for response to neoadjuvant chemotherapy.

Findings
PET/CT images show a focal area of increased FDG uptake in the midabdomen, localized to the lower part of an abdominal aortic aneurysm. A second FDG-avid focus in the left abdomen is related to physiologic tracer excretion in the small bowel.

Note on MIP: Abnormal uptake in the right lung tumor is seen.

There was no further evidence of distant metastases.

Main Teaching Point and Summary
1. Focal increased FDG uptake in aortic aneurysms has been reported and explained by an inflammatory reaction in the vascular wall. However, the precise clinical significance of this finding is not yet fully clarified.

Case 5.10.3 BENIGN AORTIC GRAFT INFECTION AND PSOAS MUSCLE ABSCESS (FIG. 5.10.3)

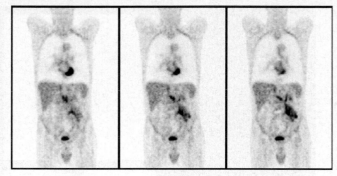

A

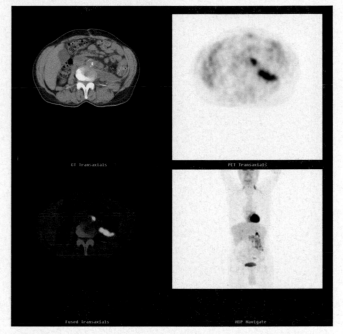

B

Brief History

A 65-year-old patient was referred for initial staging of a small lymphocytic low-grade non-Hodgkin's lymphoma. Diagnosis had been made from biopsy of retroperitoneal lymphadenopathy detected incidentally during surgery performed for resection of an aortic pseudo-aneurysm.

Findings

A. Selected coronal PET images show an inhomogeneous area of intense FDG uptake in the left paravertebral region and left lower abdomen.

B. PET/CT images localize these lesions to a thickened aortic wall and to a hypodense mass in, and anterior to the left psoas muscle. The suspicion of an infectious process related to recent surgery was raised.

Repeat surgery confirmed the diagnosis of psoas abscess and infected aortic graft.

Note on MIP image: There is increased uptake in the lower cervical region, bilateral, consistent with physiologic uptake in tense muscles. No abnormal FDG uptake was detected in the para-aortic and retroperitoneal lymphadenopathy, probably representing a non–FDG-avid lymphoma.

Main Teaching Points and Summary

1. Highly intense, inhomogeneous FDG uptake in sites of previous surgery should raise the suspicion of infection.
2. PET/CT precisely localizes the hypermetabolic lesion to the infectious process and determines its whole extent.
3. PET/CT indicates that there is no FDG uptake in the enlarged abdominal lymph nodes histologically proven for lymphomatous involvement, a more common finding in the small lymphocytic non-Hodgkin's lymphoma subtype.

5.11 BONE—LUMBAR SPINE

Case 5.11.1 BENIGN—DEGENERATIVE CHANGES IN VERTEBRAL BODY (FIG. 5.11.1)

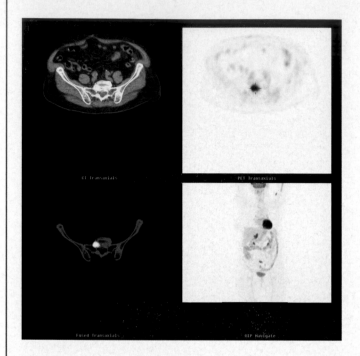

Brief History
A 73-year-old patient with low-grade non-Hodgkin's lymphoma, was assessed for suspected recurrence after a new lesion was seen on CT in the region of the upper pole of the right kidney.

Findings
PET/CT images demonstrate a focus of increased FDG uptake in degenerative changes seen on CT as a sclerotic lesion in the right anterior aspect of the S-1 vertebral body.

Note on MIP: Abnormal FDG uptake in the right upper abdomen, consistent with involvement of enlarged para-aortic lymph nodes at the upper pole of the right kidney, is seen.

There was no evidence of active lymphoma in the S-1 vertebra on clinical follow-up.

Main Teaching Points and Summary
1. PET/CT can precisely localize foci of increased FDG uptake to bony structures.
2. Structural skeletal abnormalities on the CT component of PET/CT can help define the clinical significance of foci of increased FDG uptake.
3. A small percentage of degenerative changes or other benign skeletal lesions may take up FDG.

Case 5.11.2 BENIGN—DEGENERATIVE CHANGES IN ARTICULAR FACETS (FIG. 5.11.2)

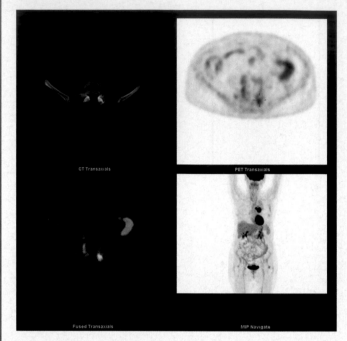

Brief History
A 73-year-old patient was referred for staging of a newly diagnosed non–small cell lung cancer. The patient also complained of back pain.

Findings
PET/CT images demonstrate a focus of moderately increased FDG uptake in degenerative changes in the left articular facet of the L-5 vertebra.

Note on MIP: Abnormally increased FDG uptake in the known primary lung tumor is seen. Low-intensity focal activity at the level of the greater trochanter, bilateral, is consistent with trochanteric bursitis.

Main Teaching Points and Summary
1. PET/CT can precisely localize foci of increased FDG uptake to bony structures.
2. In the presence of structural skeletal abnormalities on the CT component, PET/CT allows for the differential diagnosis between bone metastases and degenerative changes in the lumbar spine.
3. A positive correlation between the severity of the degenerative disease and the intensity of FDG uptake has been described.

Case 5.11.3 BENIGN—DEGENERATIVE CHANGES OF INTERVERTEBRAL DISC (FIG. 5.11.3)

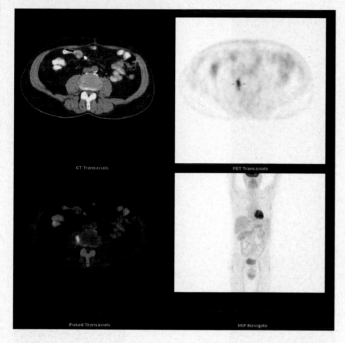

Brief History
A 66-year-old patient with colon cancer, metastatic to the liver, was referred to assess response to chemotherapy.

Findings
PET/CT images show a focus of increased FDG uptake in the right paravertebral area at the interface of L-3 and L-4 vertebrae, with corresponding calcification of the intervertebral disk seen on CT, consistent with degenerative changes.

Main Teaching Points and Summary
1. PET/CT can localize the hypermetabolic lesion to soft tissues and thus exclude involvement of the skeleton.
2. Both degenerative disk and spine disease can demonstrate increased FDG uptake, usually of low intensity, probably due to active inflammatory processes.

Case 5.11.4 TUMOR—LYTIC FDG-AVID METASTASIS (FIG. 5.11.4)

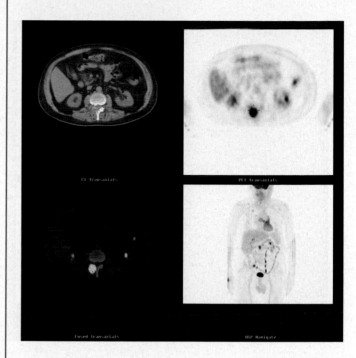

Brief History
A 77-year-old patient with non–small cell lung cancer, status post–left lower lobectomy, was referred to assess the extent of disease before radiotherapy planning.

Findings
PET/CT images show a focus of abnormal FDG uptake in the right paramedian lumbar region, localized to a lytic lesion in the right posterior arch of the L-3 vertebra, consistent with a bone metastasis.

Note on MIP: Additional abnormally increased tracer uptake is seen in residual active tumor in the mediastinum and in a lytic rib metastasis.

Main Teaching Point and Summary
1. Untreated lytic bone metastases have been reported to show a higher FDG avidity as compared with blastic lesions.

Case 5.11.5 TUMOR–SCLEROTIC FDG-NEGATIVE METASTASES (FIG. 5.11.5)

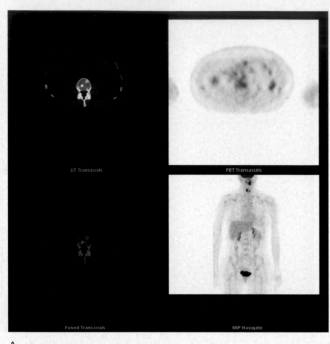

A

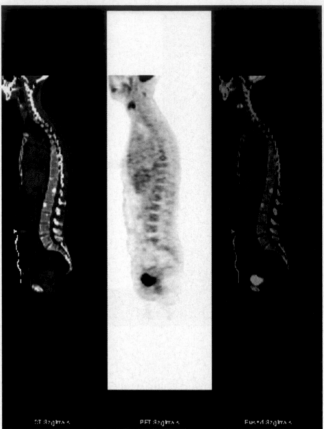

B

Brief History

A 45-year-old patient with breast cancer metastatic to bone was referred to assess response to chemotherapy.

Findings

A. Transaxial slice PET/CT images show FDG-negative osteoblastic lesions in the body of L-2 vertebra.
B. Midsagittal PET/CT images confirm the absence of FDG uptake in multiple osteoblastic lesions in the body of T-11, T-12, L-2 and L-3 vertebrae.

The findings were considered to represent previously treated and inactive vertebral metastases.

Main Teaching Points and Summary

1. Sclerotic skeletal metastases have been reported to show lower FDG avidity, both pretreatment and most notably so after treatment.
2. This may be partly related to response to chemotherapy and the lack of viable tumor.

Case 5.11.6 TUMOR—BONE AND SOFT TISSUE METASTASIS (FIG. 5.11.6)

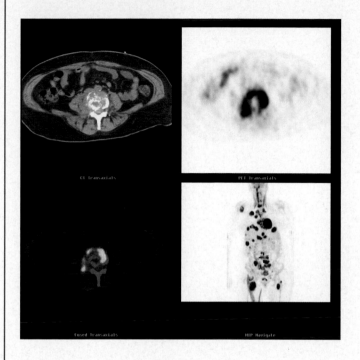

Brief History
A 45-year-old patient with advanced right upper lobe non–small cell lung cancer was referred for whole body staging before further treatment planning.

Findings
PET/CT images show abnormal FDG uptake in a lytic lesion in the body of the L-5 vertebra with extension to a right paravertebral soft tissue mass.

Note on MIP: There are multiple foci of abnormal FDG uptake throughout the body consistent with widespread metastatic disease involving lymph nodes, lungs, liver, skeleton, and soft tissues.

Main Teaching Point and Summary
1. If isolated to the vertebral body or disk space, infection would be considered, but in this patient, given the disseminated pattern, this is a typical metastatic pattern.

PET/CT of the Pelvis

Rachel Bar-Shalom

6.1 NORMAL PATTERN

Case 6.1.1 MALE PELVIS (FIG. 6.1.1)

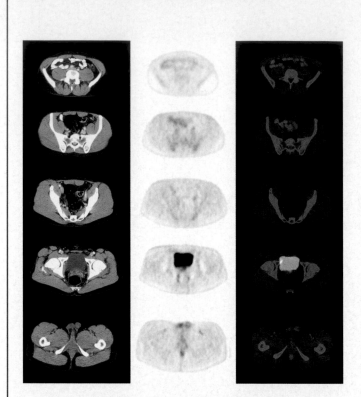

This is an example of a normal PET/CT study of the male pelvis. The use of oral contrast facilitates the ability to define and locate bowel loops and separate them from nodal or peritoneal structures. Similarly, i.v. contrast aids in separation of normal blood vessels from lymph nodes.

Physiologic regional FDG uptake in the pelvis includes tracer excretion with visualization of the bowel and urinary bladder. Normal FDG activity in the bowel can be of variable intensity and show either focal or linear patterns. Minimal to moderate FDG uptake is also seen in bone marrow and the testes.

Misinterpretation of PET/CT studies in this region can result from differences in the filling status and content of the urinary bladder between CT and PET acquisition.

Case 6.1.2 FEMALE PELVIS (FIG. 6.1.2)

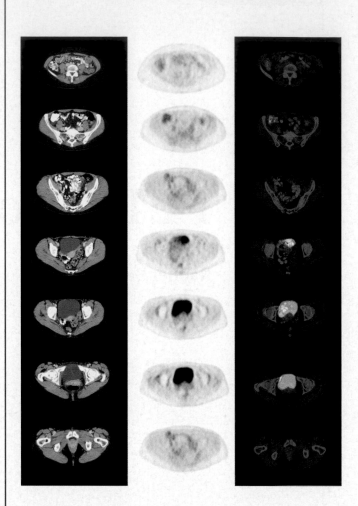

This is an example of a normal PET/CT study of the female pelvis. As in the male, the use of oral contrast facilitates the ability to define and locate bowel loops and separate them from nodal or peritoneal structures. Physiologic FDG uptake includes tracer excretion with visualization of bowel and the urinary bladder. Minimal FDG activity is seen in bone marrow.

In premenopausal women, special attention should be given to the phase of the menstrual cycle at the time of performing the PET/CT study. Increased physiologic tracer activity can normally be seen in one or both ovaries during the ovulatory and menstrual phases. This is not the case in postmenopausal women, in whom focal tracer uptake in the ovaries is concerning for malignancy.

Misinterpretation of PET/CT findings in the pelvis may result from differences in the filling status and content of the urinary bladder related to the sequential (not simultaneous) acquisition of the PET and CT components of the hybrid imaging study, as well as to bowel motion. Intravenous contrast administration can sometimes be useful.

6.2 PELVIC WALL, SOFT TISSUES, AND PERITONEUM

Case 6.2.1 PITFALL—FOCAL UPTAKE, COLOSTOMY (FIG. 6.2.1)

Case 6.2.2 PITFALL—FOCAL UPTAKE, INGUINAL HERNIA (FIG. 6.2.2)

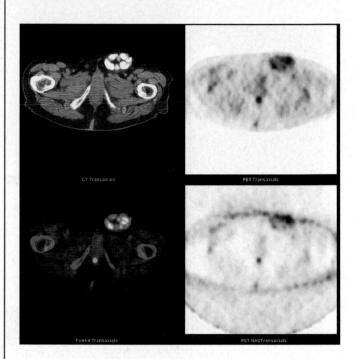

Brief History

A 58-year-old patient with rectal carcinoma, status post-radiotherapy and surgery, was referred for assessment of a presacral mass seen on CT.

Findings

PET/CT images show an area of increased FDG uptake in the anterior aspect of the left pelvic wall located at his colostomy.

No abnormal presacral FDG uptake was detected, and no evidence of disease was seen on further follow-up.

Main Teaching Points and Summary
1. Benign FDG uptake at the site of a colostomy, of mild to moderate intensity, is due to inflammatory tissue or physiologic activity in bowel loops.
2. Focally intense uptake at the site of a colostomy raises the possibility of a local tumor recurrence, but the specificity of such a finding is lowered by the substantial but variable normal tracer uptake levels.

Brief History

A 76-year-old patient with newly diagnosed lung cancer was referred for systemic staging.

Findings

PET/CT images show an area of increased FDG uptake in the left inguinal region localized to physiologic tracer activity in contrast-enhanced bowel loops within an inguinal hernia. This focal uptake is seen on both the attenuation corrected and the corresponding uncorrected slices (right bottom), excluding the possibility of a CT-based attenuation correction artifact in a region of hyperdense contrast enhancement.

Main Teaching Points and Summary
1. Physiologic FDG uptake in the gastrointestinal tract may be atypically located. This can be precisely characterized by PET/CT.
2. In this case, with PET alone, the erroneous possibility of inguinal nodal metastases would need to have been considered in the differential diagnosis.

Case 6.2.3 PITFALL—FOCAL UPTAKE, URINARY CATHETER (FIG. 6.2.3)

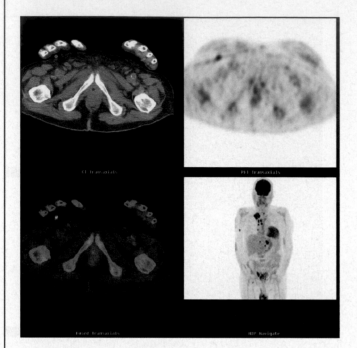

Case 6.2.4 BENIGN—SKIN GRANULOMA (FIG. 6.2.4)

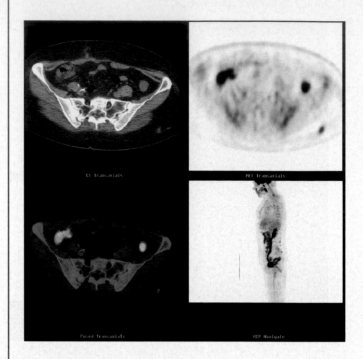

Brief History

A 72-year-old patient was referred for staging of a right upper lobe lung cancer, incidentally diagnosed during preoperative assessment for benign prostatic hypertrophy.

Findings

PET/CT images show a small focus of increased FDG uptake in the right inguinal region, localized to a urinary catheter outside the body.

Note on MIP: Multiple malignant FDG-avid foci in the primary tumor in the right lung, and mediastinal and left adrenal metastases.

Main Teaching Points and Summary

1. PET/CT prevents misinterpretations of foci of increased FDG uptake in sites of physiologic tracer activity, increasing the specificity of the study.
2. Urinary catheters should be placed between the patient's legs with the bag out of the field of view to minimize potential confusion with FDG-avid tumor.

Brief History

A 50-year-old patient with a history of cervical carcinoma was referred for assessment of disease activity and extent before vaginal reconstruction surgery.

Findings

PET/CT images show a small nodule with ill-defined borders in the subcutaneous fat of the left buttock with mildly increased FDG uptake, consistent with an inflammatory granuloma.

Note on lateral MIP: Intense physiologic FDG uptake in the bowel, linear in nature, is seen.

Main Teaching Points and Summary

1. Increased FDG uptake in granulomas has been described, especially after intramuscular injections, probably due to the presence of an inflammatory reaction.
2. In patients with known or suspected malignant skin lesions, such as melanoma or cutaneous lymphoma, the morphologic features on the CT component of PET/CT may indicate the need for biopsy.

Case 6.2.5 BENIGN—INFECTION, PILONIDAL SINUS (FIG. 6.2.5)

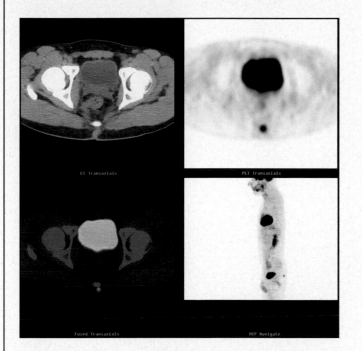

Brief History
A 21-year-old patient with cutaneous lymphoma was referred for routine follow-up during clinical remission.

Findings
PET/CT images show increased FDG uptake in a focal soft tissue density with ill-defined borders, located in the midpelvis, just posterior to, but not involving the coccyx.

The patient reported coccygeal pains of recent onset, and pilonidal sinus infection was diagnosed on physical examination.

There is no evidence for active lymphoma. The patient remained in complete remission with repeat negative FDG PET/CT studies.

Main Teaching Points and Summary
1. FDG is not a specific tracer for cancer. Acute infection and active inflammation may present intense tracer uptake that may mimic malignancy.
2. Clinical correlation is key in such cases.

Case 6.2.6 BENIGN—INFECTION, PELVIC ABSCESS (FIG. 6.2.6)

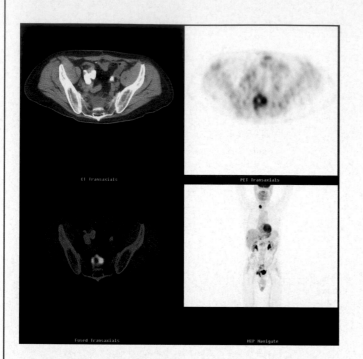

Brief History

A 64-year-old patient with rectal cancer metastatic to the liver, status post–low anterior resection 2 months before PET/CT, was referred for restaging before beginning systemic treatment.

Findings

PET/CT images show an area of intense, ringlike increased FDG uptake within a large presacral soft tissue mass with blurring of surrounding fat, seen on CT in the posterior aspect of the pelvis.

The presacral lesion was suspicious for recurrence, although an inflammatory reaction after recent surgery could not be excluded. Biopsy was negative for malignancy. Surgical resection with histopathologic examination demonstrated the presence of a pelvic abscess, with areas of chronic and acute inflammation, fibrosis, and no evidence of malignancy.

Note on MIP: A focus of increased uptake in the right neck, further diagnosed as thyroid carcinoma and multiple foci consistent with liver metastases, are seen.

Main Teaching Points and Summary

1. Intense FDG uptake may be seen in sites of infection or inflammation due to increased glucose utilization by activated macrophages and granulation tissue formation.
2. The differential diagnosis between a pelvic abscess and recurrent or metastatic disease may be impossible even on fused data sets because of similar imaging patterns.
3. PET/CT may, however, guide biopsy, which is at times the only means to provide definitive diagnosis.
4. A thyroid incidentaloma detected on FDG-PET/CT must be further evaluated because it may represent a second primary tumor, a metastasis or a benign lesion.

Case 6.2.7 TUMOR–PRESACRAL RECURRENCE, RECTAL CANCER (FIG. 6.2.7)

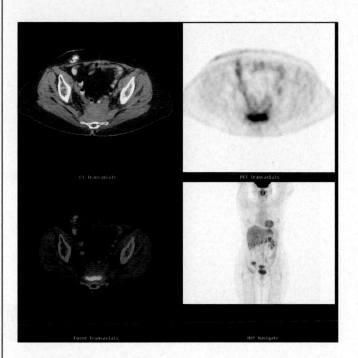

Brief History
A 69-year-old patient with rectal cancer, status post–surgery, chemotherapy, and radiation treatment to the pelvis, was referred for assessment of a new presacral soft tissue mass detected on CT.

Findings
PET/CT images show a focus of intense FDG uptake in the posterior aspect of the pelvis, localized to the posterior part of a large presacral soft tissue mass seen on CT, consistent with recurrent malignancy.

Note on MIP: Mildly increased FDG uptake in the right anterior pelvic wall, in the region of the colostomy, and multiple foci consistent with liver metastases are evident.

Main Teaching Points and Summary
1. PET/CT can provide the spatial localization of viable malignancy within larger areas related to post-therapeutic morphologic changes.
2. PET/CT can pinpoint areas of viable cancer within large fibrotic masses, guiding further invasive diagnostic procedures or radiation treatment planning.

Case 6.2.8 TUMOR–METASTASIS IN PSOAS MUSCLE (FIG. 6.2.8)

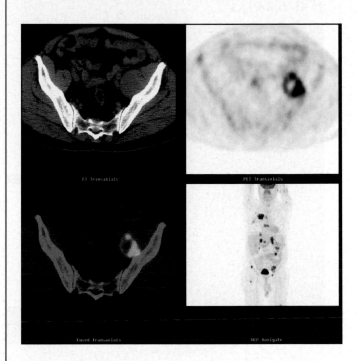

Brief History
A 66-year-old patient was referred for staging of newly diagnosed right upper lobe lung cancer.

Findings
PET/CT shows an area of inhomogeneous increased FDG uptake in a large hypodense mass involving the left iliopsoas muscle, consistent with a metastatic lesion.

Note on MIP: The primary right lung tumor and disseminated metastatic disease in the mediastinum, adrenals, upper abdomen, and skeleton are seen.

Main Teaching Points and Summary
1. Muscle metastases are not uncommon in lung cancer.
2. Heterogeneous FDG uptake in malignant lesions, in particular with a peripheral rim of increased uptake and a central area of decreased or absent activity, indicates the presence of necrosis.
3. An abscess could have a similar PET appearance. However, this patient did not have clinical symptoms of infection.

Case 6.2.9 TUMOR–METASTASIS, CUL-DE-SAC PERITONEAL NODULE (FIG. 6.2.9)

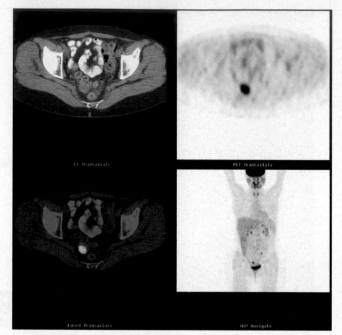

Brief History
A 54-year-old patient with ovarian cancer, 4 years after total abdominal hysterectomy and bilateral oophorectomy and chemotherapy, was referred for suspected recurrence in the presence of elevated tumor markers and a right pelvic mass on CT.

Findings
PET/CT images show abnormally increased FDG uptake within a pelvic mass located in the cul-de-sac in the right posterior pelvis, consistent with local recurrence.

Note on MIP: An additional small peritoneal metastasis in the left upper pelvis is visible.

Main Teaching Points and Summary
1. FDG-PET has been reported to have sensitivity and specificity of approximately 80% for the detection of macroscopic recurrent ovarian cancer, usually superior to that of CT.
2. FDG-PET is of value for diagnosis of distant metastases and local recurrence in the presence of equivocal or negative conventional imaging or rising serum markers.

Case 6.2.10 TUMOR–METASTASES, FOCAL PERITONEAL NODULES (FIG. 6.2.10)

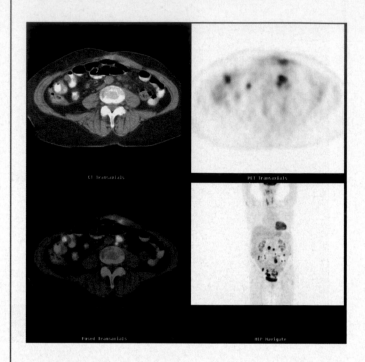

Brief History
A 67-year-old patient with a history of colon cancer, status post–surgery and chemotherapy, was assessed for suspected recurrence because of elevated serum tumor markers and retroperitoneal lymphadenopathy on CT.

Findings
PET/CT images show sites of abnormally increased FDG uptake in the pelvis, corresponding to peritoneal nodules, some adjacent to bowel loops, and a retroperitoneal lymph node, consistent with multiple metastases.

Note on MIP: Additional abdominal metastases involving para-aortic lymph nodes and peritoneal nodules are seen.

Main Teaching Points and Summary
1. PET/CT is an excellent modality for diagnosis of malignant peritoneal spread, which may appear as small implants or nodules, but may fail to detect micrometastases.
2. Peritoneal metastases may be localized in close vicinity to normal organs and may therefore not be always readily detected on CT.
3. Oral contrast is particularly useful in this case to differentiate bowel activity from FDG-avid peritoneal metastases.
4. Precise PET/CT assessment of the extent of disease in patients with recurrent colon cancer has an impact on the further therapeutic approach, preventing futile surgery in patients with advanced metastatic disease.

Case 6.2.11 TUMOR—DIFFUSE PERITONEAL INVOLVEMENT (FIG. 6.2.11)

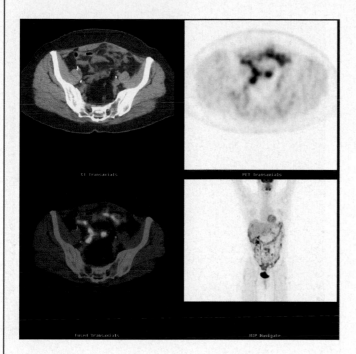

Case 6.3.1 PITFALL—PHYSIOLOGIC, FOCAL UPTAKE IN BOWEL (FIG. 6.3.1)

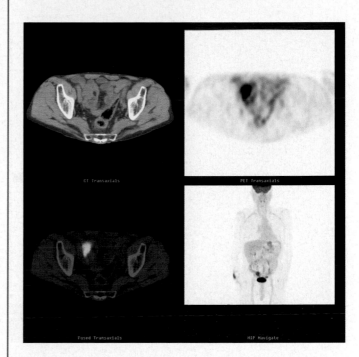

Brief History

A 48-year-old patient, 4 years after total abdominal hysterectomy and bilateral oophorectomy for ovarian cancer, was referred for suspected recurrence because of elevated serum tumor markers and equivocal CT demonstrating soft tissue strands in the peritoneum.

Findings

PET/CT images show irregular linear uptake throughout the pelvis, localized to soft tissue strands with blurring of peritoneal pelvic fat, consistent with peritoneal carcinomatosis.

Note on MIP: Heterogeneous increased FDG uptake around the periphery of the liver and in the abdomen is seen, consistent with diffuse metastatic peritoneal spread.

Main Teaching Points and Summary

1. Peritoneal carcinomatosis is a typical pattern for spread of metastatic ovarian cancer.
2. Diagnosis of peritoneal carcinomatosis by conventional imaging modalities is difficult.
3. FDG-PET pattern of intraperitoneal spread can be diffuse or focal.
4. PET/CT is useful for characterizing unclear structural findings, but both PET and PET/CT are of limited sensitivity in low-volume disease.

Brief History

A 75-year-old patient was referred 6 years after left upper lobectomy for lung cancer to assess for suspected recurrence in the presence of elevated serum carcinoembryonic antigen levels with negative CT.

Findings

PET/CT images show a focus of increased uptake in the right pelvis, localized to bowel loops, with no overt structural pathology.

The patient had a negative colonoscopy and remained without evidence of disease during a follow-up of 16 months.

Main Teaching Points and Summary

1. PET/CT facilitates the precise localization of focal pelvic uptake to the gastrointestinal tract, and within that to a particular segment, thus directing further diagnostic investigation.
2. Physiologic bowel uptake of FDG is most probably related to muscular activity and tracer accumulation in intestinal bacteria and leukocytes.
3. Physiologic FDG activity in the bowel is usually of mild intensity and has a linear pattern.

Case 6.3.2 BENIGN—RECTAL POLYP (FIG. 6.3.2)

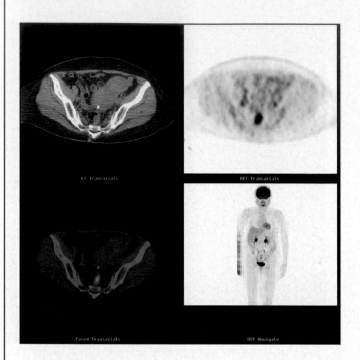

Case 6.3.3 BENIGN—INFLAMMATORY BOWEL DISEASE (FIG. 6.3.3)

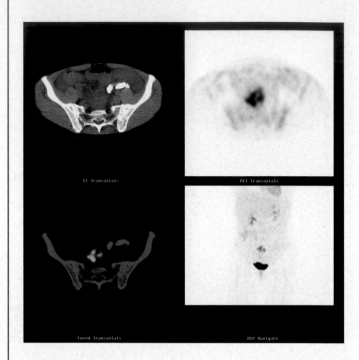

Brief History

A 49-year-old patient recently treated for recurrent non-Hodgkin's lymphoma was referred to assess response to salvage therapy.

Findings

PET/CT images show a focus of increased uptake in the posterior midpelvis, localized to a thickened rectal wall bulging intraluminally on CT.

This single lesion was new and had not been apparent on the previous PET/CT study performed before initiating treatment. A sessile rectal polyp was resected during colonoscopy, and histopathologic examination diagnosed a villous adenoma. The patient showed no evidence of active lymphoma on clinical follow-up.

Main Teaching Points and Summary
1. Focal FDG uptake located by PET/CT to the gastro-intestinal tract (GIT) was of clinical significance in present case.
2. Although it may represent physiologic tracer activity, focal FDG uptake to the GIT should be further investigated because cancer, premalignant or benign lesions may be found in up to 70% of patients.

Brief History

A 40-year-old patient with known Crohn's disease and clinically suspected partial bowel obstruction was referred to assess for the presence of active disease.

Findings

PET/CT images show an area of abnormally increased FDG uptake in the midpelvis, localized to the distal small bowel, consistent with the presence of active inflammatory bowel disease.

Main Teaching Points and Summary
1. FDG can accumulate in active infections and inflammatory processes including active inflammatory bowel disease, such as Crohn's.
2. PET/CT is not yet used as a routine test in this clinical setting, and its diagnostic accuracy is therefore not yet fully established.

(Case courtesy of Dr. P. Ginsburg and H. Jacene, Johns Hopkins Hospital, Baltimore, Maryland.)

Case 6.3.4 TUMOR–PRIMARY RECTAL CANCER (FIG. 6.3.4)

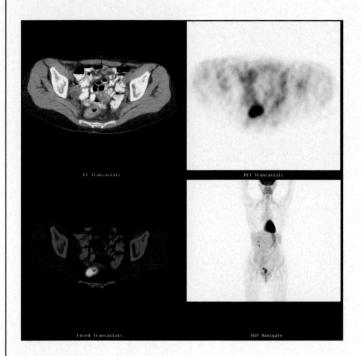

Brief History
A 53-year-old patient was referred for systemic staging of a recently diagnosed rectal cancer.

Findings
PET/CT images show a focus of abnormally increased FDG uptake in the posterior lower pelvis, localized to an area of circular thickening of the rectal wall with associated luminal narrowing on CT, consistent with the known primary tumor.

Main Teaching Points and Summary
1. FDG-PET can demonstrate uptake in primary colorectal tumors.
2. Although FDG-PET does not currently represent the modality of choice for initial screening or diagnosis of colorectal cancer, focal PET-positive findings in the colon must be considered as highly concerning for cancer and warrant further investigation or close clinical monitoring.

Case 6.3.5 TUMOR–PRIMARY RECTOSIGMOID CANCER AND PARARECTAL NODES (FIG. 6.3.5)

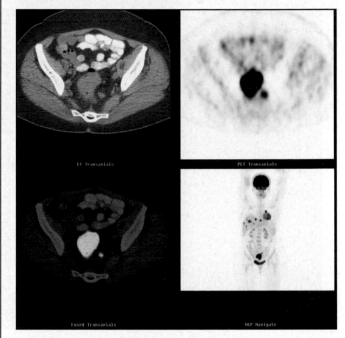

Brief History
A 48-year-old patient with recently diagnosed rectosigmoid carcinoma was referred to assess potential resectability status following equivocal hepatic lesions on CT.

Findings
PET/CT images show a large area of intense abnormal uptake in the posterior right mid-lower pelvis, localized to a rectosigmoid mass, consistent with the known primary tumor. An additional small focus of abnormally increased FDG uptake is located in an enlarged pararectal lymph node, consistent with a locoregional lymph node metastasis.

Note on MIP: Advanced metastatic disease involving the liver and left lung is evident.

Main Teaching Points and Summary
1. Intense FDG uptake has been described in primary colorectal cancer.
2. In the preoperative assessment of patients with colon cancer, FDG-PET plays a growing role in the diagnosis of distant metastases.
3. Intense tracer uptake at the site of the primary tumor has been suggested as a possible explanation for the reported low sensitivity of stand-alone FDG PET for diagnosis of local nodal staging in patients with colorectal cancer. However, very small nodal metastases would be expected to be undetectable even if background activities are low.
4. PET/CT may improve the detectability rate of small metastatic lesions in the vicinity of the primary tumor by precise localization and characterization of adjacent foci.

Case 6.3.6 TUMOR–RESPONSE TO TREATMENT, METASTATIC RECTAL CANCER (FIG. 6.3.6)

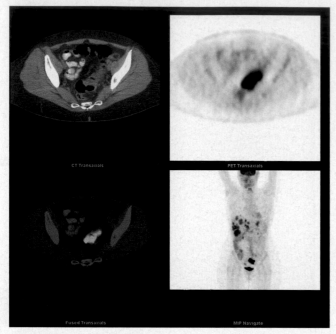

A

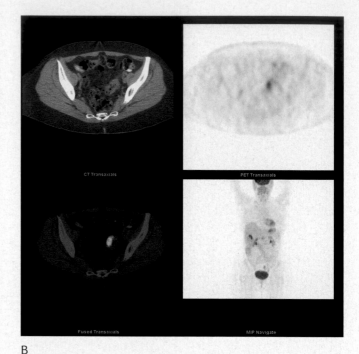

B

Brief History

A 49-year-old patient with newly diagnosed cancer of the rectosigmoid colon, metastatic to the liver, was referred for baseline assessment before chemotherapy.

Findings

A. PET/CT images at diagnosis show a large space-occupying lesion in the rectosigmoid colon with intense FDG uptake.

Note on MIP: Multiple foci of increased FDG uptake in liver and nodal metastases at the level of the hepatic hilum are seen.

Chemotherapy was started, and PET/CT was repeated after 3 months to assess response to treatment.

B. PET/CT images after treatment show significant shrinkage in the diameter of the tumor mass on CT and a substantial decrease in the intensity of FDG uptake in the primary tumor, demonstrating that the patient had achieved a partial response but still had residual viable cancer.

Note on MIP: Significant improvement in the extent of the metastatic spread, with disappearance of most hepatic and nodal tumor foci, is seen.

Main Teaching Points and Summary

1. A residual mass after treatment does not necessarily represent residual active cancer.
2. PET/CT can effectively assess response to chemotherapy by monitoring changes in both tumor volume and metabolic activity.

Case 6.3.7 TUMOR–RECURRENCE, RECTAL CANCER (FIG. 6.3.7)

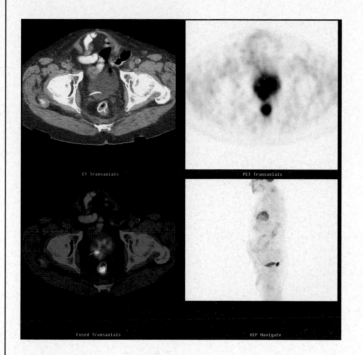

Brief History
An 89-year-old patient with rectal cancer, status post–anterior resection, was referred for restaging in the presence of local recurrence diagnosed on colonoscopy.

Findings
PET/CT images show a focus of intense uptake in the lower pelvis located in a soft tissue mass at the site of anastomosis, consistent with the known recurrence.

Main Teaching Points and Summary
1. FDG PET/CT is an accurate diagnostic modality for recurrence in regions of structural abnormalities related to previous surgery and radiotherapy.
2. Occasionally suture materials can result in an intense inflammatory reaction, and this possibility has to be included in the differential diagnosis in patients with uncertain findings.

Case 6.3.8 TUMOR–RECURRENCE, RECTAL CANCER AND ILIAC NODES (FIG. 6.3.8)

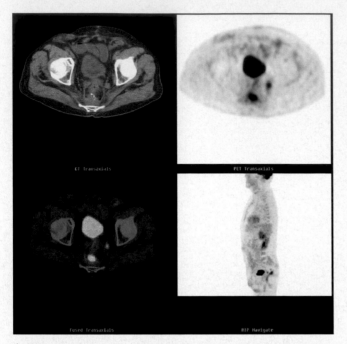

A

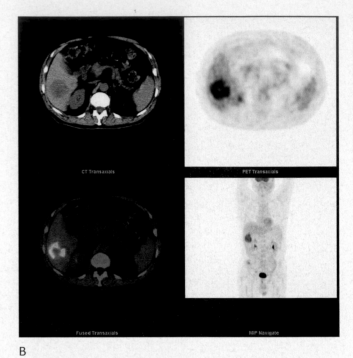

B

Brief History
A 59-year-old patient with a history of rectal carcinoma, status post–abdominoperineal resection, chemotherapy, and radiotherapy, presented with a new liver metastasis and was referred to assess the extent of disease before planned resection of the hepatic tumor. CT of the pelvis performed 30 days before PET/CT reported post-therapy soft tissue changes in the presacral region.

Findings
A. PET/CT images of the pelvis show an intense focus of abnormal FDG uptake in the posterior midpelvis in the region of the surgical anastomosis, consistent with local recurrence. There is an additional small focus of abnormal FDG uptake in the left posterior pelvis, corresponding to an 18-mm left internal iliac lymph node, not appreciated on the initial review of CT.
B. PET/CT images of the upper abdomen show a focus of intense abnormal FDG uptake in the known liver metastasis.

Based on the PET/CT diagnosis of local recurrence with nodal metastases, hepatic surgery was cancelled, and the patient was referred to chemotherapy.

Main Teaching Points and Summary
1. CT cannot differentiate post-therapy fibrosis from active disease and may fail to detect mild pelvic lymphadenopathy.
2. FDG-PET is very sensitive for the detection of local recurrence of colorectal cancer at the site of the surgical anastomosis, as well as for diagnosis of metastatic lymphadenopathy.
3. PET/CT can provide an anatomic template for separation of locoregional nodal metastases from an adjacent primary or recurrent tumor.

6.4 URINARY TRACT

Case 6.4.1 PITFALL—ECTOPIC PELVIC KIDNEY (FIG. 6.4.1)

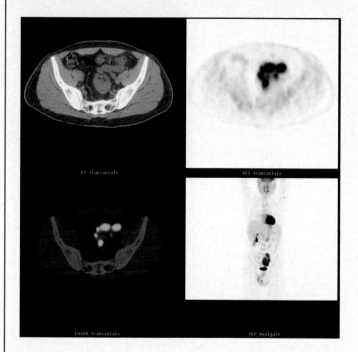

Case 6.4.2 PITFALL—RENAL TRANSPLANT (FIG. 6.4.2)

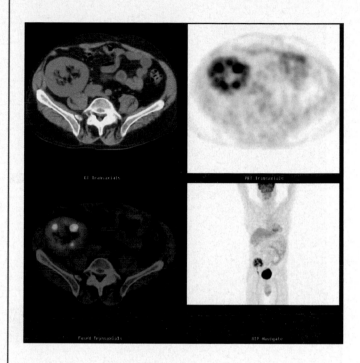

Brief History

A 48-year-old patient was referred for further assessment of a suspicious lesion in the head of the pancreas seen on CT, with an inconclusive biopsy.

Findings

PET/CT images show an area of highly intense FDG uptake in the left anterior pelvis, representing a dilated collecting system and ureter of an ectopic left pelvic kidney.

Note on MIP: No left kidney is seen in the expected anatomic location.

PET/CT was negative in the pancreas, as were endoscopic ultrasound with biopsy. The patient remained with no evidence of pancreatic malignancy for a follow-up of 8 months.

Main Teaching Points and Summary

1. Physiologic FDG uptake in normal anatomic variants must not be confused with sites of tumor.
2. PET/CT can define the nature of benign or physiologic FDG uptake within structures representing anatomic variants, such as ectopic kidneys.

Brief History

A 56-year-old patient with Hodgkin's lymphoma was referred to assess response to chemotherapy. The patient had a history of renal transplant.

Findings

PET/CT images show an area of increased FDG uptake in the right pelvis, localized to the renal transplant. No FDG uptake is seen in either native kidney because of impaired function.

PET was negative for active disease, and the patient remained in continuous clinical remission for a follow-up of 31 months.

Main Teaching Points and Summary

1. PET/CT can accurately define normal anatomic variants, such as the pelvic location of a transplanted kidney.
2. Precise anatomic localization of increased tracer activity can facilitate accurate characterization and exclude the suspicion of malignancy in these sites.

Case 6.4.3 PITFALL—FOCAL UPTAKE IN URETER (FIG. 6.4.3)

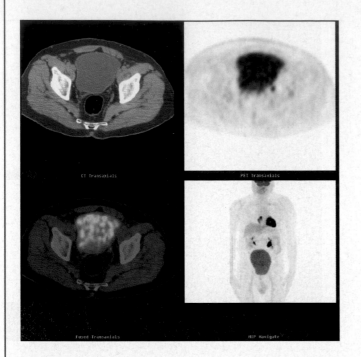

Brief History
A 72-year-old patient was referred for the assessment of a solitary pulmonary nodule in the left upper lobe. The patient had known benign prostatic hypertrophy and reported difficulty emptying his bladder before scanning.

Findings
PET/CT images show a small focus of increased FDG uptake localized in the distal left ureter adjacent to the left aspect of a full urinary bladder.

Note on MIP: Mildly increased FDG uptake in the left upper lobe lung lesion, subsequently diagnosed as non–small cell lung cancer and incidental normal visualization of the right atrium are seen.

Main Teaching Points and Summary
1. FDG activity in the ureter, a normal variant, may appear as discrete focal uptake.
2. PET/CT can usually differentiate between the physiologic nature of this suspicious site and abnormal uptake in adjacent metastatic lymph nodes or soft tissue lesions.
3. PET/CT is of particular value for imaging patients with voiding difficulties without the need for bladder catheterization.

Case 6.4.4 PITFALL–FOCAL UPTAKE IN OBSTRUCTED URETER (FIG. 6.4.4)

Brief History
A 68-year-old patient with non-Hodgkin's lymphoma was referred for routine follow-up.

Findings
A. PET/CT images shows increased FDG uptake in the right pelvis localized to a dilated ureter.

Note on MIP: There is linear uptake along the entire right ureter and in the proximal left ureter.

B and C. Selected PET/CT and CT images demonstrate a 6-mm calculus at the distal end of the right ureter, partly obstructing urine flow and FDG excretion.

Main Teaching Points and Summary
1. Intense FDG activity along the whole ureter suggests the presence of a benign or malignant process interfering with urine excretion and must not be confused with active tumor.
2. PET/CT may precisely identify the etiology of the obstruction—in this case, the calculus in the distal right ureter—which may be also an incidental finding, unrelated to the primary malignancy.

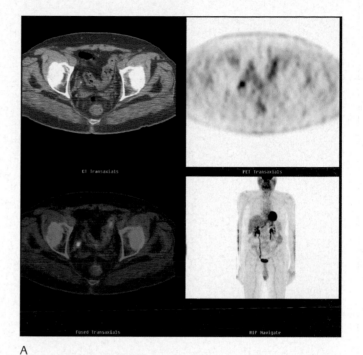

A

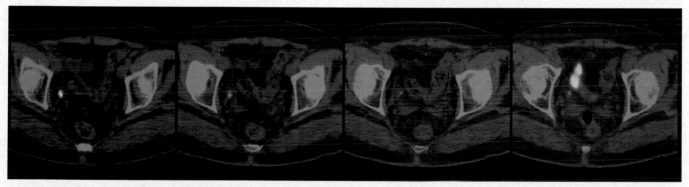

B

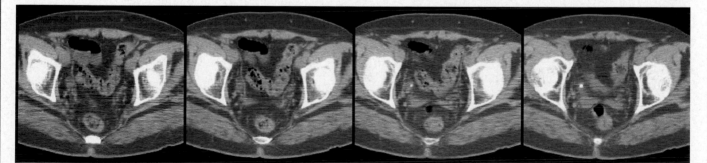

C

Case 6.4.5 PITFALL—DILATED PROSTATIC URETHRA (FIG. 6.4.5)

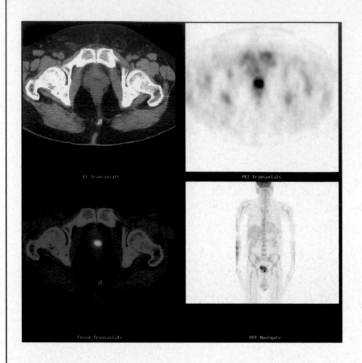

Brief History

A 71-year-old patient with aggressive non-Hodgkin's lymphoma was referred for monitoring response to therapy. The patient underwent transurethral resection of the prostate (TURP) for benign prostatic hypertrophy 4 months before the PET/CT study.

Findings

PET/CT images show a focus of increased FDG uptake below the urinary bladder, localized to the proximal part of the prostatic urethra, as is typical in patients after TURP.

No other foci of abnormal uptake are seen, indicating a good response of the lymphoma to therapy.

Main Teaching Points and Summary
1. Physiologic urinary FDG activity may appear in various pelvic locations, mimicking a malignant focus in structures such as the prostate or rectum.
2. The high intensity of FDG uptake is not typical of primary prostate cancer.
3. Knowledge of the clinical history combined with PET/CT data helps in the exclusion of disease.

Case 6.4.6 PITFALL—BLADDER DIVERTICULUM (FIG. 6.4.6)

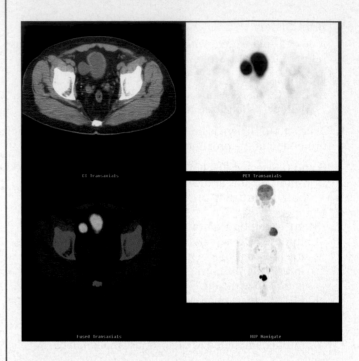

Brief History

A 67-year-old patient with Burkitt's lymphoma in complete clinical remission was referred for routine follow-up.

Findings

PET/CT images show a large area of intense FDG uptake in the right pelvis, adjacent to, but separate from, the urinary bladder, localized to a right-sided bladder diverticulum connected with a thin neck to the bladder.

Main Teaching Points and Summary
1. Physiologic urine FDG uptake in a bladder diverticulum is typically a small but highly intense focus that may show residual radioactive urine even after voiding or catheterization. The content of the bladder and the diverticulum have typically identical standardized uptake value levels.
2. PET/CT can help to avoid false-positive interpretations.

Case 6.4.7 PITFALL—BLADDER HERNIATION (FIG. 6.4.7)

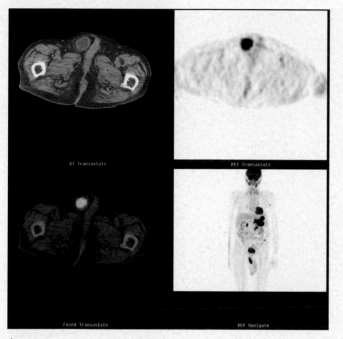

A

Brief History

A 75-year-old patient with non-Hodgkin's lymphoma was assessed for clinically suspected recurrence.

Findings

A. PET/CT images show a focus of intense FDG uptake in the urinary bladder herniated into the right inguinal canal.

B and C. Serial transaxial PET/CT (B) and CT (C) images demonstrate the full extent of the bladder herniation into the right inguinal canal.

Note on MIP: Recurrent lymphoma in multiple additional sites in the abdomen and left axilla is seen.

Main Teaching Points and Summary

1. Some sites of FDG uptake in unusual pelvic locations can be accurately defined by PET/CT as unrelated to cancer, thus avoiding erroneous or equivocal interpretations.
2. Urinary bladder herniation is relatively uncommon. This pattern could have been misread as a nodal metastasis on PET alone.

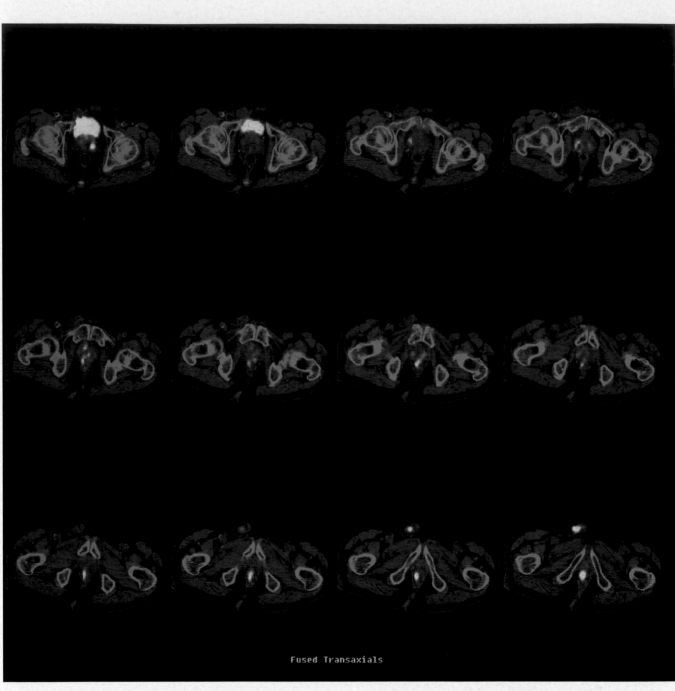

Fused Transaxials

B

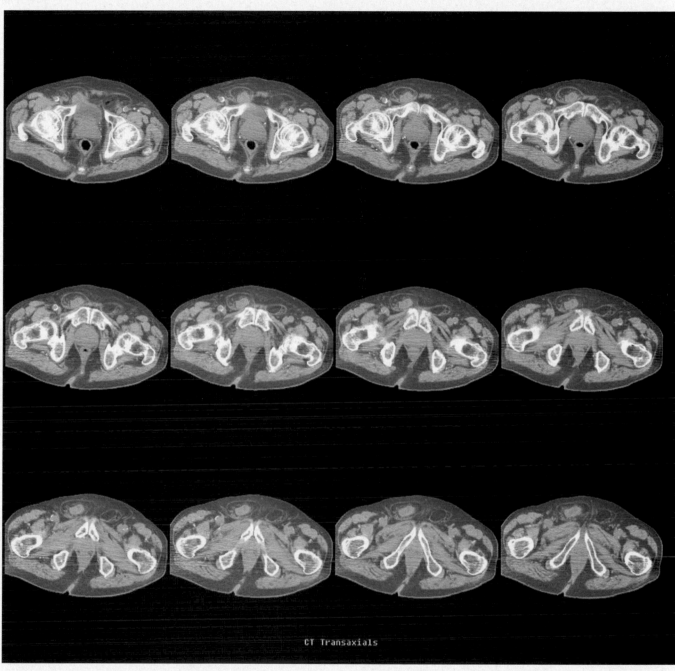

CT Transaxials

C

Case 6.4.8 TUMOR–CARCINOMA OF URETER (FIG. 6.4.8)

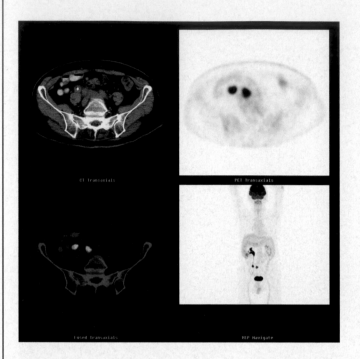

Brief History
A 77-year-old patient was referred for staging of a transitional cell carcinoma (TCC) involving the right ureter.

Findings
PET/CT images show two foci of intense abnormal uptake in the right and midpelvis, localized to the known right ureteral mass and an adjacent right lower para-aortic lymph node below the aortic bifurcation, consistent with the known primary ureteral tumor and a nodal metastasis. A stent within the obstructed ureter is seen on the CT image.

Note on MIP: There is increased tracer activity in a right hydronephrotic renal pelvis and along the course of the obstructed right proximal ureter.

Main Teaching Points and Summary
1. FDG PET diagnosis of cancer involving the urinary tract is hampered by physiologic urinary excretion of the tracer.
2. PET/CT can be used to correlate FDG biodistribution with morphologic abnormalities. Nevertheless, accurate identification of urinary tract malignancy may be impossible on PET/CT without the use of invasive procedures such as catheterization and irrigation.
3. FDG PET may be used for assessment of nodal or distant metastases of TCC.

Case 6.4.9 TUMOR—CARCINOMA OF URINARY BLADDER AND LYMPHOMA OF BONE (FIG. 6.4.9)

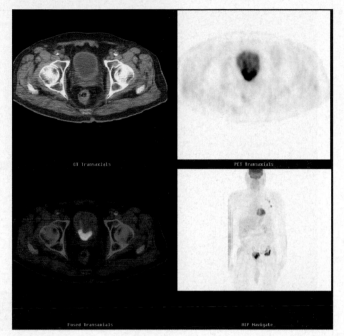

A

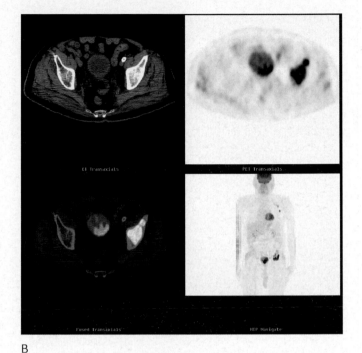

B

Brief History

An 83-year-old patient with recurrent non-Hodgkin's lymphoma and newly diagnosed bladder carcinoma was referred for assessment of the activity status of the lymphoma before receiving radiation treatment to the urinary bladder.

Findings

A. PET/CT images at the level of the mid-acetabulum show a focus of intense FDG uptake localized to a thickened posterior wall of the urinary bladder, corresponding to the site of the known primary tumor.

B. PET/CT images at a more cephalad level show intense heterogeneous FDG uptake in the left hip region, involving the left ilium and acetabulum, consistent with active lymphoma of the bone.

Note on MIP: Additional sites of active lymphoma with abnormally increased FDG uptake in the left axilla are seen.

Main Teaching Points and Summary

1. Cancer of the urinary bladder is difficult to detect on FDG-PET.
2. A focus of abnormal tracer uptake, higher in intensity than physiologic urinary FDG activity, localized by PET/CT to a structural lesion in the bladder, can improve the diagnostic accuracy of the study.

6.5 OVARY, CERVIX, AND UTERUS

Case 6.5.1 PITFALL—OVULATING OVARY (FIG. 6.5.1)

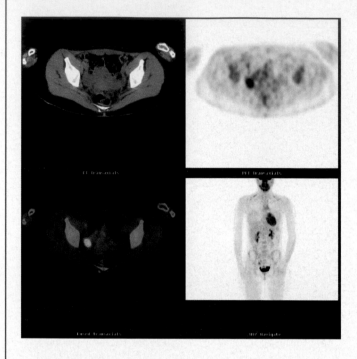

Case 6.5.2 PITFALL—MENSTRUATION (FIG. 6.5.2)

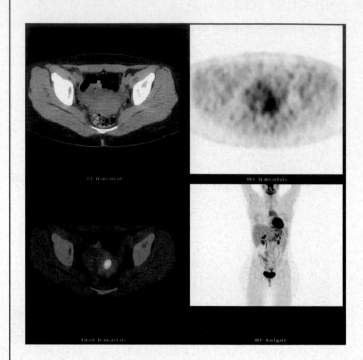

Brief History

A 19-year-old patient with Hodgkin's lymphoma was referred for routine follow-up after completion of treatment.

Findings

PET/CT images show increased FDG uptake in an enlarged hypodense right ovary.

The patient reported menstruation 2 weeks before the PET/CT study. The suspicious focus was therefore considered to represent physiologic FDG activity in an ovulating ovary.

The patient remained in continuous clinical remission.

Main Teaching Points and Summary
1. Increased FDG uptake in the ovaries during ovulation is common.
2. Increased pelvic FDG uptake in premenopausal women, localized by PET/CT to ovaries, is most commonly physiologic in etiology.
3. Intense FDG uptake post menopause is highly concerning for cancer and requires further workup.

Brief History

A 23-year-old patient with treated non-Hodgkin's lymphoma was referred for routine follow-up while in complete clinical response.

Findings

PET/CT images show an area of moderately increased FDG uptake in the left paramedian pelvis, cephalad to the urinary bladder, localized to the uterine body, with no apparent anatomic abnormality on CT.

Note on MIP: There is increased mediastinal tracer uptake representing benign thymic hyperplasia in this young patient after chemotherapy.

Clinical history revealed that the study was performed during menstruation.

The patient remained in complete remission for a follow-up of 17 months.

Main Teaching Points and Summary
1. PET/CT characterizes normal physiologic variants, such as endometrial FDG uptake during the menstrual cycle.
2. PET/CT findings need to be correlated with clinical data.

Case 6.5.3 BENIGN—MYOMA (FIG. 6.5.3)

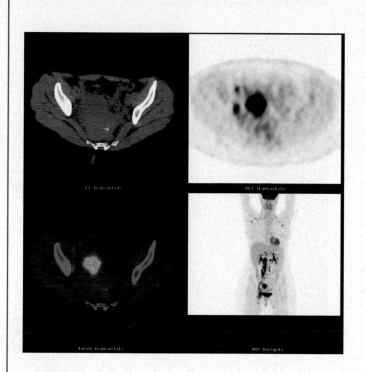

Brief History
A 41-year-old patient with non-Hodgkin's lymphoma was referred for initial staging before therapy.

Findings
PET/CT images demonstrate an intense focus of increased FDG uptake in the pelvis, located in a large hypodense exophytic mass in the right side of the uterus, consistent with a known large, probably necrotic, uterine myoma.

Note on MIP: Multiple sites of known nodal lymphoma above and below the diaphragm, with abnormal FDG uptake, are seen.

Repeat gynecologic examinations and ultrasound showed a stable large uterine myoma, FDG avid on PET/CT studies for a follow-up of 40 months.

After chemotherapy, the patient achieved complete remission with resolution with all abnormal sites of FDG uptake except for the pelvic hypermetabolic myoma.

Main Teaching Points and Summary
1. Mild to moderately increased FDG uptake has been reported in uterine leiomyoma.
2. In this case, PET/CT accurately localized the increased pelvic uptake and made the differential diagnosis between an FDG-avid myoma and malignant pelvic lymphadenopathy.
3. Despite the precise PET/CT localization of increased tracer activity to a benign lesion, the relatively high intensity of FDG uptake in this particular patient warranted the need for further evaluation to confirm the myomatous mass and exclude the presence of malignancy.

Case 6.5.4 TUMOR–LYMPHOMA IN OVARY (FIG. 6.5.4)

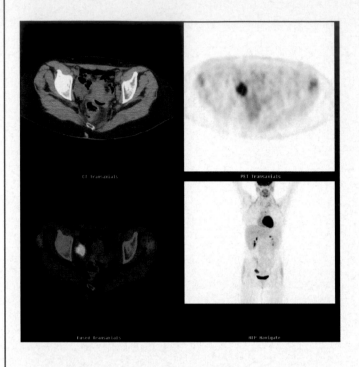

Brief History
A 22-year-old patient with high-grade non-Hodgkin's lymphoma was referred to assess response to treatment following completion of chemotherapy.

Findings
PET/CT images demonstrate increased FDG uptake in an enlarged hypodense ovary in the right pelvis. This focus had not been seen on the prior study performed at midtherapy. Of note: the patient had chemotherapy-induced amenorrhea.

Recurrent lymphoma in the right ovary was diagnosed on laparotomy.

Main Teaching Points and Summary
1. Although physiologic FDG uptake in the ovaries may be seen during ovulation, clinical patient data need to be considered for correct interpretation of PET/CT findings.
2. In this patient intense FDG uptake in the ovary and the clinical history of amenorrhea suggest the ovarian lesion to be of clinical significance.
3. Lymphoma may involve various extranodal sites including, albeit infrequently, the ovaries.

Case 6.5.5 TUMOR–PRIMARY OVARIAN CARCINOMA (FIG. 6.5.5)

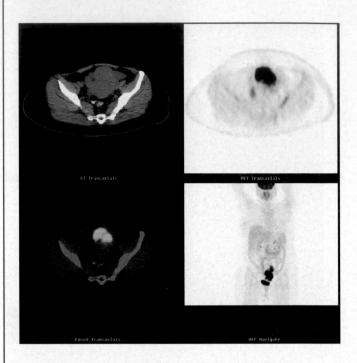

Brief History
A 47-year-old patient diagnosed with peritoneal carcinomatosis during surgery for an abdominal mass was referred after chemotherapy to assess resectability of a single left ovarian mass seen on CT.

Findings
PET/CT images show a large heterogeneous mass with abnormally increased FDG uptake within the left ovary. No additional foci of increased tracer uptake are seen elsewhere in the body.

A primary ovarian carcinoma in the large left ovarian mass was diagnosed during exploratory laparotomy, which was followed by total abdominal hysterectomy and bilateral oophorectomy for maximal volume reduction of the tumor mass.

Main Teaching Points and Summary
1. Accurate staging of ovarian carcinoma is important for appropriate selection of patients and planning of surgery.
2. FDG-PET has a better sensitivity and accuracy compared with conventional imaging modalities for staging of ovarian cancer.
3. However, exploratory surgery is the only adequate tool for initial staging of these patients because microscopic disease may be missed by all imaging modalities.

Case 6.5.6 TUMOR—OVARIAN CARCINOMA, RECURRENCE AT SITE OF SURGERY (FIG. 6.5.6)

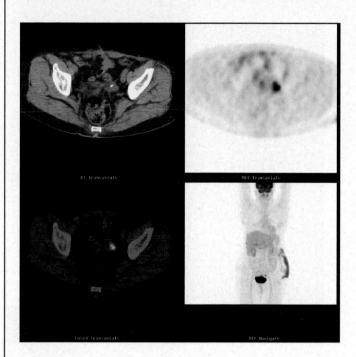

Brief History
A 66-year-old patient with a history of ovarian cancer, status post–surgery and chemotherapy, was referred for restaging of pelvic recurrence.

Findings
PET/CT images show focal FDG uptake in the left pelvis, superior to the urinary bladder, localized to a soft tissue mass in the region of the surgical clips seen on CT, consistent with recurrent disease.

Note on MIP: Tracer activity overlying the left lateral abdomen is seen, consistent with radioactive urine excreted into a nephrostomy bag.

Main Teaching Point and Summary
1. PET/CT differentiated the potential etiology of the suspicious pelvic site as being related to a malignant lesion rather that focal physiologic bowel activity.

Case 6.5.7 TUMOR—PRIMARY CERVICAL CANCER (FIG. 6.5.7)

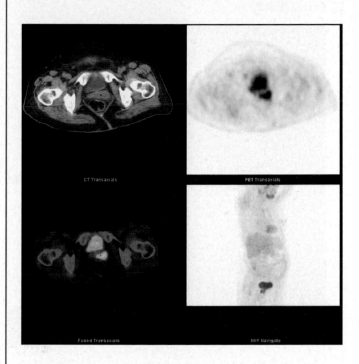

Brief History
A 74-year-old patient was referred for staging of a newly diagnosed squamous cell carcinoma of the uterine cervix.

Findings
PET/CT images show a focus of abnormally increased FDG uptake in the left lower pelvis, posterior to the urinary bladder, localized to a thickened uterine cervix, consistent with the primary tumor.

Main Teaching Points and Summary
1. PET/CT can help define the precise localization of the increased FDG uptake in the posterior pelvis.
2. PET/CT can separate physiologic tracer activity in organs such as the rectum and bladder from cervical cancer.

Case 6.5.8 TUMOR–PRIMARY CERVICAL CANCER, INHOMOGENEOUS UPTAKE (FIG. 6.5.8)

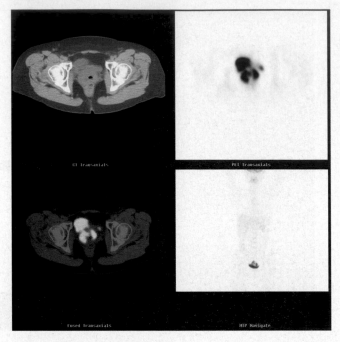

Brief History
A 59-year-old patient was referred for staging of a newly diagnosed carcinoma of the cervix.

Findings
PET/CT images show heterogeneous abnormal FDG uptake in the known, extensive tumor in the uterine cervix.

Main Teaching Points and Summary
1. FDG PET is highly sensitive for the detection of cervical cancer.
2. FDG PET is less accurate for the assessment of local tumor spread, such as involvement of the parametrium.

Case 6.5.9 TUMOR–PRIMARY CERVICAL CANCER AND ILIAC NODES (FIG. 6.5.9)

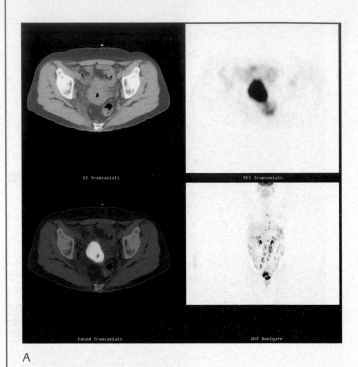

A

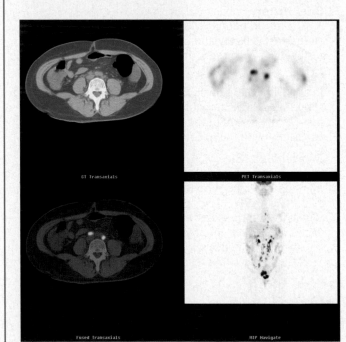

B

Case 6.5.10 TUMOR–RECURRENCE, CERVICAL CANCER (FIG. 6.5.10)

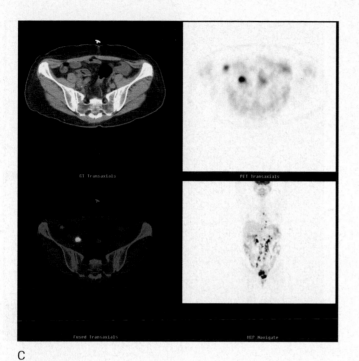

C

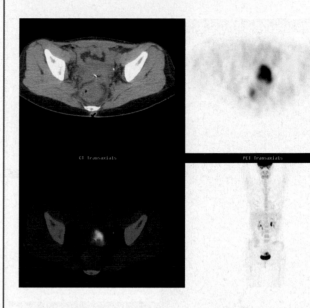

Brief History

A 45-year-old patient was referred for staging of a newly diagnosed cervical cancer in the presence of retroperitoneal lymphadenopathy on CT.

Findings

A. PET/CT images show intense FDG uptake in the primary cervical cancer in the lower pelvis.

B and C. PET/CT images at cephalad levels show multiple additional foci of abnormally increased FDG uptake in the pelvis, localized to various retroperitoneal nodal groups, including bilateral common iliac nodes (B) and external iliac nodes (C), more prominent on the right.

Note on MIP: Additional sites of mediastinal nodal metastases are seen.

Main Teaching Points and Summary

1. FDG PET is avidly taken up by primary cervical cancer, with a reported sensitivity of about 90%.
2. Cervical cancer metastasizes in a reasonably predictable pattern from pelvic to para-aortic nodes and also to other distant sites.
3. FDG PET/CT is an accurate modality for nodal staging by precise anatomic definition of involved stations in and outside the pelvis.

Brief History

A 36-year-old patient with a history of cancer of the uterine cervix, status post–surgery and radiotherapy, presented with a new pelvic mass detected on ultrasound. Biopsy performed before PET/CT showed only acute and chronic inflammation with granulation tissue related to prior surgery and radiation.

Findings

PET/CT images show heterogeneous FDG uptake in the midpelvis, localized to a soft tissue mass near surgical clips, consistent with recurrent disease at the vaginal stump.

Tumor recurrence was subsequently proved pathologically.

Main Teaching Points and Summary

1. Precise localization of suspicious findings by PET/CT can direct diagnostic biopsy to hypermetabolic foci because of precise CT coordinates.
2. This is of particular significance in the presence of fibrosis and anatomic distortion related to previous treatment, which can lead to false-negative biopsy results because of sampling errors.

6.6 PROSTATE AND TESTIS

Case 6.6.1 BENIGN—PROSTATIC HYPERTROPHY (FIG. 6.6.1)

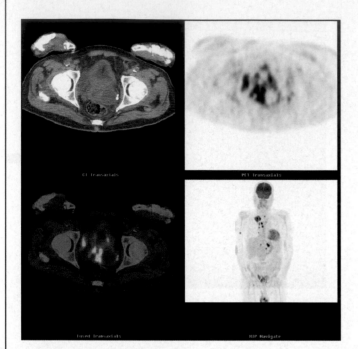

Case 6.6.2 BENIGN—INFECTION, ORCHIEPIDYDIMITIS (FIG. 6.6.2)

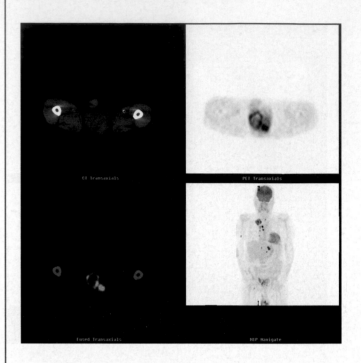

Brief History
A 63-year-old patient was referred for staging of a newly diagnosed lung cancer diagnosed incidentally during preoperative assessment for benign prostatic hypertrophy.

Findings
PET/CT images show an area of increased, heterogeneous FDG uptake in the lower midpelvis in an enlarged prostate, consistent with benign prostatic hypertrophy.

Note on MIP: Abnormal FDG uptake in the right lung cancer and in multiple metastases in the mediastinum, abdomen, and the right humerus are seen.

Main Teaching Points and Summary
1. PET/CT enables separation and localization of FDG uptake to specific anatomic structures, even when in close proximity, such as the prostate and urinary bladder.
2. The presence of increased FDG uptake in the prostate cannot be used to differentiate benign from malignant disease. Although benign prostatic hypertrophy and prostate cancer may both be FDG avid of variable intensity, prostate cancer is often not particularly FDG avid, especially in its earlier stages.

Brief History
A 63-year-old patient was referred for staging of lung cancer, diagnosed during preoperative assessment before prostatectomy.

Findings
PET/CT images show an area of increased heterogeneous uptake below the anatomic pelvis, localized to the periphery of the thickened capsule of an enlarged right testis and to the posterior aspect of the left testis.

Note on MIP: Abnormal FDG uptake in the right lung tumor and in multiple metastases in the mediastinum, abdomen, and right humerus are seen.

During hospitalization, the patient complained of pain and swelling of both testes. Ultrasound and clinical and laboratory tests diagnosed bilateral orchiepididymitis, more prominent on the right.

Main Teaching Points and Summary
1. Increased FDG uptake in infectious processes is a well-recognized cause of false-positive PET results in cancer patients.
2. Some testicular uptake is a normal variant, but the extent and distribution are very abnormal in this case.

Case 6.6.3 TUMOR—LYMPHOMA IN TESTIS (FIG. 6.6.3)

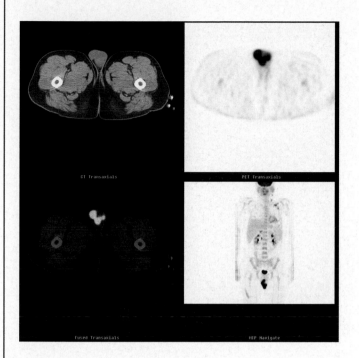

Brief History
A 37-year-old patient was referred for initial staging of Hodgkin's lymphoma, diagnosed by biopsy of a left axillary lymph node.

Findings
PET/CT images show several foci of intense inhomogeneous FDG uptake in enlarged testes in the midanterior aspect of the lower pelvis.

Note on MIP: Abnormal FDG uptake in known sites of lymphoma involving the left neck and axilla and the right upper abdomen is seen.

Ultrasound confirmed the presence of bilateral testicular enlargement compatible with lymphomatous infiltration. Symptoms disappeared with chemotherapy, and follow-up imaging studies were negative.

Main Teaching Points and Summary
1. The peripheral anterior midline location of the foci of increased FDG uptake may be misleading on PET alone, suggesting urinary contamination.
2. Precise PET/CT localization to specific lesions or to areas outside the body enables the distinction between malignant disease and artifactual, clinically nonsignificant findings.
3. Testicular FDG uptake can be moderate in normal patients, but the intense uptake in this case is most consistent with active tumor.

6.7 LYMPH NODES

Case 6.7.1 COMMON AND EXTERNAL ILIAC LYMPH NODES (FIG. 6.7.1)

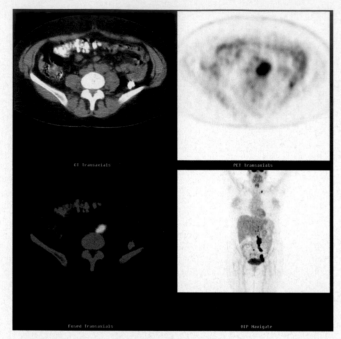

A

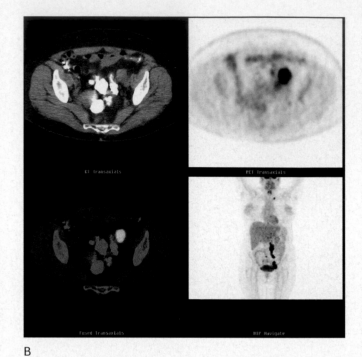

B

Brief History
A 53-year-old patient with newly diagnosed cervical cancer was referred for initial staging.

Findings
A and B. PET/CT images at the level of the upper (A) and mid (B) pelvis show multiple foci of abnormal FDG activity in the mid and left pelvis, located to enlarged lymph nodes of the common iliac (A) and left external iliac (B) chain, consistent with metastatic lymphadenopathy.

Note on MIP: Metastatic adenopathy in the left supraclavicular region is seen.

Main Teaching Points and Summary
1. PET/CT is useful for precise localization of pelvic foci to different nodal stations.
2. Following PET/CT, this patient will require systemic chemotherapy for disseminated disease. FDG PET has been found to be more accurate that CT in this setting.
3. Disease remote from the pelvis carries a poor prognosis.

Case 6.7.2 INTERNAL ILIAC LYMPH NODES (FIG. 6.7.2)

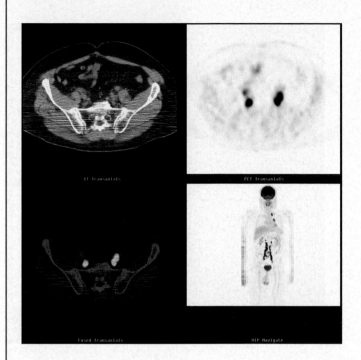

Brief History
A 59-year-old patient with recurrent Merkel cell carcinoma was referred to assess response to chemotherapy and radiotherapy.

Findings
PET/CT images show multiple foci of abnormal FDG uptake in the pelvis bilaterally, located in borderline enlarged lymph nodes of the internal iliac chain, consistent with metastatic lymphadenopathy.

Note on MIP: Metastatic para-aortic and mediastinal lymph nodes in the left chest are seen.

Main Teaching Points and Summary
1. Malignant adenopathy can be accurately localized by PET/CT to a specific pelvic nodal group. This information may be important for planning surgical lymph node dissections or radiation treatment.
2. In this case, widely disseminated disease precluded surgical therapies.

Case 6.7.3 INTERNAL ILIAC LYMPH NODES IN LOWER PELVIS (FIG. 6.7.3)

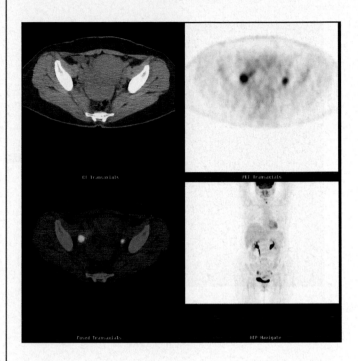

Brief History
A 44-year-old patient was referred for staging of newly diagnosed cervix carcinoma.

Findings
PET/CT images show abnormal FDG uptake localized to bilateral slightly enlarged internal iliac nodes, consistent with nodal metastases, further confirmed by surgery.

Note on MIP: Abnormal FDG uptake of moderate intensity in the primary cervical cancer in the posterior pelvis is seen.

Main Teaching Points and Summary
1. FDG PET/CT is useful for precise nodal staging of cervical cancer, which represents a major factor for treatment planning and prognosis.
2. Separation of abnormal nodal uptake from normal ureter activity can be challenging in some cases.

Case 6.7.4 INGUINAL LYMPH NODES AND PRIMARY CERVICAL CANCER (FIG. 6.7.4)

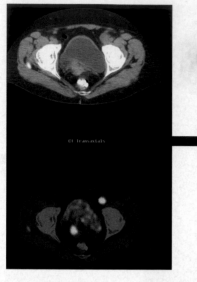
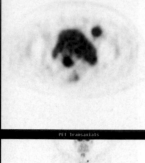

Brief History
A 53-year-old patient with newly diagnosed cervical cancer was referred for initial staging.

Findings
PET/CT images show a focus of abnormally increased FDG uptake in the left lower pelvis, localized to enlarged left inguinal lymph nodes, consistent with metastatic lymphadenopathy. There is also intense focal activity in the primary cervical cancer located behind the urinary bladder.

Note on MIP: Sites of abnormal FDG uptake in pelvic, abdominal, and supraclavicular nodal metastases are seen.

Main Teaching Points and Summary
1. PET/CT is useful for the precise localization of pelvic foci of increased FDG uptake to involved lymph nodes and their differentiation from tracer activity in adjacent normal structures.
2. Because pelvic anatomy can be highly variable, this morphologic information is critical for accurate diagnosis.

Case 6.7.5 INGUINAL LYMPH NODES AND METASTATIC MELANOMA IN GLUTEAL MASS (FIG. 6.7.5)

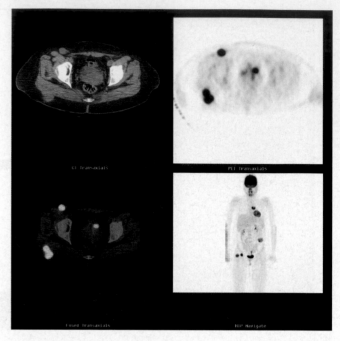

Brief History
A 34-year-old patient with metastatic melanoma was referred to assess response to immunotherapy.

Findings
PET/CT images show a focus of abnormal FDG uptake in the anterior aspect of the right lower pelvis, located in an enlarged inguinal lymph node, consistent with metastatic lymphadenopathy. In addition intense FDG uptake is demonstrated in a right gluteal mass.

Note on MIP: Abnormally increased uptake in a soft tissue mass in the left pelvis and in the mediastinum, consistent with metastatic disease, is seen.

Main Teaching Points and Summary
1. PET/CT localization of pelvic FDG accumulation provides accurate characterization of disease as soft tissue metastases, malignant adenopathy, or normal structures.
2. Muscle metastases are relatively common in melanoma.

6.8 VASCULAR

Case 6.8.1 PITFALL—NONINFECTED AORTOBIFEMORAL BYPASS (FIG. 6.8.1)

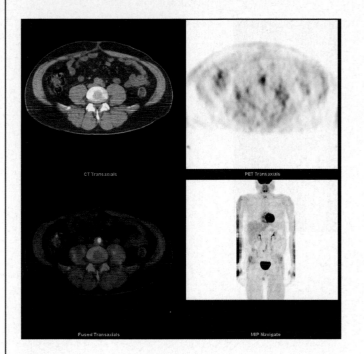

Brief History

A 50-year-old patient with Hodgkin's lymphoma involving the cervical and supraclavicular region was referred for assessing response to treatment 2 months after completing chemotherapy. The patient had vascular bypass surgery 4 months pre-PET/CT, with no symptoms or signs of graft infection.

Findings

PET/CT images show a focal area of moderately increased FDG uptake localized to the aortobifemoral vascular graft in the mid upper pelvic region, consistent with inflammatory reaction after recent surgery.

The PET/CT study was reported as negative for malignancy, and the patient achieved a continuous clinical remission.

Main Teaching Points and Summary

1. Increased FDG uptake has been described in regions of stent or graft implants following the surgical procedure, probably due to an inflammatory reaction. This uptake is usually linear and of mild to moderate intensity.
2. PET/CT can define the benign nature of focal FDG uptake in locations outside the tracer biodistribution by localizing the suspicious sites to areas of prior nononcologic surgical interventions, detected on the CT component of the study.

Case 6.8.2 BENIGN—INFECTED AORTIC VASCULAR GRAFT (FIG. 6.8.2)

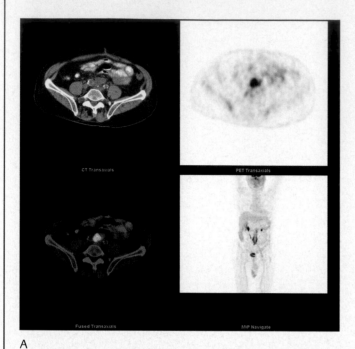

A

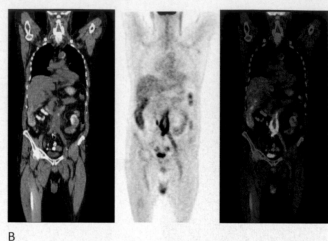

B

Brief History

An 80-year-old patient, 7 months after vascular surgery of an abdominal aortic aneurysm with left aortofemoral and right aortoiliac grafts, was referred with a clinically suspected graft infection due to fever, elevated sedimentation rate, and leukocytosis, unexplained by conventional imaging.

Findings

A and B. Transaxial (A) and coronal (B) PET/CT images show increased FDG uptake in the left pelvis, located along the left aortofemoral graft. The most prominent uptake is seen in the region of the aortic bifurcation on CT. There is also increased tracer uptake in the mid-lower abdomen, along the distal aortic segment of the vascular graft.

The findings were considered to represent an infectious process involving the graft.

Following intensive prolonged intravenous antibiotic treatment, the patient remained stable and systemic fever and signs of infection resolved for a follow-up of 7 months.

Main Teaching Points and Summary

1. FDG PET has been suggested as a tool for the assessment of infection in vascular grafts, a diagnosis that may have significant clinical and therapeutic consequences.
2. Precise pinpointing of increased FDG uptake to the involved graft is not possible on PET alone, especially in the presence of postsurgical soft tissue edema and infiltration.

6.9 BONE

Case 6.9.1 PITFALL—RADIATION-INDUCED "COLD" SACRUM (FIG. 6.9.1)

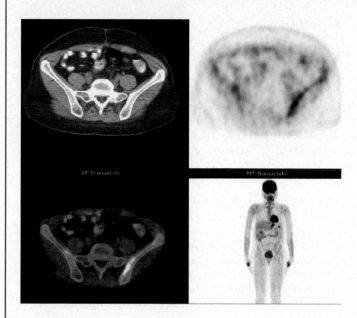

Case 6.9.2 BENIGN—SACRAL FRACTURE (FIG. 6.9.2)

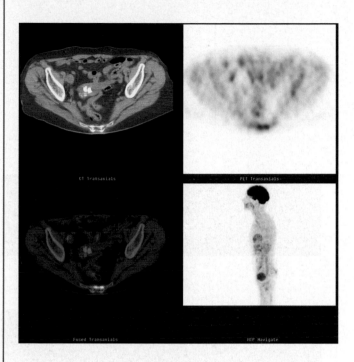

Brief History

A 45-year-old patient, 2 years after chemotherapy and radiotherapy of recurrent ovarian carcinoma, was referred for suspected second recurrence indicated by elevated serum tumor markers.

Findings

PET/CT images show asymmetric FDG uptake in pelvic bones, reduced in the sacrum and the right hemipelvis, with no associated skeletal abnormalities on CT, consistent with changes induced by radiotherapy administered to the pelvis 2 years before current examination.

Note on MIP: Focal abnormal uptake in the left upper abdomen, consistent with a new peritoneal metastasis, is seen.

Main Teaching Points and Summary

1. Decreased skeletal tracer uptake may be seen as a late sequela of radiotherapy to bone and is characterized by its sharp borders corresponding to the radiation treatment portals.
2. This benign uptake pattern should be recognized to prevent misinterpretation of asymmetric normal contralateral or adjacent bone uptake.

Brief History

An 83-year-old patient with non-Hodgkin's lymphoma, in complete remission for the last 4 years, was referred for suspected recurrence indicated by elevated lactate dehydrogenase (LDH) levels.

Findings

PET/CT images show an area of increased FDG uptake in the posterior pelvis localized by fused images to the sacral bone, with no definite lesion seen on CT.

The patient reported falling on her buttock 5 days before the PET/CT study. Following this examination, the patient remained in continuous clinical remission for the lymphoma for a follow-up of 10 months.

Main Teaching Points and Summary

1. Recent fractures can show variable degrees of FDG uptake and mimic malignant disease.
2. PET/CT can exclude the presence of soft tissue lesions, localizing PET findings to bone.
3. In the absence of a skeletal abnormality on CT, the mere localization of increased tracer uptake to bone, combined with detailed patient history of trauma, can direct further diagnosis toward benign causes of skeletal FDG uptake. Recent fractures can be very subtle on CT until bone resorption occurs, which can be weeks after the original event.
4. Increased FDG uptake has also been reported to occur in sclerotic stress fractures.

Case 6.9.3 BENIGN—PAGET'S DISEASE (FIG. 6.9.3)

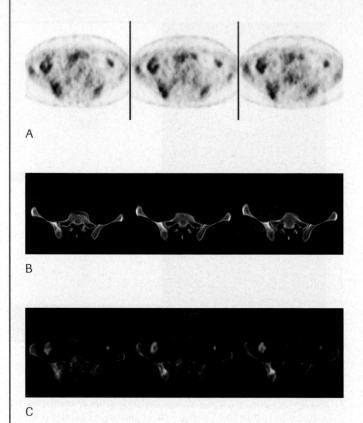

A

B

C

Brief History

A 55-year-old patient was referred for the evaluation of a solitary pulmonary nodule in the right lower lobe, incidentally found on CT.

Findings

A–C. Serial transaxial PET (A), CT (B), and PET/CT (C) images show increased FDG uptake in the right posterior aspect of the pelvis, localized to a heterogeneous mixed sclerotic and lytic lesion with bone expansion and deformation in the right ilium, consistent with Paget's disease.

There was no uptake in the lung nodule, and the patient had no evidence of lung malignancy on further follow-up.

Main Teaching Points and Summary

1. Benign bone disease may show increased FDG uptake of variable intensity and should be considered in the differential diagnosis of skeletal lesions during the interpretation of PET/CT studies in cancer patients.
2. Increased or normal FDG uptake in Paget's disease of the bone has been previously described, with the intensity of tracer uptake suggested to correlate with the degree of disease activity.
3. The presence of morphologic findings characteristic of Paget's disease on the CT component of the study generally enables the characterization of the suspicious lesion as benign.

Case 6.9.4 TUMOR–METASTASIS IN SACRUM AND EPIDURAL SPACE (FIG. 6.9.4)

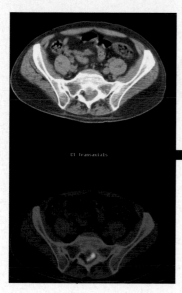
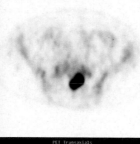
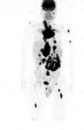

Brief History
A 38-year-old patient was referred for initial staging of non-Hodgkin's lymphoma diagnosed from a mediastinal mass.

Findings
PET/CT images show an intense focus of increased FDG uptake in the posterior upper pelvis, localized to an epidural mass at the level of the S1 vertebra, consistent with intraspinal involvement of lymphoma.

Note on MIP: Multiple foci of intense FDG uptake in lymphoma involving the chest, abdomen, and the axial and appendicular skeleton are seen.

Main Teaching Point and Summary
1. PET/CT can differentiate intraspinal involvement of lymphoma from vertebral disease.

Case 6.9.5 TUMOR–METASTASIS IN ILIUM AND SOFT TISSUES (FIG. 6.9.5)

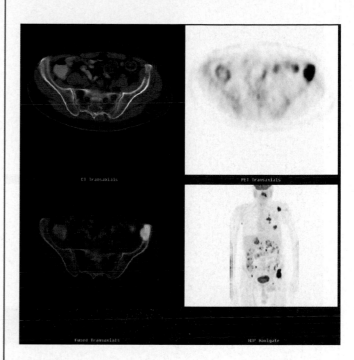

Brief History
A 77-year-old patient was referred for staging of a newly diagnosed lung cancer.

Findings
PET/CT images show an area of intense FDG uptake in the anterior aspect of the left pelvis, localized to a lytic lesion in the left ilium and an adjacent soft tissue mass.

Note on MIP: Multiple foci of abnormal uptake in the left lung cancer and in mediastinal, abdominal, and skeletal metastases are seen.

Main Teaching Points and Summary
1. Skeletal metastases can demonstrate soft tissue extension.
2. Both soft tissue and bone CT windows may be needed to evaluate these lesions optimally.
3. Bone metastases may be associated with normal CT scans of the skeleton.

Case 6.9.6 TUMOR—LYMPHOMA, INVOLVEMENT OF THE ISCHIUM (FIG. 6.9.6)

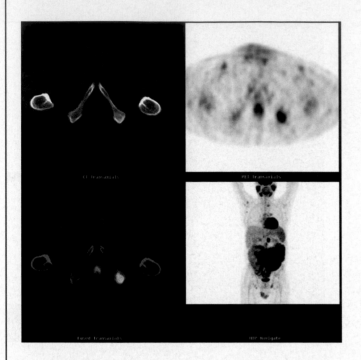

Brief History
A 56-year-old patient was referred for initial staging of low-grade non-Hodgkin's lymphoma, which presented as bowel obstruction and was diagnosed by laparoscopic biopsy of an abdominal mass.

Findings
PET/CT images show a focus of increased FDG uptake in a subtle sclerotic lesion in the left ischium, consistent with lymphomatous bone involvement.

Note on MIP: Diffuse abdominal FDG uptake in the known, extensive, intestinal lymphoma is seen.

Main Teaching Points and Summary
1. Diagnosis of extranodal lymphoma is of clinical significance for accurate staging and follow-up after therapy.
2. Pelvic FDG uptake in the bone may mimic nodal lesions but is accurately localized and characterized by PET/CT.
3. Lymphoma involving the bone is most commonly negative on CT even when evaluated with bone windows.

PET/CT of the Extremities

Ora Israel • Daniela Militianu

7.1 SKIN

Case 7.1.1 BENIGN—HEALING SURGICAL SCAR, THIGH (FIG. 7.1.1)

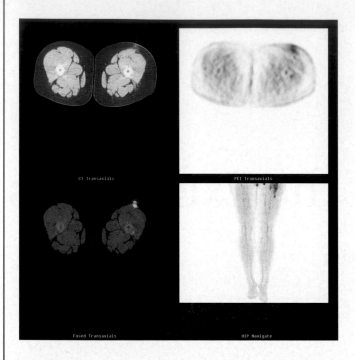

Brief History
A 33-year-old patient was referred for systemic staging 5 weeks after the complete excision of a malignant melanoma from the anterior left thigh.

Findings
PET/CT images show an area of increased 2-[18F] fluoro-2-deoxy-D-glucose (FDG) activity of moderate intensity in the anterior aspect of the left proximal thigh, in a subcutaneous surgical scar.

Main Teaching Points and Summary
1. Increased FDG activity can be found in sites of an inflammatory reaction, such as the healing process of recent surgical scars.
2. In the presence of equivocal findings (moderate intensity, not well circumscribed), PET/CT can differentiate between a malignant lesion and a benign reactive process.

Case 7.1.2 BENIGN—INFECTED SURGICAL SCAR, THIGH (FIG. 7.1.2)

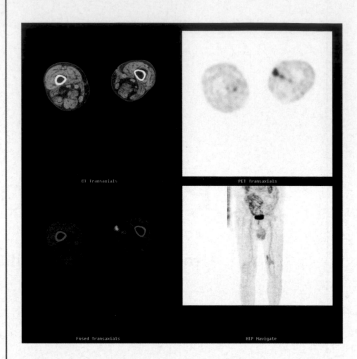

Brief History
A 67-year-old patient, status post–left femoropopliteal graft 7 months pre-PET/CT, was referred with the clinical suspicion of an infectious process in the left inguinal region, following recent drainage of a left thigh abscess.

Findings
PET/CT images show an area of increased FDG activity in the medial aspect of the left distal thigh, located in an infected sinus tract along an infected surgical scar.

Main Teaching Points and Summary
1. PET/CT can fuse sites of increased FDG activity due to an active infectious process to soft tissues or infected scars.
2. This rather intense uptake is greater than would be expected in the normal postoperative setting at 7 months postsurgery.

Case 7.1.3 BENIGN–INFECTED SKIN ULCERS, LEGS (FIG. 7.1.3)

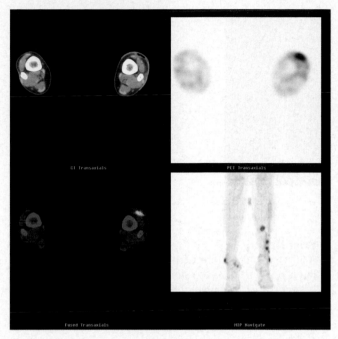

A

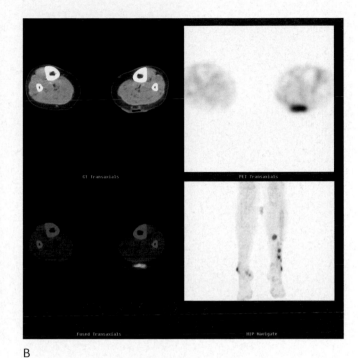

B

Brief History

An 18-year-old patient with vasculitis and infected skin ulcers in both legs was referred with the clinical suspicion of lymphoma because of the presence of splenomegaly and abnormal laboratory test results, including lympho-cytosis, anemia, and elevated LDH.

Findings

A and B. PET/CT images show multiple areas of abnormally increased FDG uptake in the anterior (A) and posterior (B) aspect of the distal half of the left leg, in areas of thickening of the skin and necrotizing ulcers.

Note on MIP (lower limbs): Multiple additional foci of increased tracer uptake in the right ankle and left distal leg and ankle are seen, consistent with known extensive cutaneous vasculitis-related lesions.

On biopsy, the lesions were not found to represent cutaneous lymphoma.

Main Teaching Point and Summary

1. PET/CT can detect the presence and precisely localize lesions to skin or soft tissue and guide biopsy when clinically indicated.

Case 7.1.4 TUMOR—MALIGNANT MELANOMA, NODULES IN THIGH AND CALF (FIG. 7.1.4)

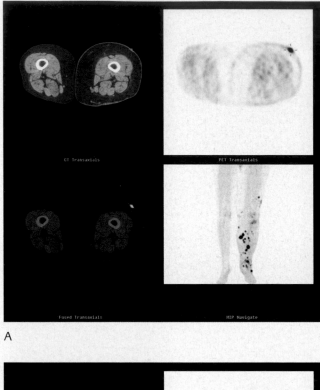

A

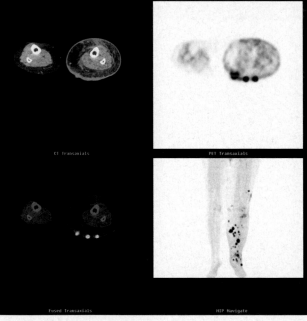

B

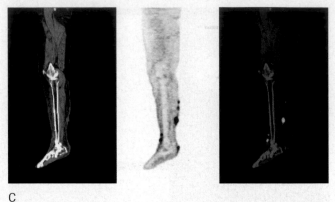

C

Brief History

A 58-year-old patient with malignant melanoma of the left leg and thigh was referred with the clinical suspicion of recurrence because of pain and swelling of the left leg and the presence of nodules in the same region on palpation.

Findings

A. PET/CT images, transaxial slices at the level of the distal thigh, show a focal area of abnormally increased FDG uptake located in a small exophytic skin nodule adjacent to findings suggestive of lymphedema of the skin and of the subcutaneous fat.

B. PET/CT images, transaxial slices at a lower level, demonstrate multiple focal areas of abnormally increased FDG uptake in the posterior aspect of the midcalf in discrete nodules located in thickened skin, with associated extensive edematous changes of the subcutaneous fat.

C. Sagittal slice PET/CT images confirm the presence and superficial localization of the hypermetabolic foci in addition to the morphologic changes seen on CT, consistent with multiple sites of recurrent melanoma and impaired lymphatic drainage.

Main Teaching Point and Summary

1. In the presence of extensive diffuse structural changes due to impaired lymphatic drainage, CT alone cannot accurately diagnose nodular malignant involvement, in contrast to the effectiveness of superimposition of hypermetabolic lesions on PET/CT images.

7.2 SOFT TISSUE

Case 7.2.1 BENIGN—ABSCESS, LEG (FIG. 7.2.1)

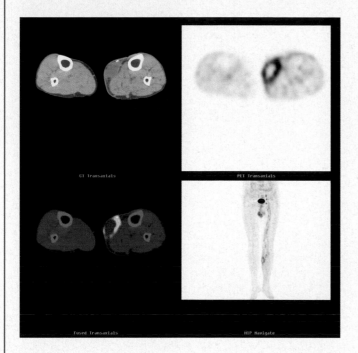

Case 7.2.2 TUMOR—SUBCUTANEOUS LYMPHOMA, NODULE IN ARM (FIG. 7.2.2)

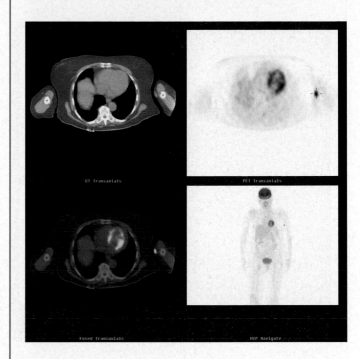

Brief History
A 54-year-old patient, status post–left femoropopliteal bypass 6 weeks before PET/CT, was referred for further assessment because of clinical suspicion of vascular graft infection due to the presence of an infected surgical wound at the medial aspect of the left calf.

Findings
PET/CT images demonstrate an area showing a hyper-metabolic rim of abnormally increased FDG uptake and a central focus of decreased activity in the medial aspect of the mid-third of the left leg, corresponding to a subcutaneous fluid collection.

A soft tissue abscess was drained in this region.

Note on the MIP (lower limbs): Increased linear FDG activity along the vascular graft, consistent with a non-specific inflammatory process, and focal abnormal tracer uptake in reactive left inguinal lymph nodes are seen.

Main Teaching Point and Summary
1. PET/CT can diagnose the presence of a soft tissue infection and guide local therapeutic drainage procedures.

Brief History
An 81-year-old patient with low-grade lymphoma of the skin was referred to monitor response to treatment.

Findings
PET/CT images show a focus of abnormally increased FDG uptake in a subcutaneous nodule in the medial aspect of the left arm, consistent with residual viable lymphoma.

Main Teaching Points and Summary
1. After treatment of cancer PET/CT can define equivocal findings as residual active tumor in the presence of congruent hypermetabolic tracer activity and persistent morphologic abnormalities.
2. In this case, the focal lesion in the arm could easily have been mistaken for FDG uptake in a vein or a site of extravasation at the injection site. Knowledge of the injection site and of the clinical history are critical to the correct diagnosis in addition to physical examination.

Case 7.2.3 TUMOR—SUBCUTANEOUS MELANOMA, NODULE IN THIGH (FIG. 7.2.3)

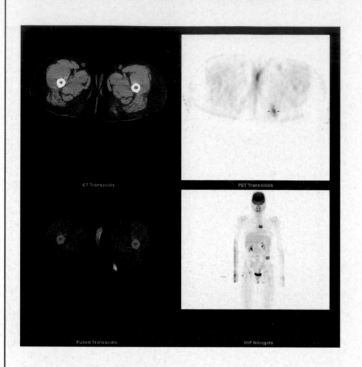

Brief History

A 33-year-old patient with recurrent malignant melanoma was referred for monitoring response to immunotherapy.

Findings

PET/CT images show a focus of slightly increased FDG uptake in a subcutaneous nodule in the medial aspect of the proximal left thigh, consistent with residual melanoma.

Note on MIP: Increased FDG uptake in the right inguinal region consistent with metastatic lymphadenopathy is seen.

Main Teaching Point and Summary

1. After treatment, PET/CT can define the presence of residual viable tumor by superimposition of foci with low intensity FDG uptake to small residual anatomic lesions.

Case 7.2.4 TUMOR—SOFT TISSUE SARCOMA, HAND, WITH BONE INVOLVEMENT (FIG. 7.2.4)

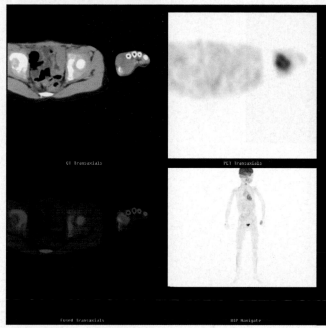

A

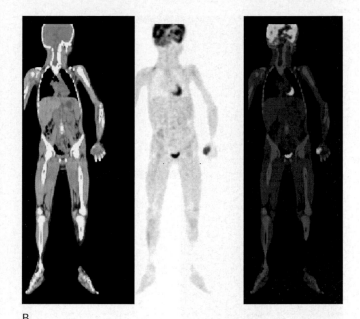

B

Brief History
A 5-year-old patient with newly diagnosed alveolar rhabdomyosarcoma of the left hand was referred for whole body staging with PET/CT.

Findings
A. PET/CT images, transaxial slices, show an area of increased FDG uptake in a soft tissue mass located between the first and second finger of the left hand, involving also the first metacarpal bone, as seen on CT.
B. Coronal slice PET/CT images confirm the presence and localization of the hypermetabolic lesion to the primary tumor in the left hand.

Main Teaching Points and Summary
1. Aggressive soft tissue sarcomas typically have intense FDG uptake prior to therapy.
2. PET/CT allows whole body staging of newly diagnosed patients.
3. PET/CT, but not PET alone, precisely resolves the location of primary lesions in the extremities and their relationship to normal bony anatomy.

7.3 JOINTS

Case 7.3.1 ARTIFACT—METAL-INDUCED PERIPROSTHETIC ACTIVITY AND REACTIVE PROCESS, HIP (FIG. 7.3.1)

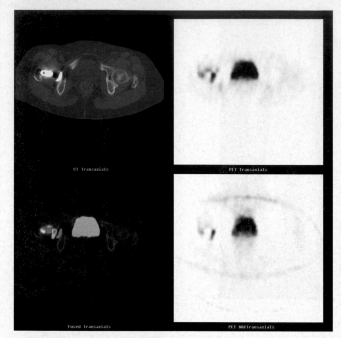

A

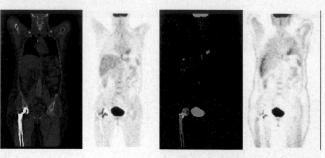

B

Brief History
A 57-year-old patient with a history of recurrent breast cancer 3 years pre-PET/CT, status post–surgery, chemotherapy, and radiotherapy to the left axilla, was referred for assessment of a newly diagnosed single pulmonary lesion in the left upper lobe and whole body staging. The patient had a right total hip replacement 6 years earlier.

Findings
A. Transaxial slice PET/CT images at the level of the hips show an area of increased FDG activity surrounding the metal prosthetic implant, less prominent on the uncorrected images (lower right panel).
B. PET/CT images, coronal slices including uncorrected images (far right), confirm the presence and localization of the increased tracer uptake around the right hip prosthesis, related in part to a reactive inflammatory process following previous surgery, as well as to attenuation-corrected reconstruction artifacts.

Main Teaching Points and Summary
1. Evaluation of attenuation corrected PET images only in areas adjacent to metal implants can lead to false positive interpretation of increased FDG uptake due to the presence of metal artifacts.
2. The intensity of tracer uptake is reduced, but not absent, on the non–attenuation corrected images near the metallic prosthesis because there is no "overcorrection" due to the high absorption of x-ray photons.
3. Homogenous FDG uptake of moderate intensity in regions of previous surgery and following insertion of prosthetic devices can be related to a reactive inflammatory process.
4. Some degree of tracer uptake about a prosthetic joint is quite common and does not necessarily indicate the presence of infection.

Case 7.3.2 BENIGN–PERIARTICULAR UPTAKE, TROCHANTERIC BURSITIS (FIG. 7.3.2)

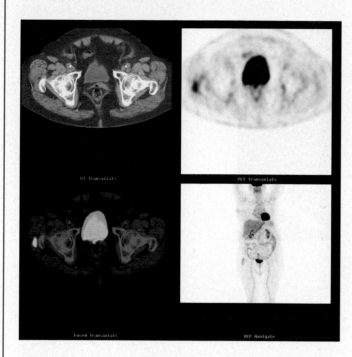

Case 7.3.3 BENIGN–PERIARTICULAR UPTAKE, SYNOVITIS OF KNEES (FIG. 7.3.3)

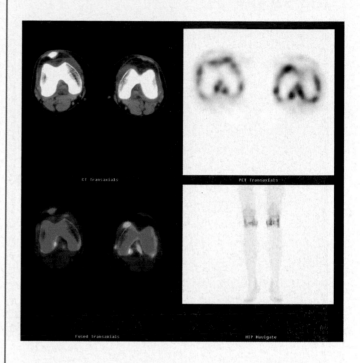

Brief History

A 76-year-old patient with low-grade non-Hodgkin's lymphoma, status postchemotherapy 5 years before the current study, was referred for routine follow-up during continuous clinical remission.

Findings

PET/CT images show an area of increased FDG uptake in the lateral aspect of the right proximal thigh corresponding to soft tissue swelling adjacent to the lateral part of the greater trochanter, consistent with trochanteric bursitis.

Note on MIP: Foci of moderately intense abnormal FDG uptake in the right mediastinal region, most probably due to a granulomatotic process, are seen.

The patient had no evidence of active lymphoma on clinical follow-up.

Main Teaching Points and Summary
1. Asymmetric FDG uptake of moderate intensity can be related to an inflammatory process.
2. Precise PET/CT localization to anatomic lesions with a characteristic benign pattern can exclude the presence of cancer.
3. Trochanteric bursitis is common and demonstrates often moderately increased FDG uptake that is physically separate from the hip joint as seen on PET/CT.

Brief History

A 53-year-old patient, status post–wide excision of malignant melanoma of the back and right axillary lymph node dissection, was referred for whole body PET/CT for further assessment of equivocal findings on chest CT. The patient also complained of pain in the lower limbs.

Findings

PET/CT images demonstrate diffusely increased FDG uptake in both knees, localized to bilateral knee effusion and thickened synovia, consistent with acute synovitis.

Main Teaching Points and Summary
1. Diffuse increased intra-articular FDG uptake following the anatomy of the joints can indicate the presence of an active inflammatory arthritic process.
2. Although most commonly due to an inflammatory process such as rheumatoid arthritis, a similar pattern can be also caused by inflammation related to hemarthrosis associated with hemophilia.

Case 7.3.4 BENIGN—TENOSYNOVITIS AND TENDON TEAR, FOOT AND DISTAL LEG (FIG. 7.3.4)

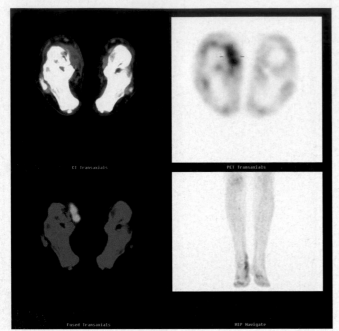

A

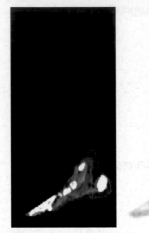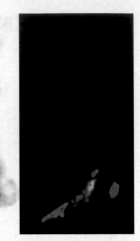

B

Brief History

A 70-year-old patient, status post–excision of malignant melanoma of the back and right axillary node dissection, was referred for PET/CT for suspected tumor recurrence due to the presence of equivocal CT findings in the right axilla. The patient had a history of osteoarthritis, calcified plantar fasciitis, and Achilles' tendonitis.

Findings

A. Transaxial PET/CT images demonstrate increased FDG uptake along the medial aspect of the midfoot, localized to a soft tissue mass in the site of the tibialis posterior and flexor digitorum longus tendon.

B. Sagittal PET/CT images confirm the presence and localization of the abnormally increased FDG uptake to the aforementioned morphologic changes, consistent with tear and inflammatory healing of the tibialis posterior and a partial tear of the flexor digitorum longus tendons, and surrounding tenosynovitis.

Main Teaching Points and Summary

1. The presence of increased FDG uptake on the PET component and of morphologic changes on the CT component of the PET/CT study enables a single-test diagnosis of an active inflammatory process and its precise localization.

2. Although PET/CT can show the location of the mass and the inflammation, fused images do not reveal the tendon tear directly. Magnetic resonance imaging or ultrasound are the anatomic imaging modalities of choice for diagnosis of such abnormalities.

Case 7.3.5 BENIGN—LOW-GRADE INFECTION, HIP (FIG. 7.3.5)

Case 7.4.1 PHYSIOLOGIC—TENSE MUSCLES, THIGHS (FIG. 7.4.1)

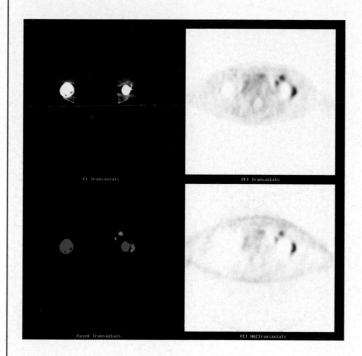

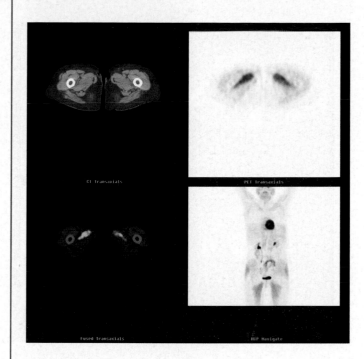

Brief History
A 58-year-old patient with squamous cell carcinoma of the cervix was referred to assess response to chemotherapy and radiotherapy to the pelvis. The patient had a left total hip replacement 15 years earlier and a right total hip replacement 1 year before the current PET/CT.

Findings
Transaxial PET/CT images demonstrate an irregular area of abnormally increased FDG uptake, surrounding the head of the left hip prosthesis, showing a similar pattern on the attenuation corrected (upper right) and uncorrected (lower right) slices, consistent with a low-grade infectious or inflammatory process extending to soft tissues separate from the prosthesis.

Note: There is no increased FDG uptake in the region of the right hip joint prosthesis.

Main Teaching Points and Summary
1. Irregular intense FDG uptake following insertion of prosthetic devices can be related to low-grade infection or inflammation.
2. In this case, the fact that the findings were in a site where surgery was performed 15 years earlier make postoperative inflammatory changes less likely, although this type of findings can persist for a certain period of time.
3. This level of tracer uptake should not be related to inaccurate attenuation correction because findings on attenuation-corrected and uncorrected images are very similar in appearance.

Brief History
A 63-year-old patient was referred for routine follow-up of a gastric non-Hodgkin's lymphoma. Clinically, the patient had remained in complete remission following chemotherapy.

Findings
PET/CT images show bilateral symmetrically increased FDG uptake in the adductor muscles in the medial aspect of the proximal thighs.

Note on MIP: Increased FDG uptake in additional muscles in the hip girdle and shoulder musculature.

This pattern of diffuse, symmetric increased FDG uptake in muscles was considered to represent physiologic tracer activity related to a short fasting period. The study was reported as negative for recurrent lymphoma, and the patient remained in continuous clinical remission for a follow-up of 14 months.

Main Teaching Points and Summary
1. Increased FDG uptake in skeletal muscles can be physiologic and should not be confused with cancer-related findings.
2. Muscle uptake of FDG may occur diffusely if the patient has fasted inadequately and insulin levels are elevated or in a more local pattern following increased physical stress.
3. Asymmetric, intense, focal FDG uptake located by PET/CT to muscles needs to be evaluated carefully to exclude the presence of pathology, although it is only rarely related to active malignancy.

Case 7.4.2 TUMOR–METASTASIS, ARM (FIG. 7.4.2)

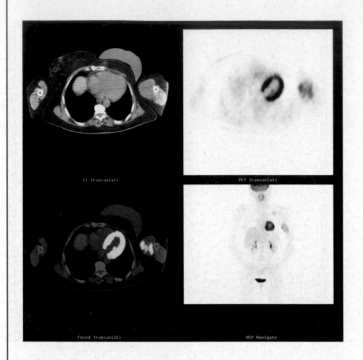

Case 7.4.3 TUMOR–METASTASES, THIGH (FIG. 7.4.3)

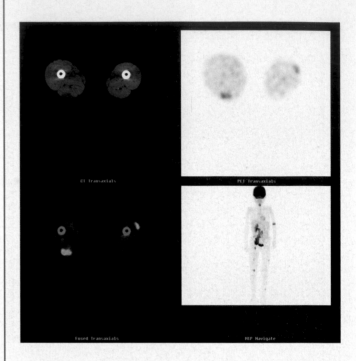

Brief History

A 59-year-old patient with a history of breast cancer 19 years before the current examination was referred to assess a mass in the medial aspect of the left arm and to evaluate for systemic recurrent cancer.

Findings

PET/CT images show an area of inhomogeneous, abnormally increased FDG uptake in a soft tissue mass involving the biceps and brachial muscles in the medial aspect of the left midarm.

Note on MIP: An additional site of increased FDG uptake in the left axilla, localized by PET/CT (not shown) to the pectoralis muscle, was seen.

The patient was referred for biopsy of the larger mass, which confirmed the presence of metastatic breast cancer.

Main Teaching Points and Summary

1. In this case, the differential diagnosis included recurrent breast cancer as well as a soft tissue sarcoma of the proximal arm musculature.
2. Suspicious lesions in an unusual location can be further investigated using PET/CT to pinpoint the optimal focus for invasive tissue sampling.
3. The ability to assess the entire body is an advantage of PET/CT and can be useful in soft tissue tumor assessments.

Brief History

A 6-year-old patient with a metastatic alveolar rhabdomyosarcoma of the left hand, status post–surgery, chemotherapy, and radiotherapy, was referred to assess response to treatment.

Findings

PET/CT images show hypodense masses in both thighs on CT involving the semimembranous (right) and the vastus lateralis (left) muscles, with corresponding foci of abnormally increased FDG uptake, consistent with metastases.

Note on MIP: Multiple additional sites of abnormally increased FDG uptake in lymph nodes, soft tissues, and the skeleton are seen, consistent with extensive metastatic disease.

Main Teaching Points and Summary

1. PET/CT can define the location of a metastatic process, including structures that are uncommonly involved by malignancy as in the present case.
2. Further invasive diagnostic procedures, as well as treatment strategy, can be guided by results of fused images.

7.5 LYMPH NODES

Case 7.5.1 EPITROCHLEAR LYMPH NODES (FIG. 7.5.1)

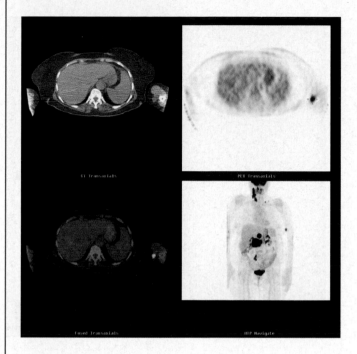

Case 7.5.2 POPLITEAL LYMPH NODES (FIG. 7.5.2)

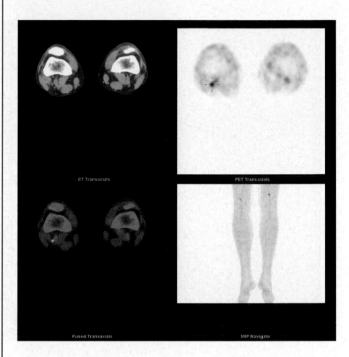

Brief History

A 64-year-old patient with newly diagnosed aggressive gastric lymphoma was referred for whole body staging.

Findings

PET/CT images show a small focus of increased FDG uptake in an epitrochlear lymph node in the left arm.

Note on MIP: Foci of increased tracer uptake in the distal portion of the stomach, the oropharynx, right cervical, and left supraclavicular lymph nodes and peritoneal nodules in the lower abdomen, indicating the presence of extensive supra- and infradiaphragmatic lymphoma involvement.

Main Teaching Points and Summary

1. Foci of FDG uptake in the region of the elbows are commonly related to slight extravasation of the radiotracer at the site of the injection.
2. Assessment of PET/CT slices may enable the detection of previously unknown sites of peripheral lymph node involvement.
3. Although inclusion of the arms may diminish the quality of the thoracic CT, it does allow a more complete assessment of the entire body.

Brief History

A 36-year-old patient with newly diagnosed aggressive non-Hodgkin's lymphoma with known nodal and skeletal involvement was referred for systemic staging.

Findings

PET/CT images show a small focus of low-intensity FDG uptake in a popliteal lymph node in the right distal thigh.

Note on MIP: An additional site of disease involvement in a left popliteal lymph node in a more cephalad location is seen.

Main Teaching Points and Summary

1. FDG uptake in the lower limbs can be due to a variety of etiologies. CT images provide confidence that tracer uptake is in a lymph node and not in a vein or other anatomic structure.
2. PET/CT can localize equivocal low-intensity, small FDG foci to lymphadenopathy and therefore induce upstaging of disease to sites of previously unknown lymphomatous involvement.

Case 7.5.3 POPLITEAL LYMPH NODES (FIG. 7.5.3)

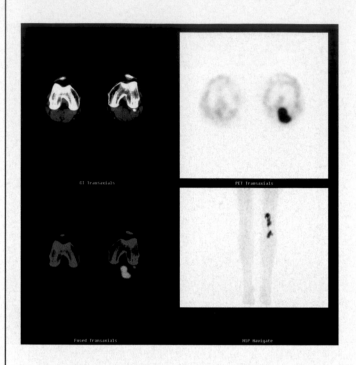

Case 7.6.1 PITFALL—VASCULAR UPTAKE (FIG. 7.6.1)

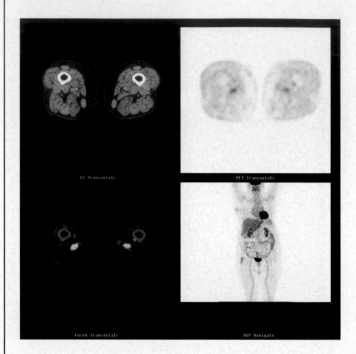

Brief History

A 69-year-old patient with low-grade non-Hodgkin's lymphoma was referred to assess response to treatment.

Findings

PET/CT images show a focus of abnormally increased FDG uptake in a markedly enlarged left popliteal lymph node, consistent with a site of persistent active lymphoma.

Note on MIP (lower limbs): An additional site of disease involvement in a large soft tissue mass in the left distal thigh.

Main Teaching Points and Summary

1. PET/CT allows precise localization of foci of lymphoma anywhere in the body.
2. PET/CT can also differentiate between lymphadenopathy and involvement of adjacent soft tissue.

Brief History

A 76-year-old patient with low-grade non-Hodgkin's lymphoma, status–post chemotherapy 5 years pre-PET/CT, was referred for routine follow-up during continuous clinical remission.

Findings

PET/CT images show slightly increased FDG uptake in the medial aspect of both thighs localized intravascular, in close proximity to small calcifications in the femoral arteries.

Note on MIP: Increased tracer activity in the lateral aspect of the right proximal thigh, overlying the right hip joint is seen consistent with trochanteric bursitis.

Main Teaching Points and Summary

1. FDG can localize to blood vessels, either in the vascular wall, with or without congruent calcifications seen on CT, or because of some retention of FDG within the blood pool itself.
2. When asymmetric and focal, vascular uptake needs to be precisely localized by PET/CT to vessels to differentiate accurately benign increased tracer activity from malignant processes.
3. Vascular wall FDG uptake may be a marker of early atherosclerosis.

Case 7.6.2 BENIGN—INFECTED VASCULAR GRAFT (FIG. 7.6.2)

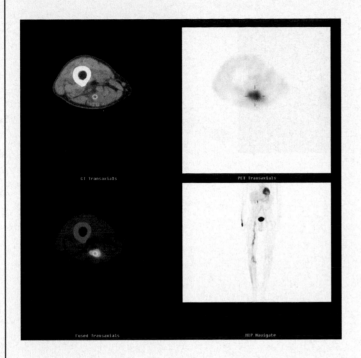

Brief History

A 52-year-old man who underwent right femoropopliteal bypass 4 months before the current study was referred for suspected graft infection in the presence of a known superficially infected surgical scar in the right midcalf.

Findings

PET/CT images show abnormally increased FDG uptake along the medial aspect of the right thigh and proximal leg, fused to the vascular graft and surrounding soft tissue edema, consistent with graft and soft tissue infection.

The patient was started on intensive intravenous antibiotic therapy. Graft infection was confirmed at surgery performed 6 weeks later.

Main Teaching Points and Summary

1. FDG is taken up by acute infectious processes that demonstrate hypermetabolic activity.
2. PET/CT diagnosis or exclusion of involvement of a vascular graft by an adjacent soft tissue infectious process may have a significant clinical impact on further patient management, referring patients to, or sparing unneeded surgery with high morbidity.

7.7 BONE AND BONE MARROW

Case 7.7.1 BENIGN—OSTEOMYELITIS, PHALANX OF FOOT (FIG. 7.7.1)

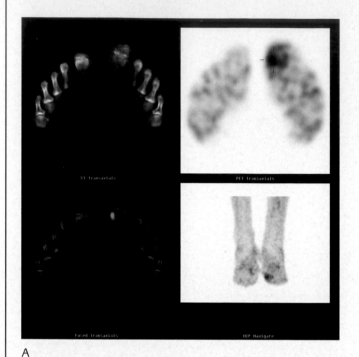

A

B

Brief History

A 51-year-old patient with an ingrown toenail of the first toe of the left foot presented with local pain, swelling, and edematous changes, persisting for more than 1 month, with normal x-rays of the region. PET/CT was performed because of suspicion of osteomyelitis.

Findings

A. Transaxial PET/CT images show a focal area of abnormally increased FDG uptake in the distal, medial aspect of the left foot, localized to a destructive lesion at the apex of the left first proximal phalanx.

B. Sagittal PET/CT images confirm the presence and localization of the abnormally increased FDG focus to morphologic changes representing osteomyelitis of the first proximal phalanx of the left foot.

Main Teaching Points and Summary

1. In anatomic regions with close proximity of soft tissues and small bones, PET/CT can help separate soft tissue from skeletal lesions of various etiologies, thus further directing patient management.

2. Active infectious processes typically show increased FDG uptake. In the presence of simultaneous structural changes, PET/CT can provide a single-step diagnosis of osteomyelitis.

Case 7.7.2 TUMOR–BONE METASTASIS, SCAPULA (FIG. 7.7.2)

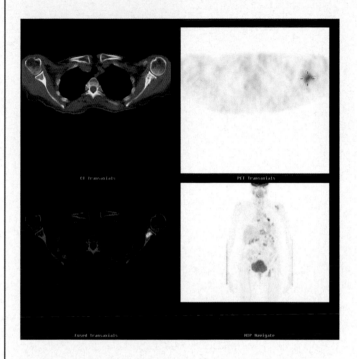

Brief History
A 74-year-old patient with a history of breast cancer 7 years pre-PET/CT was referred for restaging before surgery for a newly diagnosed single brain metastasis.

Findings
PET/CT images show a focus of abnormally increased FDG uptake in the left shoulder, localized to a predominantly sclerotic lesion with periosteal reaction in the lateral aspect of the scapula, consistent with a bone metastasis.

Note on MIP: Multiple additional metastases in the axial and appendicular skeleton are seen.

Based on diagnosis of disseminated bone metastases, craniotomy was cancelled, and systemic treatment was instituted.

Main Teaching Points and Summary
1. PET/CT can precisely localize foci of increased tracer uptake to bony structures.
2. FDG uptake has been reported as more frequent in untreated osteolytic lesions than in osteoblastic bone metastases.
3. In many instances, the CT component is essentially normal despite the positive PET study, probably because FDG in early metastases is taken up mainly in tumor within the bone marrow.

Case 7.7.3 TUMOR–BONE METASTASIS, HUMERUS (FIG. 7.7.3)

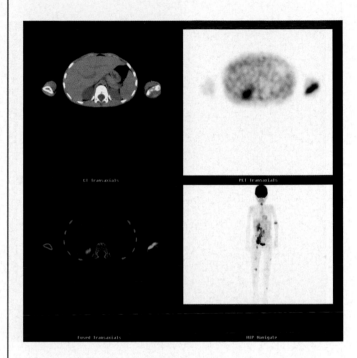

Brief History
A 6-year-old patient with metastatic alveolar rhabdomyosarcoma of the left hand, status post–surgery, chemotherapy, and radiotherapy, was referred for assessing response to treatment.

Findings
PET/CT images show abnormally increased FDG uptake in the left elbow, localized to a lytic lesion in the distal left humerus.

Note on MIP: Extensive metastatic disease involving lymph nodes, soft tissue, and skeleton. Physiologic but asymmetric renal activity is seen.

Main Teaching Point and Summary
1. PET/CT can differentiate between artifactual increased FDG uptake at the site of tracer injection and malignant lesions in soft tissue or bone in the elbow region.

Case 7.7.4 TUMOR–BONE METASTASIS, FEMUR (FIG. 7.7.4)

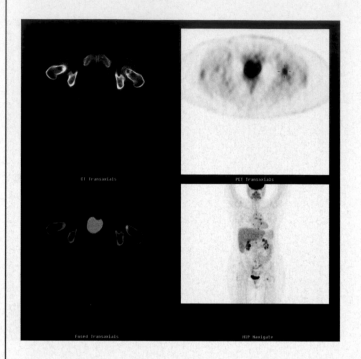

Brief History

A 53-year-old patient with a history of breast cancer diagnosed 9 years before the current investigation was referred for PET/CT with a suspicion of tumor recurrence due to rising serum tumor markers.

Findings

PET/CT images show a focal area of abnormally increased FDG uptake in a predominantly osteolytic lesion in the femoral neck seen on CT.

Note on MIP: Metastatic disease involving mediastinal lymphadenopathy and the L1 vertebra is seen.

Main Teaching Point and Summary

1. PET/CT can precisely localize foci of abnormal FDG uptake to bony structures and also indicate the presence of previously unknown structural lesions, which may require particular tailoring of further treatment procedures including palliative radiotherapy.

Case 7.7.5 TUMOR–LYMPHOMA, HUMERUS AND SOFT TISSUES (FIG. 7.7.5)

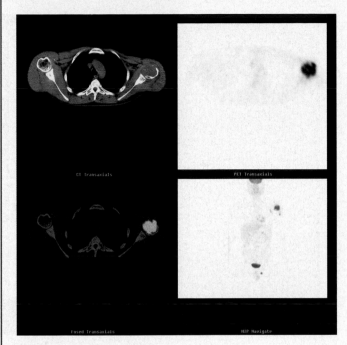

A

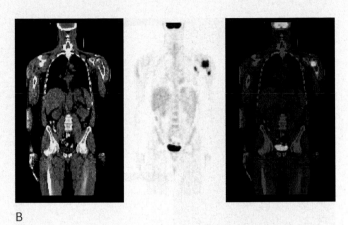

B

Brief History

A 39-year-old patient with newly diagnosed peripheral T-cell lymphoma was referred for staging 1 month after biopsy of a pathologic fracture of the left proximal humerus.

Findings

A. Transaxial PET/CT images show a focal area of increased FDG uptake in a large osteolytic lesion involving the left humeral head (with destruction of the cortex) and adjacent soft tissues.

B. Coronal PET/CT images confirm the presence and localization of the abnormal FDG focus and the structural changes on CT, consistent with a site of lymphomatous involvement. There are additional foci of abnormal FDG uptake in the proximal third of the left humeral shaft and left axillary lymph nodes, suggestive of additional sites of lymphomatous involvement or a reactive process following recent surgery.

Note on MIP: Focal intense uptake in the left ischium (with a corresponding lytic lesion on the CT component, not shown), representing another site of bone lymphoma, is seen.

Main Teaching Points and Summary

1. PET/CT can define the etiology and extent of involvement of malignant lesions and therefore improve treatment planning of lymphoma without the need for additional invasive diagnostic procedures.

2. Although CT is abnormal in this case, the most common CT appearance associated with active lymphoma of the bone is an unremarkable (normal) CT scan because lymphoma infiltrates primarily the marrow space until the disease is quite advanced.

Case 7.7.6 TUMOR–BONE MARROW INVOLVEMENT, MULTIPLE MYELOMA, FEMUR (FIG. 7.7.6)

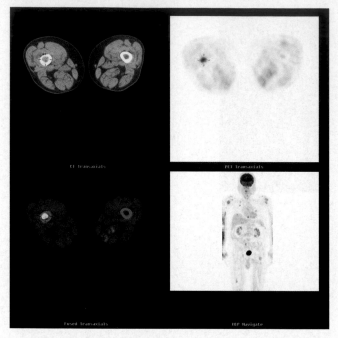

Brief History
A 59-year-old patient with multiple myeloma in complete remission after chemotherapy and bone marrow transplantation was assessed for new onset of diffuse skeletal pain.

Findings
PET/CT images show a focal area of mildly intense FDG uptake in an intramedullary infiltration in the mid-third of the right femoral shaft.

Note on MIP: Multiple additional foci of disease involving the axial and appendicular skeleton are seen.

Main Teaching Points and Summary
1. PET/CT can precisely localize foci of abnormal FDG uptake to the cortex of the bone or to the intramedullary space.
2. Intramedullary localization of increased tracer activity can provide a noninvasive diagnosis of bone marrow involvement in equivocal cases despite negative biopsy results.
3. False-negative biopsies are not uncommon in marrow-infiltrating malignancies because the disease can have a scattered distribution pattern that can be missed on a single biopsy.

Case 7.7.7 TUMOR–BONE MARROW AND SOFT TISSUE LYMPHOMA, HUMERUS (FIG. 7.7.7)

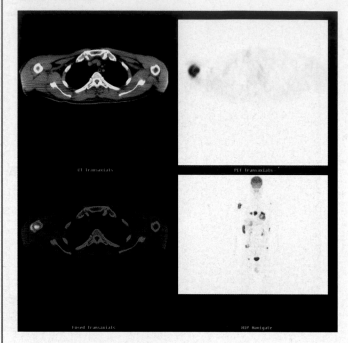

Brief History
A 36-year-old patient with newly diagnosed aggressive non-Hodgkin's lymphoma involving the skeleton and lymph nodes was referred for staging.

Findings
PET/CT images show abnormally increased FDG uptake in an intramedullary infiltration in the right proximal humeral shaft and an adjacent soft tissue mass.

Note on MIP: Multiple additional sites of lymphoma involving the axial and appendicular skeleton are seen.

Main Teaching Points and Summary
1. PET/CT can precisely localize foci of abnormal FDG uptake to the cortex of the bone or the intramedullary space.
2. Localization of increased FDG uptake can facilitate diagnosis of bone marrow involvement, even in cases of equivocal or negative biopsy, which are not uncommon because of sampling errors.

Case 7.7.8 TUMOR–BONE MARROW AND SOFT TISSUE LYMPHOMA, TIBIA AND LEG (FIG. 7.7.8)

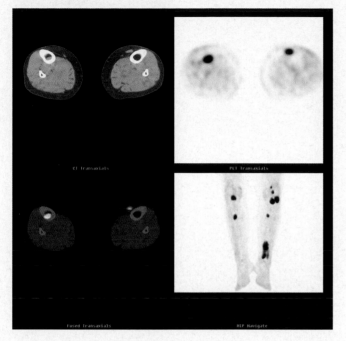

Brief History

A 68-year-old patient with recurrent low-grade non-Hodgkin's lymphoma involving lymph nodes, soft tissues, and bone was referred for restaging before second-line chemotherapy.

Findings

PET/CT images show foci of abnormal FDG uptake in both legs localized to an intramedullary infiltration in the tibial shaft (right) and a subcutaneous nodule (left).

Note on MIP (lower limbs): Multiple additional sites of bone and soft tissue lymphoma in both knees and the lower left leg.

Main Teaching Points and Summary

1. Melanoma and lymphoma are two of the more common entities to produce FDG-avid soft tissue masses. The bilaterality of this case suggests lymphoma as the etiology.
2. PET/CT can precisely localize foci of abnormal FDG uptake with similar patterns on PET to different anatomic structures located in close vicinity.

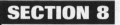

SPECT/CT

Zohar Keidar

8.1 In111-PENTETREOTIDE SPECT/CT

Case 8.1.1 PHYSIOLOGIC—BOWEL AND KIDNEY UPTAKE (FIG. 8.1.1)
In111-PENTETREOTIDE SPECT/LOW-DOSE CT

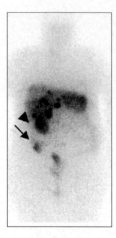
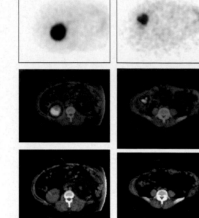

Case 8.1.2 PITFALL—UPTAKE IN GALLBLADDER (FIG. 8.1.2)
In111-PENTETREOTIDE SPECT/MULTISLICE CT

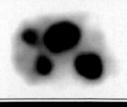
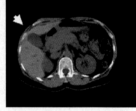
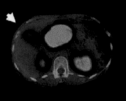
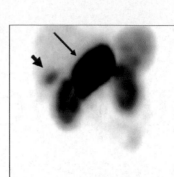

Brief History
A 55-year-old patient with newly diagnosed duodenal carcinoid was referred for whole body staging before surgery.

Findings
Whole body In111-pentetreotide scintigraphy, anterior view (left), shows multiple lesions consistent with liver metastases and additional suspicious foci in the mid-right abdomen (arrowhead) and the right lower quadrant (arrow).

SPECT/CT demonstrates that the right midabdominal focus represents physiologic tracer uptake within a large single right kidney (center column, arrowhead), whereas the right lower abdominal focus is due to physiologic activity in the bowel (right column).

Main Teaching Points and Summary
1. Physiologic In111-pentetreotide bowel activity is common, mainly on scintigraphy performed at 24 hours postinjection. Focal uptake can mimic tumor.
2. Anatomic localization to bowel using SPECT/CT may define the cause of tracer uptake and exclude additional sites of disease.
3. The kidneys are part of the normal biodistribution of In111-pentetreotide. In cases of abnormal or postsurgical distorted anatomy, misinterpretation may be avoided using SPECT/CT.

Brief History
A 48-year-old patient with pancreatic islet cell tumor and no anatomic evidence for distant metastatic disease on CT was referred for whole body assessment after chemotherapy, before surgery.

Findings
Planar In111-pentetreotide scan of the abdomen, anterior view (left), shows two foci of increased tracer uptake in the upper midabdomen (arrow) and in the right aspect of the abdomen (arrowhead).

SPECT/CT (right) localizes the mid-abdominal focus to the lesion in the pancreas and the suspicious right lateral lesion to normal activity in the gallbladder (arrowhead).

Main Teaching Points and Summary
1. The main route of In111-pentetreotide clearance is through renal excretion rather than the hepatobiliary system. Tracer accumulation in the gallbladder may occur, however, most probably related to the fasting state, and may be more extensive if there is reduced renal function.
2. Anatomic localization using SPECT/CT clarifies this unusual site of physiologic accumulation as normal gallbladder, thus avoiding a false-positive report of a liver metastasis.

Case 8.1.3 TUMOR–RESIDUAL CARCINOID (FIG. 8.1.3)
In111-PENTETREOTIDE SPECT/LOW-DOSE CT

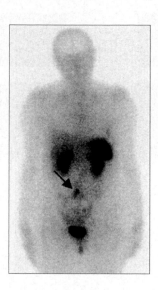
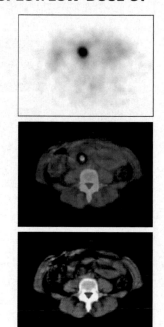

Brief History
A 42-year-old patient, status post–surgical removal of small bowel carcinoid, was referred in search of residual tumor after histologic examination of the surgical specimen revealed positive margins for tumor.

Findings
Whole body In111-pentetreotide scintigraphy, anterior planar view (left), shows an area of focally increased tracer uptake in the midabdomen (arrow).

SPECT/CT (right) localizes the suspicious focus to a small bowel loop, indicating the presence of residual active disease.

Main Teaching Points and Summary
1. Assessing the presence of residual tumor, mainly after surgery, may be difficult because of postoperative anatomic changes.
2. SPECT/CT enhances the detectability rate of residual active tumor and helps in re-explorative surgery planning. In the present case, the focal pattern of uptake weighed against this being excreted activity in the gut.

Case 8.1.4 TUMOR–METASTATIC CARCINOID (FIG. 8.1.4)
In111-PENTETREOTIDE SPECT/LOW-DOSE CT

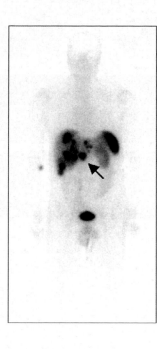
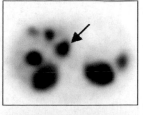
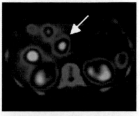
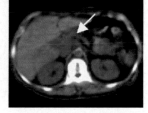

Brief History
A 77-year-old patient with carcinoid, metastatic to the liver, was referred for whole body assessment in search of the primary tumor site.

Findings
Whole body In111-pentetreotide scintigraphy, anterior view (left), shows multiple foci of tracer uptake in the upper right abdomen projecting over the liver.

SPECT/CT (right) localizes one focus to the head of the pancreas (arrow), representing the primary tumor. All additional lesions are consistent with liver metastases.

Main Teaching Points and Summary
1. Carcinoid may present as metastatic disease. Detection of the primary tumor may affect patient management and alter the treatment strategy.
2. Hepatic carcinoid is treated differently in the presence of additional extrahepatic disease (systemic therapy versus liver chemoembolization).
3. It can be difficult on planar imaging alone to separate left hepatic lobe metastases from lesions in the head of the pancreas.
4. SPECT/CT can exclude or confirm the presence of extrahepatic disease. However, even with SPECT/CT, it can sometimes be difficult to separate duodenal wall lesions from involvement of the pancreas.

Case 8.1.5 TUMOR–DISSEMINATED CARCINOID (FIG. 8.1.5) In111-PENTETREOTIDE SPECT/LOW-DOSE CT

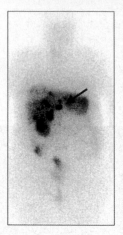
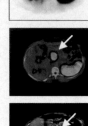
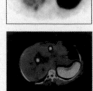
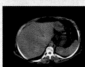

Case 8.1.6 TUMOR–VERTEBRAL METASTASIS, NEUROENDOCRINE TUMOR (FIG. 8.1.6) In111-PENTETREOTIDE SPECT/LOW-DOSE CT

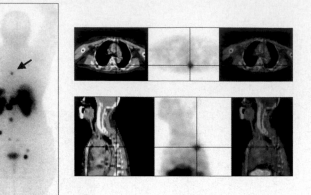

Brief History
A 55-year-old patient with newly diagnosed duodenal carcinoid and no evidence of metastatic disease on CT was referred for whole body assessment before surgery.

Findings
Whole body In111-pentetreotide scintigraphy, anterior view (left), shows multiple foci of tracer uptake in the upper right and midabdomen.

SPECT/CT localizes the primary lesion to the duodenum (center column, arrow) adjacent to the pancreatic head and demonstrates that the additional foci represent multiple liver metastases (right column).

Main Teaching Points and Summary
1. SPECT/CT can accurately demonstrate the extent of disease involvement in the whole body and, specifically, clarify the complex anatomy of the upper abdomen.
2. SPECT/CT also easily separates tracer activity in the left lobe of liver from splenic uptake.

Brief History
A 53-year-old patient, status post–surgical removal of a neuroendocrine tumor from the head of the pancreas, was referred for further assessment of new onset of back pain in the presence of recently diagnosed liver metastases.

Findings
Whole body In111-pentetreotide scintigraphy, posterior view (left) shows a suspicious focus of abnormal uptake projecting over the mid-chest (arrow).

SPECT/CT (right, transaxial slices upper row, sagittal slices lower row) precisely localizes the thoracic lesion to the left costovertebral junction of T6.

Note on planar scintigraphy: Multiple additional lesions in abdomen and pelvis, consistent with disseminated disease to liver and bones, are seen.

The patient was treated with a Lu177-labeled somatostatin analog, with partial regression of the liver metastases and improvement of back pain.

Main Teaching Points and Summary
1. SPECT/CT can accurately localize the tumor spread and improve further patient care.
2. SPECT/CT is helpful in separating foci in the posterior lung from lesions in the posterior mediastinum or spine.

(Case courtesy of Dr. Y. Krausz, Hadassah, Hebrew University Medical Center, Jerusalem, Israel.)

8.2 IODINE131 SPECT/CT

Case 8.2.1 PHYSIOLOGIC—REMNANT THYROID (FIG. 8.2.1)
I131 SPECT/MULTISLICE CT

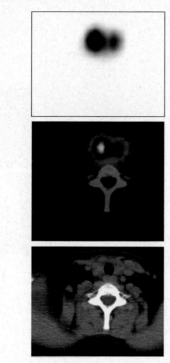

Brief History
A 28-year-old patient with papillary thyroid cancer was evaluated 4 weeks after subtotal thyroidectomy in search of occult metastatic foci.

Findings
Whole body I131 scintigraphy, anterior view (left), shows a focus of increased tracer uptake in the mid-neck.

SPECT/CT (right) localizes this focus to the remnant tissue in the thyroid bed in the anterior aspect of the neck. No pathologic findings are demonstrated on the corresponding CT.

Main Teaching Points and Summary
1. Iodine uptake in remnant thyroid tissue is common after surgery.
2. SPECT/CT can differentiate this pattern from pathologic uptake in metastatic cervical lymphadenopathy.

Case 8.2.2 PHYSIOLOGIC—BOWEL UPTAKE (FIG. 8.2.2)
I131 SPECT/MULTISLICE CT

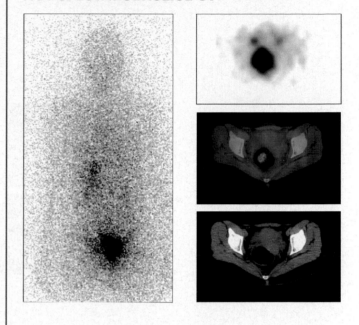

Brief History
A 40-year-old patient with multifocal papillary thyroid cancer, status post–total thyroidectomy, was assessed 6 months after ablative therapy.

Findings
Whole body I131 scintigraphy, posterior view (left), shows an area of increased tracer uptake in the mid-pelvis, of unclear location, representing either a tumor site in the bone or physiologic activity in bowel or possibly bladder.

SPECT/CT (right) localizes the suspicious focus to rectal excretion of I131.

Main Teaching Points and Summary
1. The physiologic biodistribution of I131 includes bowel excretion.
2. Intense and focal bowel accumulation can mimic malignant uptake and requires further investigation. Separating bowel uptake from the urinary bladder may be difficult.
3. Precise SPECT/CT localization may define the etiology of this suspicious site and exclude the need for delayed imaging or other diagnostic procedures.

Case 8.2.3 PITFALL–THYMIC UPTAKE (FIG. 8.2.3)
I131 SPECT/LOW-DOSE CT

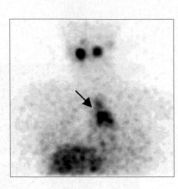

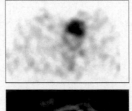

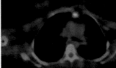

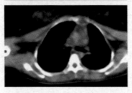

Brief History
A 20-year-old patient with papillary thyroid cancer and cervical lymph node metastases, status post–total thyroidectomy, lymph node dissection, and radioiodine therapy, was assessed after the administration of a therapeutic dose of 5.5 GBq (150 mCi) I131.

Findings
Planar I131 scintigraphy, anterior view (left) shows an area of increased tracer uptake in the left anterior mediastinal region (arrow).

SPECT/CT (right) localizes this focus of increased tracer uptake to the thymus.

Main Teaching Points and Summary
1. Increased radioiodine uptake by the normal thymus can occasionally be found in the posttreatment I131 scan of patients younger than 50 years.
2. These findings are more prominent on the 7-day scan and can be a potential cause of false-positive scintigraphy.
3. Localization of suspicious foci by SPECT/CT may exclude other causes for I131 uptake in the same area, such as mediastinal metastases.

Case 8.2.4 PITFALL–DENTAL AND UTERINE INFLAMMATORY PROCESS (FIG. 8.2.4)
I131 SPECT/MULTISLICE CT

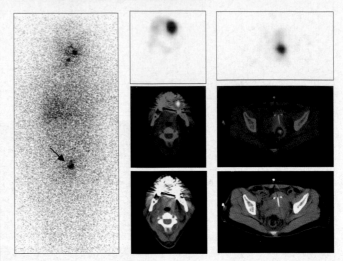

Brief History
A 51-year-old patient with a history of papillary thyroid cancer, status post–near-total thyroidectomy and radioiodine ablation, was assessed following the administration of a therapeutic dose of 3.7 GBq (100 mCi) of I131.

Findings
Whole body I131 scintigraphy, anterior view (left), shows two foci of increased tracer uptake in the mid- and left upper neck, and an additional focus in the midpelvis (arrow).

SPECT/CT at the level of the neck localizes the proximal cervical focus (center column) to a recently performed dental procedure in the left mandible.

Note: The lower cervical focus (not shown) represents remnant thyroid tissue.

SPECT/CT at the level of the pelvis (right column) localizes the suspicious pelvic lesion to the uterine cervix, close to the tip of an intrauterine device seen on CT.

Main Teaching Points and Summary
1. I131 can accumulate in areas of inflammation and infection, potentially leading to false-positive results when investigating thyroid cancer.
2. Accurate localization using SPECT/CT can define a benign etiology and thus eliminate false-positive reports.

Case 8.2.5 PITFALL—UPTAKE IN ECTOPIC STOMACH (FIG. 8.2.5) I131 SPECT/LOW-DOSE CT

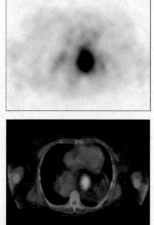

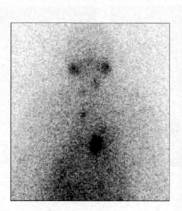

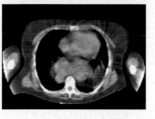

Brief History

A 73-year-old patient with a history of papillary thyroid cancer, status post–near-total thyroidectomy and radio-iodine ablation, was assessed after receiving a therapeutic dose of 3.7 GBq (100 mCi).

Findings

Planar I131 scintigraphy, anterior view (left) shows highly intense tracer uptake in the left mediastinum.

SPECT/CT (right) localizes the increased uptake to an intrathoracic stomach due to diaphragmatic hernia seen on CT.

Note on planar scintigraphy: A focus of increased activity in the upper mediastinum, most probably low thyroid remnant.

Main Teaching Points and Summary

1. The biodistribution of I131 includes accumulation and excretion by the gastric mucosa, commonly demonstrated on scintigraphy.
2. In cases of altered anatomy, gastric uptake may be misinterpreted as disease-related pathology. SPECT/CT can eliminate such false-positive results.

Case 8.2.6 TUMOR—MEDIASTINAL NODAL METASTASIS, THYROID CANCER (FIG. 8.2.6) I131 SPECT/LOW-DOSE CT

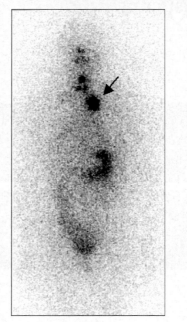

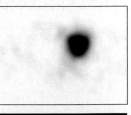

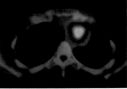

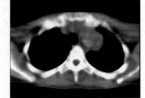

Brief History

A 40-year-old patient with multifocal papillary thyroid cancer, status post–subtotal thyroidectomy, was referred for whole body evaluation at 4 weeks after surgery.

Findings

Whole body I131 scintigraphy, anterior view (left) shows a focus of increased tracer uptake in the left mediastinum (arrow).

SPECT/CT (right) localizes the thoracic lesion to an anterior upper mediastinal mass.

Note on planar scintigraphy: Additional foci of increased tracer uptake in the anterior neck, consistent with thyroid remnant uptake, are seen.

On re-exploration, the mediastinal lesion was confirmed to represent metastatic thyroid cancer.

Main Teaching Points and Summary

1. Thyroid cancer may metastasize to mediastinal lymph nodes, although this is uncommon.
2. I131 SPECT/CT can help in differentiation between mediastinal and pulmonary metastases.

Case 8.2.7 TUMOR–CERVICAL AND SUPRACLAVICULAR NODAL METASTASES, THYROID CANCER (FIG. 8.2.7) I131 SPECT/MULTISLICE CT

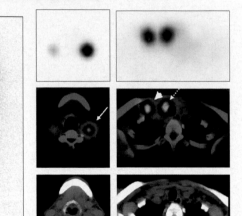

Case 8.2.8 TUMOR–LUNG METASTASIS, THYROID CANCER (FIG. 8.2.8) I131 SPECT/LOW-DOSE CT

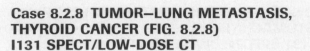

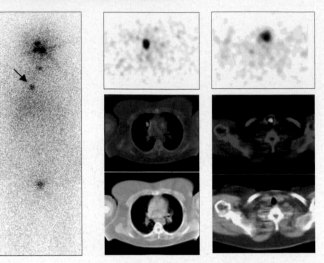

Brief History

A 20-year-old patient with invasive papillary thyroid cancer and multiple cervical lymph node metastases, status post–subtotal thyroidectomy and ablation, was referred for radioiodine treatment. Scintigraphy was performed after receiving the treatment dose of 5.5 GBq (150 mCi) I131.

Findings

Whole body I131 scintigraphy, anterior view (left) shows multiple foci of increased tracer uptake in the neck.

SPECT/CT (right) localizes the abnormal foci as demonstrated in selected sites to cervical (center column) and supraclavicular (right column, arrowhead) metastatic lymph nodes and to the thyroid bed (dotted arrow).

Main Teaching Points and Summary
1. Lymph node involvement can affect the management of thyroid cancer.
2. In most cases SPECT/CT differentiates I131 uptake in lymph nodes from remnant thyroid tissue.
3. SPECT/CT may further define the precise localization of involved lymph nodes of clinical significance when further surgical or radiation treatment is planned.

Brief History

A 64-year-old patient with local recurrence of papillary thyroid cancer, status post–radioiodine treatment, was assessed after the administration of the therapeutic dose of 5.5 GBq (150 mCi) I131.

Findings

Whole body I131 scintigraphy, anterior view (left) shows a site of focal uptake in the lower right chest (arrow).

SPECT/CT localizes the suspicious thoracic lesion to the medial aspect of the lower lobe of the right lung, suggesting the presence of a previously unknown lung metastasis (center column), despite the fact that no anatomic lesion is seen on the corresponding low-dose CT.

A 6-mm pulmonary nodule was found on subsequently performed high-resolution CT.

Note: Additional foci of increased tracer uptake in the neck are localized by SPECT/CT (right column) to tracer activity in remnant thyroid tissue.

Main Teaching Points and Summary
1. Small lung metastases from thyroid cancer can be I131-avid.
2. SPECT/CT can diagnose small, previously undetected pulmonary lesions, with implications for further surgery or radioiodine therapy.
3. In cases in which the quality of CT is inadequate to achieve optimal lesion detection, a full diagnostic CT may be required.

Case 8.2.9 TUMOR–BONE METASTASIS, THYROID CANCER (FIG. 8.2.9) I131 SPECT/MULTISLICE CT

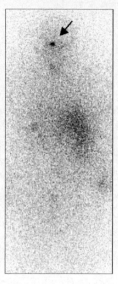
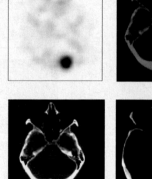

Brief History
A 59-year-old patient with recurrent papillary thyroid cancer, status post–radioiodine treatment, was assessed after receiving the therapeutic dose of 5.5 GBq (150 mCi) of I131.

Findings
Whole body I131 scintigraphy, posterior view (left) shows a focus of increased tracer uptake in the region of the head (arrow).

SPECT/CT (right, upper row) localizes the suspicious focus to the occipital bone.

Matched CT slices assessed with bone window setting (right, lower row) show a small lytic lesion in the same location, confirming the suspicion of a bone metastasis (arrow).

Main Teaching Points and Summary
1. Diagnosis of bone metastases may affect prognosis and treatment of patients with thyroid cancer.
2. Localization of focal uptake to a lesion in the skull is critical because the scalp is a common site of external contamination, which can occasionally cause a false-positive scan for bone metastases.
3. SPECT/CT localizes focal I131 uptake within the bone and helps in planning the treatment of localized disease.

Case 8.2.10 TUMOR–BONE METASTASES, THYROID CANCER (FIG. 8.2.10) I131 SPECT/LOW-DOSE CT

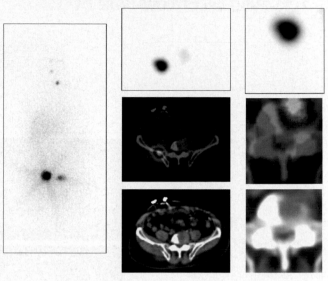

Brief History
A 55-year-old patient with mixed follicular and papillary thyroid cancer, status post–subtotal thyroidectomy, was referred for whole body evaluation after surgery.

Findings
Whole body I131 scintigraphy, posterior view (left) shows two foci of abnormal activity in the pelvic area.

SPECT/CT localizes the prominent right focus to the iliac bone (center column) and the second midline lesion to the body of the S1 vertebra (right column), in areas showing corresponding lytic lesions on CT, consistent with bone metastases are seen.

Note on planar scintigraphy: Two additional foci of increased uptake in the neck, consistent with thyroid remnant and lymph node metastases.

Main Teaching Points and Summary
1. Diagnosis of bone metastases may affect thyroid cancer management.
2. SPECT/CT can identify I131 uptake within the bone and differentiate this from adjacent soft tissue or physiologic sites (e.g., bowel).

8.3 IODINE123-METAIODOBENZYL-GUANIDINE (MIBG) SPECT/CT

Case 8.3.1 PHYSIOLOGIC—CARDIAC UPTAKE (FIG. 8.3.1)
I123-MIBG SPECT/LOW-DOSE CT

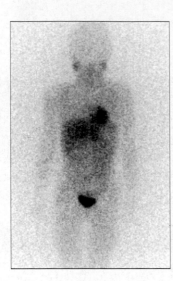

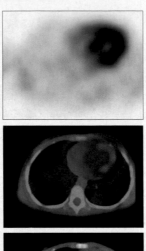

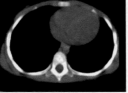

Brief History

A 12-year-old patient with a history of neuroblastoma was referred to assess response to treatment.

Findings

Whole body I123-MIBG scintigraphy, anterior view (left) shows increased tracer uptake in the lower left midchest.

SPECT/CT (right) localizes the area of homogenously increased activity to the heart. The study was interpreted as negative for tumor recurrence.

Main Teaching Points and Summary

1. MIBG is taken up by the myocardium because of its adrenergic innervation. Tracer uptake in the heart may be particularly high in young children.
2. The paracardiac region needs to be examined carefully to avoid false-negative reports when pathology is masked by physiologic tracer uptake.

Case 8.3.2 PHYSIOLOGIC—INHOMOGENEOUS CARDIAC UPTAKE, ISCHEMIC HEART DISEASE AND PHEOCHROMOCYTOMA (FIG. 8.3.2)
I123-MIBG SPECT/LOW-DOSE CT

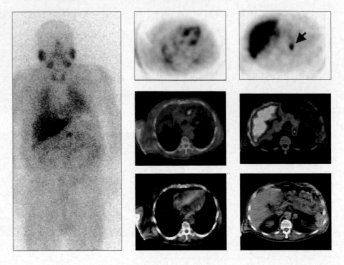

Brief History

A 70-year-old patient with ischemic heart disease, congestive heart failure, and uncontrolled hypertension was found to have elevated serum catecholamine levels and was referred with the clinical suspicion of pheochromocytoma.

Findings

Whole body I123-MIBG scintigraphy, anterior view (left), shows mildly increased tracer uptake in both lungs and in the lower left chest. Focal uptake is demonstrated on whole body scintigraphy in the upper left abdomen.

SPECT/CT shows inhomogeneous myocardial uptake (center column). The focus of tracer uptake in the upper left abdomen localizes to the left adrenal and represents a pheochromocytoma (right column, arrow).

Main Teaching Point and Summary

1. A pattern of inhomogeneous or a segmental decrease in myocardial uptake of MIBG in patients with ischemic heart disease and congestive heart failure is associated with a poor prognosis.

Case 8.3.3 PHYSIOLOGIC—RENAL UPTAKE (FIG. 8.3.3)
I123-MIBG SPECT/MULTISLICE CT

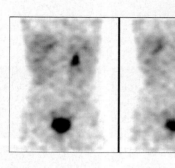

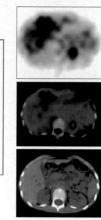

Brief History
An 8-year-old patient with stage 4 neuroblastoma involving the right adrenal and bone marrow was referred to assess response to treatment.

Findings
Selected coronal SPECT slices (left) show focally increased tracer uptake in the region of the left adrenal.

SPECT/CT (right) localizes the suspicious focus to the left renal pelvis that appears enlarged on CT.

Ultrasound and renal scintigraphy confirmed the presence of moderate left hydronephrosis, unrelated to the primary disease.

Main Teaching Points and Summary
1. MIBG is excreted by the kidneys. In the presence of hydronephrosis or renal obstruction, tracer uptake may be asymmetric and focal, of moderate to high intensity.
2. SPECT/CT can accurately localize a suspicious focus to enlarged renal calyces or the renal pelvis, thus avoiding misinterpretation of urinary activity as tumor.

Case 8.3.4 PHYSIOLOGIC—ADRENAL UPTAKE (FIG. 8.3.4)
I123-MIBG SPECT/MULTISLICE CT

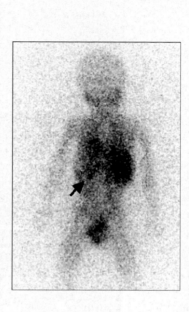

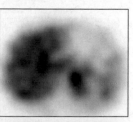

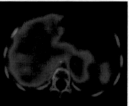

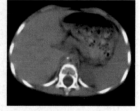

Brief History
A 4-year-old patient with a history of stage 4 neuroblastoma involving the right adrenal and bone marrow was referred for routine follow-up 1 year after completion of treatment.

Findings
Whole body I123-MIBG scintigraphy, posterior view (left) shows focally increased tracer uptake in the left upper abdomen (arrow).

SPECT/CT (right) localizes the suspicious focus to a normal sized left adrenal gland.

The patient remained in complete remission for a clinical follow-up of 24 months.

Main Teaching Points and Summary
1. MIBG is taken up by normal adrenal glands, showing a characteristic pattern of symmetric, faint uptake.
2. In cases of a missing adrenal gland (such as surgical removal in this case) unilateral uptake can be misinterpreted as active tumor.

Case 8.3.5 TUMOR—BILATERAL PHEOCHROMOCYTOMA (FIG. 8.3.5) I123-MIBG SPECT/MULTISLICE CT

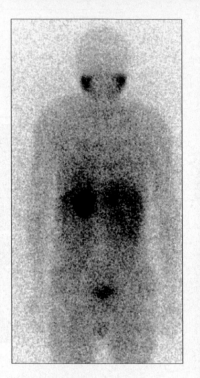
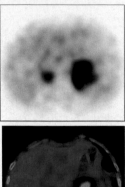
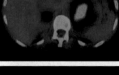

Brief History
A 38-year-old patient with neurofibromatosis was referred for a clinically suspected pheochromocytoma.

Findings
Whole body I123-MIBG scintigraphy, posterior view (left), shows two foci of increased tracer uptake in the upper abdomen, more prominent in the left flank.

SPECT/CT (right) localizes the lesions to an extremely enlarged and inhomogeneous left adrenal and a mildly enlarged right adrenal gland, consistent with bilateral pheochromocytoma.

Main Teaching Points and Summary
1. Neurofibromatosis is an autosomal-dominant disorder that affects the bone, nervous system, soft tissues, and skin.
2. Neurofibromatosis may be associated with pheo-chromocytoma involving either one or both adrenals.
3. SPECT/CT can separate renal from adrenal tracer activity and allow precise localization of extraadrenal pheochromocytomas.

Case 8.3.6 TUMOR—NEUROBLASTOMA AND BONE MARROW INVOLVEMENT (FIG. 8.3.6) I123-MIBG SPECT/LOW-DOSE CT

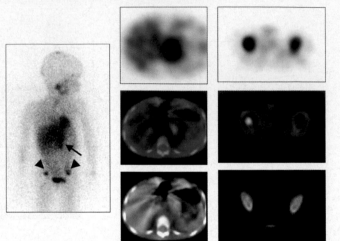
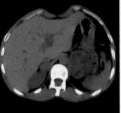

Brief History
A 4-year-old patient with newly diagnosed neuroblastoma was referred for staging.

Findings
Whole body I123-MIBG scintigraphy, anterior view (left), shows an area of increased tracer uptake in the mid-abdomen (arrow) and two suspicious sites in the pelvis on both sides (arrowheads). Additional foci are demonstrated in the skull.

SPECT/CT localizes the midabdominal focus (center column) to the known primary neuroblastoma and demonstrates the intramedullary location of the pelvic foci in the iliac bones (right column), indicating bone marrow involvement.

Stage 4 disease was confirmed histologically.

Main Teaching Points and Summary
1. In patients with newly diagnosed neuroblastoma, MIBG SPECT/CT is performed to optimize initial staging and treatment planning.
2. Follow-up SPECT/CT studies after surgery can assess for the presence of residual tumor.
3. MIBG SPECT/CT is of value in patients with stage 4 and 4s disease for diagnosis of a subclinical relapse, especially in the bone marrow, and for evaluation of new onset of bone pain.
4. SPECT/CT can differentiate between a retroperito-neal tumor and metastases in the left lobe of the liver.

8.4 GALLIUM67 SPECT/CT

Case 8.4.1 PHYSIOLOGIC—THYMIC UPTAKE (FIG. 8.4.1)
Ga67 SPECT/LOW-DOSE CT

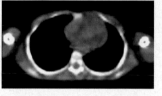
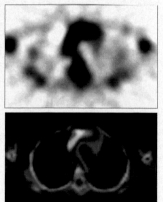
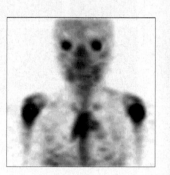

Brief History

An 11-year-old patient, 6 months after the completion of chemotherapy for Hodgkin's lymphoma involving the cervical lymph nodes, was referred for routine follow-up.

Findings

Planar Ga67 scintigraphy, anterior view (left), shows an area of increased radiotracer uptake in the anterior mediastinum.

SPECT/CT (right) localizes this focus of increased tracer uptake to the thymus.

No evidence for active tumor was found during long-term follow-up.

Main Teaching Points and Summary
1. Ga67 uptake can be commonly demonstrated in the thymus of young children.
2. In patients after chemotherapy, thymic hyperplasia (thymic "rebound") may result in variable degrees of tracer uptake, unrelated to the presence of active lymphoma.

Case 8.4.2 BENIGN—INFECTION, OSTEOMYELITIS (FIG. 8.4.2)
Ga67 SPECT/MULTISLICE CT

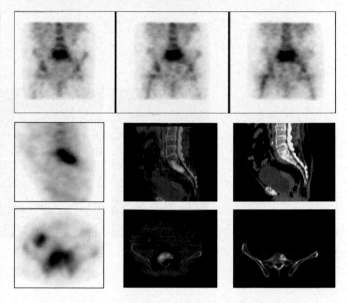

Brief History

A 63-year-old patient with fever and pelvic pain was referred with the clinical suspicion of a pelvic abscess. Ultrasound and CT of the abdominopelvic region had been reported as normal.

Findings

Selected coronal Ga67 SPECT slices (upper row) show an area of intense uptake in the posterior aspect of the midpelvis.

Sagittal (center row) and transaxial (lower row) SPECT/CT slices localize this abnormal uptake to the sacrum, consistent with osteomyelitis with no soft tissue involvement.

Note on transaxial SPECT/CT images: Increased activity in the cecum, a normal site of Ga67 excretion, is seen.

Main Teaching Points and Summary
1. SPECT/CT can define the precise localization of an infectious process and diagnose osteomyelitis.
2. A comparative bone scan could also be helpful but unnecessary when uptake is localized to the skeleton by SPECT/CT.

Case 8.4.3 BENIGN–INFECTION, BONE AND SOFT TISSUE, AND BOWEL UPTAKE (FIG. 8.4.3) Ga67 SPECT/LOW-DOSE CT

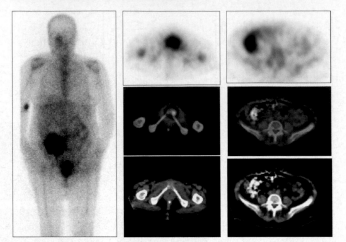

Case 8.4.4 BENIGN–INFECTION, PARAVERTEBRAL ABSCESS (FIG. 8.4.4) Ga67 SPECT/LOW-DOSE CT

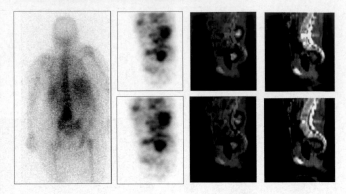

Brief History

A 60-year-old patient with fever of unknown origin, weight loss, and lower abdominal pain was referred in search of an occult abscess. Abdominal ultrasound was reported to be normal.

Findings

Whole body Ga67 scintigraphy, anterior view (left), performed 24 hours after tracer injection shows an area of abnormal uptake in the midpelvis and an additional site of intense activity in the right lower abdomen.

SPECT/CT localizes the pelvic uptake (center column) to a soft tissue mass located anterior to the symphysis pubis also involving the pubic bones, with a corresponding lytic lesion on the left, on CT. The abdominal focus (right column) represents physiologic bowel activity.

On follow-up, the patient had a soft tissue abscess in the anterior pelvis and osteomyelitis of the pubis and was treated with prolonged intravenous antibacterial therapy.

Main Teaching Points and Summary
1. SPECT/CT can determine the precise extent of an infectious process, define all involved structures, and thus optimize further treatment planning.
2. Physiologic Ga67 bowel uptake is very common, mainly in early studies performed less than 72 hours after injection. Physiologic urinary activity is not common.
3. If focal, physiologic Ga67 uptake can mimic an abscess or tumor. SPECT/CT localization may provide the differential diagnosis, without the need for repeat delayed scintigraphy.

Brief History

A 73-year-old patient, status post–lumbar spine surgery 8 months before the current study, presented with fever and complaints of severe back pain. He was assessed for clinically suspected osteomyelitis.

Findings

Whole body Ga67 scintigraphy, posterior view (left) shows an area of increased tracer uptake in the lower back.

Sagittal SPECT/CT slices at two levels (right) localize the suspicious lesion to soft tissues posterior to the lumbar spine. Metallic screws are demonstrated on the CT component at the level of L3–L4 vertebra.

Based on SPECT/CT data, soft tissue infection without bone involvement was diagnosed. No evidence for osteomyelitis was found on further clinical and imaging follow-up.

Main Teaching Points and Summary
1. Differentiation between soft tissue and bone infection is critical for accurate patient management.
2. In this patient, conventional imaging including CT, magnetic resonance imaging, and bone scintigraphy, is made difficult by the presence of postoperative changes and metallic devices.

Case 8.4.5 BENIGN—INFECTION, LIVER ABSCESS (FIG. 8.4.5) Ga67 SPECT/LOW-DOSE CT

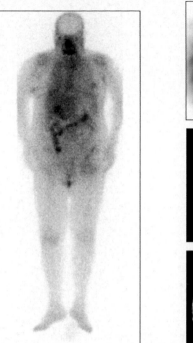

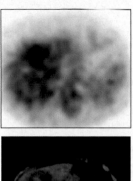

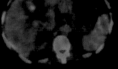

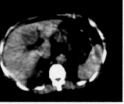

Brief History
A 64-year-old diabetic patient with pyelonephritis, unresponsive to broad-spectrum antibiotic therapy, was referred to rule out the presence of an intra-abdominal abscess. Abdominal ultrasound was reported as normal, but contrast-enhanced CT was not performed because of the patient's impaired renal function.

Findings
Whole body scintigraphy, anterior view (left) shows a focus of mildly increased tracer uptake in the right upper abdomen.

SPECT/CT (right) localizes the suspicious focus in the right upper abdomen to a space-occupying lesion in the liver.

High-resolution contrast-enhanced CT (following thorough nephrologic preparation and supervision) confirmed the SPECT/CT findings, and drainage of a liver abscess was further performed.

Main Teaching Points and Summary
1. The physiologic biodistribution of Ga-67 is characterized by variable degrees of liver uptake. Focal uptake within the liver may be difficult to detect.
2. SPECT/CT can localize suspicious foci with abnormally increased uptake and guide diagnostic and therapeutic procedures.
3. In this case, without SPECT/CT, focal liver uptake could have been confused with activity in the gallbladder without SPECT/CT.

Case 8.4.6 TUMOR—LYMPHOMA INVOLVING THE HEAD AND NECK AND MEDIASTINUM (FIG. 8.4.6) Ga67 SPECT/LOW-DOSE CT

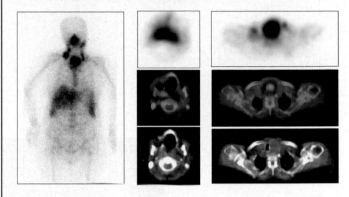

Brief History
A 70-year-old patient with newly diagnosed large-cell non-Hodgkin's lymphoma was referred for a baseline study to establish Ga67 avidity.

Findings
Whole body Ga67 scintigraphy, anterior view (left) shows multiple areas of increased tracer uptake in the region of the head, neck, and upper mediastinum.

Transaxial SPECT/CT slices at two levels localize the lesions to the nasopharynx (center column) and to a large paratracheal mass at the thoracic inlet with deviation of the trachea (right column).

Main Teaching Point and Summary
1. Accurate localization of scintigraphic findings through anatomic correlation may be further used to guide tissue sampling biopsy and radiation treatment planning.

Case 8.4.7 TUMOR–LYMPHOMA IN PELVIC MASS (FIG. 8.4.7)
Ga67 SPECT/LOW-DOSE CT

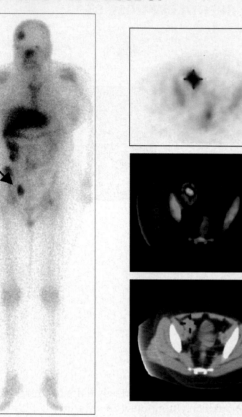

Brief History

A 24-year-old patient with a history of Hodgkin's lymphoma, 2 years after the end of therapy, was referred for routine follow-up.

Findings

Whole body Ga67 scintigraphy, anterior view (left) shows intense tracer uptake in the right abdomen and pelvis (arrow) which may represent physiologic bowel excretion.

SPECT/CT (right) localizes the lesion in the right pelvis to a soft tissue mass and not to bowel activity. Additional foci of increased uptake in the right abdomen were localized by SPECT/CT (not shown) to physiologic bowel activity.

Note on planar scintigraphy: A lesion in the right lateral aspect of the head, consistent with brain involvement, was further confirmed on magnetic resonance imaging.

Main Teaching Points and Summary

1. Accurate localization of scintigraphic findings avoided misinterpretation of right lower quadrant activity as physiologic bowel excretion of the tracer.
2. The pelvis is a challenging area for Ga67 scintigraphy to assess without SPECT/CT.

Case 8.4.8 TUMOR–LYMPHOMA IN MUSCLE, PITFALLS: RIB FRACTURE AND LUNG INFILTRATE (FIG. 8.4.8) Ga67 SPECT/LOW-DOSE CT

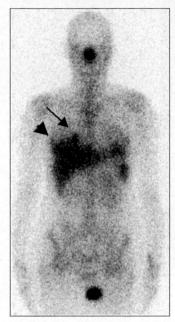

A

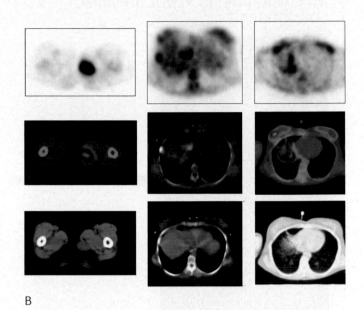

B

Brief History

A 39-year-old patient with a history of Hodgkin's lymphoma, status post–bone marrow transplantation, was referred for clinically suspected recurrence following new onset of left groin pain.

Findings

A. Whole body Ga67 scintigraphy, anterior view, shows an area of intense tracer uptake in the medial aspect of the left sub-pubic region. In addition, there are two areas of focal tracer uptake in the anterior (arrow) and lateral aspect (arrow head) of the lower right chest.

B. SPECT/CT at the level of the thighs (left column) localizes the inguinal lesion to a soft tissue mass at the medial aspect of the left thigh, adjacent to the gracilis muscle.

SPECT/CT at the level of the thorax localizes the lateral chest focus (center column) to a sclerotic bone lesion in a right lower rib, related to a recent fracture, and the anterior chest finding (right column) to a pulmonary infiltrate related to intercurrent inflammatory lung disease.

Note on SPECT/CT (B, center column): Diffuse, moderately increased symmetrical uptake in the breast tissue.

Recurrent Hodgkin's lymphoma was diagnosed histologically from biopsy of the lesion in the thigh. There was no evidence for recurrent Hodgkin's in the thorax on clinical and imaging follow-up.

Main Teaching Points and Summary

1. SPECT/CT may accurately localize and define suspicious foci in unusual locations, thus guiding further invasive procedures for histopathologic confirmation.

2. Ga67 is also a bone-seeking agent and therefore accumulates in benign lesions such as fractures and degenerative or arthritic changes unrelated to lymphoma. SPECT/CT can establish the benign etiology of skeletal lesions, thus reducing false-positive interpretations.

8.5 In111 CAPROMAB PENDETIDE (PROSTASCINT)—SPECT/CT

Case 8.5.1 NORMAL STUDY (FIG. 8.5.1) In111-CAPROMAB PENDETIDE SPECT/ LOW-DOSE CT

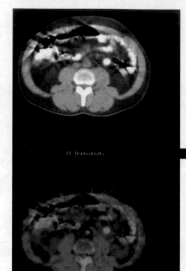
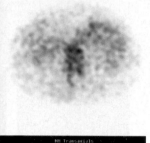
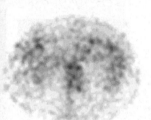

A

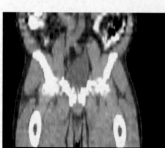
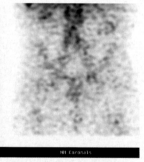

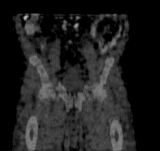
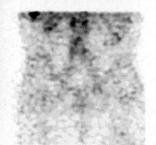

B

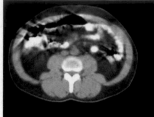
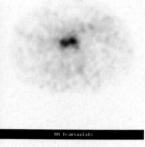

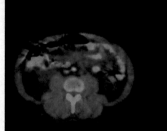
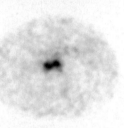

C

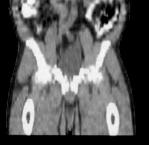
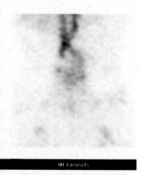

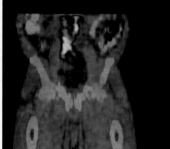
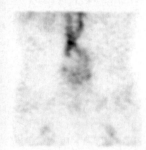

D

Brief History

A 68-year-old patient with a history of prostate cancer, after prostatectomy, presented with increasing prostate specific antigen levels (last measured value 0.8) following CT and bone scintigraphy reported as negative. The patient was referred to In111-capromab pendetide scintigraphy to evaluate for the presence of active tumor.

Findings

A and B. In111-capromab pendetide SPECT/CT images, transaxial (A) and coronal (B) slices of the abdomen and pelvis, show normal physiologic tracer activity within the blood pool, liver, spleen, bone marrow, bowel, kidney, and genitalia. No areas of abnormal radiotracer uptake suggestive of metastases are identified.

C and D. Tc99m-RBC SPECT/CT images, transaxial (C) and coronal (D) slices of the abdomen and pelvis, show physiologic blood pool activity within the heart, vascular space, liver, spleen, kidneys, and bladder.

Main Teaching Points and Summary

1. Although a prostate specific agent, this tracer has considerable normal tissue uptake because of the slow biologic clearance rates of intact IgG.
2. Gut excretion of the tracer can be variable.
3. Precise localization and characterization of findings is important to achieve diagnostic accuracy.
4. Blood pool scintigraphy has been traditionally added, providing functional landmarks that may facilitate to some extent the interpretation of the study. With the use of SPECT/CT, this additional procedure becomes less relevant.

Case 8.5.2 TUMOR—ABDOMINAL LYMPHADENOPATHY, PROSTATE CANCER (FIG. 8.5.2)
In111-CAPROMAB PENDETIDE SPECT/MULTISLICE CT

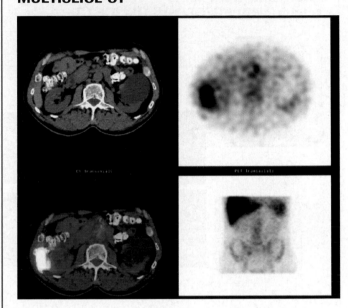

Brief History

A 65-year-old patient with a history of prostate cancer received brachytherapy 6 months before the scan with implantation of 116 seeds. CT and bone scintigraphy performed 3 months prior were reported as negative. Rising prostate specific antigen levels prompted an In111 capromab pendetide study to evaluate for the presence of active tumor.

Findings

SPECT/CT images taken on day 6 after injection of 5 mCi show two foci of abnormally increased tracer uptake that fuse to normal-sized mesenteric and aortocaval lymph nodes, highly suspicious for metastatic prostate cancer. Normal intense hepatic tracer uptake represents physiologic activity because of metabolism of In111 labeled antibodies by the liver. An incidental left renal cyst is not tracer-avid.

Main Teaching Points and Summary

1. Optimal imaging of In111-capromab pendetide requires SPECT, and ideally SPECT/CT, to localize lesions.
2. Because the radiolabeled antibody accumulates in normal tissues, SPECT/CT is critical to separate pathologic from physiologic activity.

8.6 Tc99m-METHOXYISOBUTYL ISONITRILE (MIBI) SPECT/CT (PARATHYROID IMAGING)

Case 8.6.1 PITFALL—ASYMMETRIC SALIVARY GLAND UPTAKE AND PARATHYROID ADENOMA (FIG. 8.6.1)
Tc99m-MIBI SPECT/MULTISLICE CT

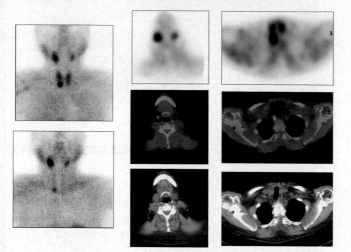

Case 8.6.2 TUMOR—PARATHYROID ADENOMA, RIGHT NECK (FIG. 8.6.2)
Tc99m-MIBI SPECT/MULTISLICE CT

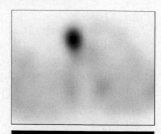
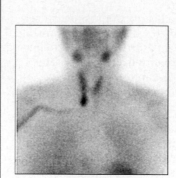
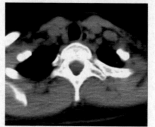
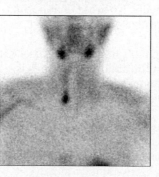

Brief History
A 60-year-old osteoporotic patient with biochemically suspected hyperparathyroidism was referred in search of a parathyroid adenoma.

Findings
Planar Tc99m-MIBI images at 10 (top left) and 120 (bottom left) minutes after tracer injection show focal uptake at the lower pole of the right thyroid lobe consistent with a parathyroid adenoma. Asymmetrically increased tracer uptake is demonstrated in the right submandibular area.

SPECT/CT localizes the increased right submandibular uptake (center column) to an enlarged salivary gland and a left hypoplasic gland, representing compensatory right hyperplasia. The adenoma is localized to the right posterior paratracheal region (right column).

Main Teaching Points and Summary
1. There is physiologic uptake of Tc99m-MIBI by the salivary glands. Asymmetric uptake should be reported with caution.
2. SPECT/CT differentiates these benign variants from findings related to an ectopic superior parathyroid adenoma.

Brief History
A 51-year-old patient with biochemically suspected hyperparathyroidism was referred in search of a parathyroid adenoma.

Findings
Planar Tc99m-MIBI scintigraphy (left) at 10 (top left) and 120 (bottom left) minutes after tracer injection show focal uptake below the lower pole of the right thyroid lobe.

SPECT/CT (right) localizes the suspicious focus to a right posterior paratracheal lesion, 8 mm in diameter.

Diagnosis, localization, and size of the adenoma were further confirmed at surgery.

Main Teaching Point and Summary
1. Accurate SPECT/CT localization of parathyroid adenomas is important for planning minimally invasive surgery.

Case 8.6.3 TUMOR–PARATHYROID ADENOMA, LEFT NECK (FIG. 8.6.3) Tc99m-MIBI SPECT/LOW-DOSE CT

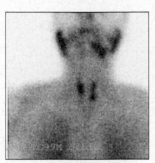
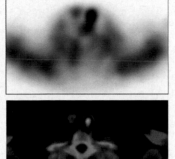
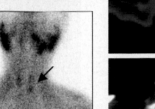
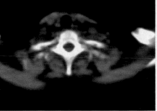

Brief History
A 67-year-old patient with a history of parathyroid adenoma surgically removed 1 year before scintigraphy presented with recurrent biochemical hyperparathyroidism and was evaluated prior to re-exploration.

Findings
Planar Tc99m-MIBI scintigraphy (left) at 10 (top left) and 120 (bottom left) minutes after tracer injection show mild focal uptake at the lower pole of the left thyroid lobe (arrow).

SPECT/CT (right) localizes the suspicious focus to a small left paratracheal lesion, consistent with a recurrent anterior parathyroid adenoma.

Main Teaching Points and Summary
1. Accurate localization of suspected parathyroid adenoma is important for successful minimally invasive surgery.
2. In patients with recurrent disease, distorted anatomy and tissue adhesions may complicate and prolong the surgical procedure. Precise localization of suspicious findings using SPECT/CT may be mandatory in this specific clinical setting.

Case 8.6.4 TUMOR–ECTOPIC PARATHYROID ADENOMA (FIG. 8.6.4) Tc99m-MIBI SPECT/LOW-DOSE CT

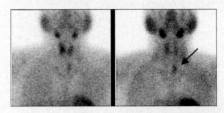
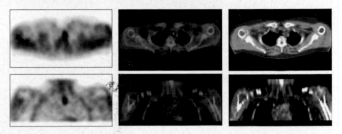

Brief History
A 65-year-old patient with biochemically suspected hyperparathyroidism was referred for diagnosis and localization of a parathyroid adenoma before surgery.

Findings
Planar Tc99m-MIBI scintigraphy (top row) at 10 (left) and 120 (right) minutes after tracer injection show focal uptake in the upper midchest at the level of the suprasternal notch (arrow).

SPECT/CT, transaxial (center row) and coronal (bottom row) slices, demonstrates the precise localization of the upper mediastinal, paratracheal lesion above the aortic arch.

Main Teaching Points and Summary
1. Diagnosis of an ectopic parathyroid adenoma is generally difficult, as is planning the optimal surgical approach.
2. SPECT/CT contributes to precise localization and surgical planning in patients with deep-seated and ectopic adenomas.

8.7 Tc99m-METHYLENE DIPHOSPHONATE (MDP) SPECT/CT

Case 8.7.1 PITFALL—UPTAKE RELATED TO A RENAL CALCULUS (FIG. 8.7.1)
Tc99m-MDP SPECT/LOW-DOSE CT

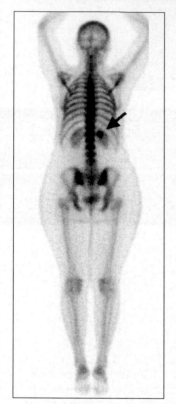
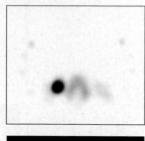
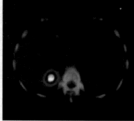
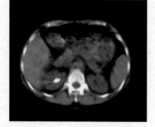

Brief History
A 45-year-old patient with newly diagnosed breast cancer was referred for metastatic workup.

Findings
Planar Tc99m-MDP scintigraphy, posterior view (left), shows intense tracer uptake in right lower rib area (arrow).

SPECT/CT (right) localizes this focus to the region of a calcified renal calculus in the right renal pelvis.

Main Teaching Points and Summary
1. Exclusion of skeletal metastases in cancer patients is of clinical significance.
2. In this case, SPECT/CT accurately localized Tc99m-MDP uptake to the renal pelvis, most likely because of urinary retention caused by local obstruction as well as possibly some uptake into the stone itself.

Case 8.7.2 BENIGN—FACET JOINT DISEASE (FIG. 8.7.2)
Tc99m-MDP SPECT/LOW-DOSE CT

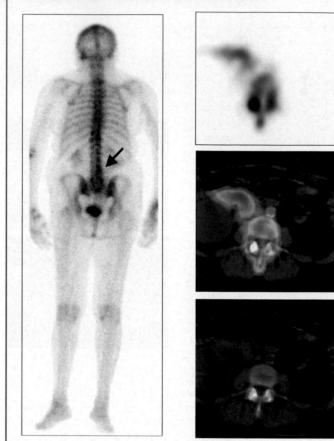

Brief History
A 76-year-old patient with newly diagnosed breast cancer was referred in search for bone metastases.

Findings
Planar Tc99m-MDP scintigraphy, posterior view (left), shows an area of increased tracer uptake in the lower lumbar spine (arrow).

SPECT/CT (right) localizes this focus to the right articular facet joint consistent with arthritic changes.

No evidence for bone metastasis was found in long-term follow-up.

Main Teaching Points and Summary
1. Diagnosis or exclusion of bone metastases in patients with cancer is important for further treatment decisions.
2. SPECT/CT accurately localizes tracer uptake to a specific region within the vertebrae and facilitates diagnosis of benign skeletal lesions, as well as their separation from malignancy.

Case 8.7.3 BENIGN—OSTEOARTHRITIS IN HIP (FIG. 8.7.3)
Tc99m-MDP SPECT/LOW-DOSE CT

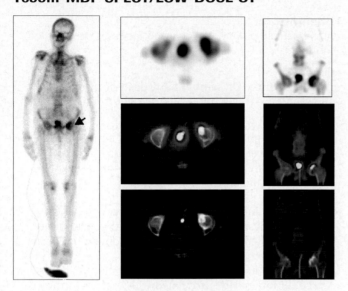

Brief History
A 75-year-old patient with newly diagnosed transitional cell carcinoma (TCC) of the urinary bladder was referred for exclusion of bone metastases.

Findings
Planar Tc99m-MDP scintigraphy, anterior view (left) shows an area of intense tracer uptake in the region of the left hip (arrow).

SPECT/CT, transaxial (center column) and coronal (right column) slices, localizes this lesion to the left acetabulum. On CT, there are severe degenerative changes characterized by subchondral cysts and joint-space narrowing in the same location.

No evidence for bone metastases was found in long-term follow-up.

Main Teaching Points and Summary
1. Highly intense tracer uptake has been described in severe osteoarthritic changes.
2. SPECT/CT demonstrates associated anatomic lesions on the CT component and thus excludes the presence of malignancy.

Case 8.7.4 BENIGN—FIBROUS DYSPLASIA (FIG. 8.7.4)
Tc99m-MDP SPECT/LOW-DOSE CT

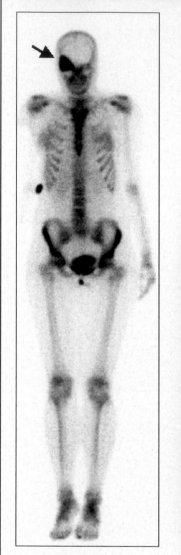

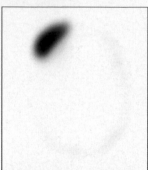

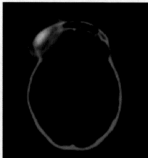

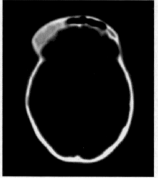

Brief History
A 19-year-old patient was referred for assessment of left foot pain.

Findings
Planar Tc99m-MDP scintigraphy, posterior view (left), shows intense tracer uptake in the right frontal bone (arrow).

SPECT/CT (right) localizes this focus of abnormally increased tracer uptake to a ground glass lesion on CT, consistent with fibrous dysplasia involving the right frontal bone and sinus.

Main Teaching Points and Summary
1. Fibrous dysplasia is a chronic disorder, with bone expanding due to abnormal development of fibrous tissue.
2. Although it can be asymptomatic in nature, this condition may be associated with bone deformity and pain, and growing tumor must be excluded.

Case 8.7.5 BENIGN—MYOSITIS OSSIFICANS (FIG. 8.7.5)
Tc99m-MDP SPECT/LOW-DOSE CT

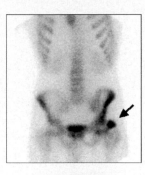

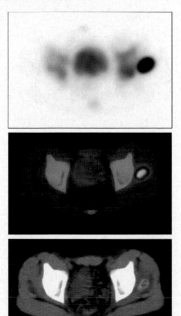

Brief History
A 17-year-old athlete was evaluated for left hip pain.

Findings
Planar Tc99m-MDP scintigraphy (left), anterior (top left) and posterior (bottom left) view of the pelvis, shows an area of intense tracer uptake in the left hip area (arrow).

SPECT/CT (right) localizes this focus to a calcified lesion in the soft tissue adjacent to but not involving the proximal left femur. The CT pattern is highly suggestive for myositis ossificans.

No specific treatment was initiated, and the pain resolved spontaneously.

Main Teaching Points and Summary
1. Myositis (or hematoma) ossificans is a benign condition usually related to previous trauma. As a rule, the lesion is self-limiting and shows spontaneous resolution.
2. SPECT/CT is helpful in localizing increased Tc99m-MDP uptake to bone or soft tissue calcifications.

Case 8.7.6 BENIGN—HEMATOMA AT PRIOR INJECTION SITE (FIG. 8.7.6)
Tc99m-MDP SPECT/LOW-DOSE CT

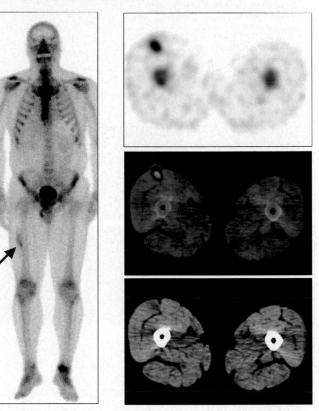

Brief History
A 37-year-old patient with a history of chronic osteochondritis dissecans of the left talus, status post–osteotomy of the left medial malleolus, was referred for assessment of persistent left ankle pain.

Findings
Planar Tc99m-MDP scintigraphy, anterior view (left) shows an incidentally found area of mildly increased tracer activity in the mid-third of right thigh (arrow). In addition, there is intense tracer uptake in left ankle due to previous surgery.

SPECT/CT (right) localizes the lesion in the thigh to a hypodense soft tissue intramuscular lesion.

Review of the patient's file and focused physical examination demonstrated the presence of a hematoma in this area, related to intramuscular injection of analgesics.

Main Teaching Point and Summary
1. Granulomatous tissues and calcifications can appear after intramuscular injections and can accumulate Tc99m-MDP.

8.8 In111-LABELED LEUKOCYTES SPECT/CT

Case 8.8.1 DIABETIC FOOT—OSTEOMYELITIS AND SOFT TISSUE INFECTION (FIG. 8.8.1) In111–WHITE BLOOD CELL (WBC) SPECT/LOW-DOSE CT

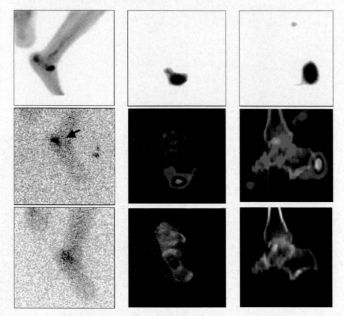

Brief History

A 65-year-old diabetic patient, status post–below left knee amputation, presented with a nonhealing infected wound in the right heel, without any evidence for bone involvement on plain x-ray imaging. The patient was assessed for suspected osteomyelitis.

Findings

Planar scintigraphy of the right foot, lateral view (left column, Tc99m-MDP top, In111-WBC center, Tc99m-sulfur colloid bottom), shows an area of increased tracer uptake in the right heel (arrow).

SPECT/CT with In111-WBC, transaxial (center column) and sagittal (right column) slices, localizes this lesion to the posterior aspect of the calcaneus and the adjacent soft tissue.

Note on planar scintigraphy: An additional focus of increased uptake is demonstrated on bone scintigraphy

only in the tarsal region, most probably due to severe diabetic arthropathy changes.

Main Teaching Points and Summary

1. Diabetic foot osteomyelitis is a challenging diagnosis and occurs, as a rule, as the result of direct contamination from a soft tissue lesion.
2. Even with the combined use of bone, bone marrow, and infection-seeking agents, scintigraphic studies in the diabetic foot can be complex.
3. Early diagnosis of osteomyelitis is crucial because antibiotic therapy can be curative and may prevent amputation.
4. The precise SPECT/CT localization of the abnormal infection-seeking tracer uptake enables an accurate differential diagnosis between osteomyelitis and soft tissue infection.

Case 8.8.2 DIABETIC FOOT—SOFT TISSUE INFECTION (FIG. 8.8.2)
In111-WBC SPECT/LOW-DOSE CT

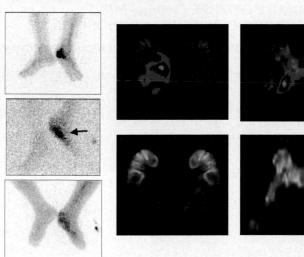

Case 8.8.3 DIABETIC FOOT—SOFT TISSUE INFECTION (FIG. 8.8.3)
In111-WBC SPECT/LOW-DOSE CT

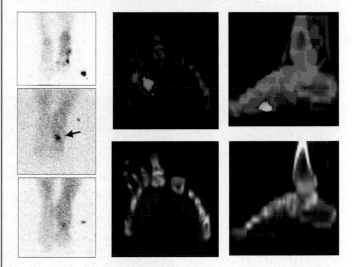

Brief History
A 72-year-old diabetic patient presented with a nonhealing wound in the plantar aspect of the right foot and was assessed for suspected osteomyelitis.

Findings
Planar images of the right foot, lateral view (left column, Tc99m-MDP top, In111-WBC center, Tc99m-sulfur colloid bottom), show an area of increased tracer uptake in the right foot (arrow).

SPECT/CT, transaxial (middle column) and sagittal (right column) slices, localizes this lesion to soft tissues in the plantar aspect of the right foot, with no evidence for bone involvement.

Note on planar scintigraphy: An additional area of intense uptake is demonstrated on bone scintigraphy only in the right calcaneus, most probably representing severe diabetic arthropathy changes.

Main Teaching Points and Summary
1. Osteomyelitis of the diabetic foot is a challenging diagnosis.
2. The precise localization of the In111-WBC focus to soft tissues provided by SPECT/CT allowed for optimized treatment tailoring.

Brief History
An 83-year-old diabetic patient, status post–fifth digit amputation on the right foot, presented with fever and local tenderness at the fourth digit. Osteomyelitis in the fourth metatarsal bone was suspected.

Findings
Planar scintigraphy of the right foot, plantar view (left column, Tc99m-MDP top, In111-WBC center, Tc99m-sulfur colloid bottom), shows an area of increased tracer uptake in the right foot (arrow).

SPECT/CT, transaxial (center column) and sagittal (right column) slices, localizes this lesion to the soft tissue at the plantar aspect of the right foot with no evidence for bone involvement.

Note on planar scintigraphy: An additional area of increased uptake is demonstrated on bone scintigraphy only along the right fourth metatarsus, most probably representing postoperative changes.

Main Teaching Point and Summary
1. Combined information provided by scintigraphy using bone- and infection-seeking agents, associated with SPECT/CT imaging, can facilitate the differential diagnosis between bone and soft tissue involvement by the infectious process, with significant therapeutic implications.

Case 8.8.4 BACTEREMIA–INFECTED AORTIC PLAQUE (FIG. 8.8.4)
In111-WBC SPECT/MULTISLICE CT

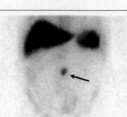
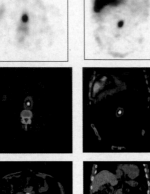
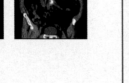

Brief History
A 86-year-old patient, status post–removal of infected aortic bypass graft complicated with aortoenteric fistula, presented with persistent bacteremia that was not responsive to antibiotic therapy. The patient was assessed in search of the source of infection.

Findings
Planar In111-WBC scintigraphy of the abdomen, anterior view (left), shows a focal area of increased tracer uptake in the midabdomen (arrow).

SPECT/CT, transaxial (right, mid column) and coronal (right column) slices, localizes this focus to an aortic plaque adjacent to the infrarenal vascular stump.

Main Teaching Points and Summary
1. The source for persistent bacteremia may be difficult to trace, especially in patients who have had major blood vessel surgery.
2. SPECT/CT enabled the precise localization of the infectious process and thus accurate diagnosis of the infection site.

8.9 CARDIAC SPECT/CT

Case 8.9.1 NORMAL STUDY (FIG. 8.9.1)
SPECT, MYOCARDIAL PERFUSION, AND CT, ATTENUATION CORRECTION
SINGLE ISOTOPE (Tc99m-MIBI), STRESS/REST SPECT/LOW-DOSE CT

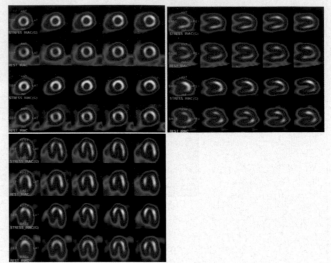

Brief History
A 64-year-old hypertensive patient was referred for suspected ischemic heart disease, following positive stress ergometry.

Findings
Stress (odd rows) and rest (even rows) myocardial perfusion SPECT slices (left, short; center, vertical long axis; right, horizontal long axis) show normal myocardial perfusion both on the attenuation-corrected images (two upper rows in each view) and uncorrected images (two lower rows in each view).

Main Teaching Points and Summary
1. The value of stress/rest SPECT myocardial perfusion imaging (MPI) for assessing the presence and extent of myocardial ischemia is well established.
2. The diagnostic accuracy of MPI may be adversely affected by attenuation, scatter, and blur.
3. SPECT/CT may overcome these technical limitations by photon attenuation correction, which will lead to improved image quality and diagnostic accuracy.
4. MPI should be interpreted using both attenuation corrected and uncorrected image sets.

Case 8.9.2 BREAST ARTIFACT (FIG. 8.9.2) SPECT, MYOCARDIAL PERFUSION AND CT, ATTENUATION CORRECTION
SINGLE ISOTOPE (Tc99m–MIBI), STRESS/REST SPECT/LOW–DOSE CT

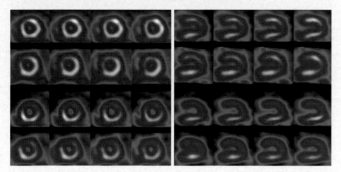

Brief History
A 58-year-old female patient with chest pain was assessed for suspected ischemic heart disease.

Findings
Stress (odd rows) and rest (even rows) myocardial perfusion SPECT slices (left-short, right-vertical long axis), show normal myocardial perfusion on attenuation-corrected images (two upper rows in each view), whereas uncorrected images (two lower rows in each view) show a fixed perfusion defect in the anterior wall.

These findings are consistent with attenuation by breast tissue. The study was reported as normal. There was no evidence of ischemic heart disease on further workup and clinical follow-up.

Main Teaching Points and Summary
1. Large breast tissue may cause attenuation of tracer activity in the anterior wall, leading to false-positive results.
2. Attenuation correction eliminates this artifact in the majority of patients, thus avoiding misinterpretation and the consequence of unnecessary diagnostic procedures and treatment.

Case 8.9.3 DIAPHRAGM ARTIFACT (FIG. 8.9.3) SPECT, MYOCARDIAL PERFUSION, AND CT–ATTENUATION CORRECTION
SINGLE ISOTOPE (Tc99m–MIBI), STRESS/REST SPECT/LOW–DOSE CT

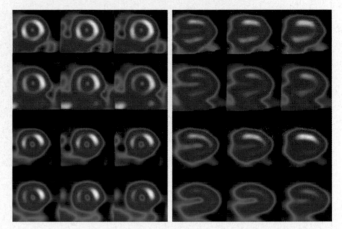

Brief History
A 53-year-old male diabetic patient was evaluated for shortness of breath and atypical chest pain.

Findings
Stress (odd rows) and rest (even rows) myocardial perfusion SPECT slices (left-short, right-vertical long axis) show normal myocardial perfusion on attenuation-corrected images (two upper rows in each view), whereas uncorrected images (two lower rows in each view) demonstrate a fixed perfusion defect in the inferior wall.

These findings are consistent with attenuation of the inferior wall by the diaphragm. The study was reported as normal. There was no evidence of ischemic heart disease on further workup and clinical follow-up.

Main Teaching Points and Summary
1. The diaphragm may cause attenuation to the inferior wall, mainly when a patient breathes heavily.
2. Attenuation correction generally eliminates this artifact and therefore decreases the rate of false-positive interpretations of MPI.

Case 8.9.4 SCAR AND ISCHEMIA (FIG. 8.9.4) SPECT, MYOCARDIAL PERFUSION, AND CT—ATTENUATION CORRECTION
SINGLE ISOTOPE (Tc99m–MIBI), STRESS/REST SPECT/LOW-DOSE CT

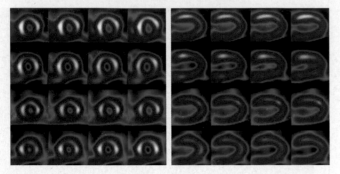

Brief History

A 61-year-old patient with a history of inferior wall myocardial infarction presented with new onset of chest pain.

Findings

Stress (odd rows) and rest (even rows) myocardial perfusion SPECT slices (left-short, right-vertical long axis) show a partially reversible perfusion defect in the inferior wall, both on attenuation-corrected (two upper rows in each view) and uncorrected images (two lower rows in each view).

The study was considered to represent ischemia within inferior wall scar tissue.

Main Teaching Points and Summary

1. Ischemic myocardium in the presence of scar is associated with a worsened patient prognosis and can be the source for arrhythmias.
2. Accurate diagnosis of ischemia and scar, mainly in the anterior and inferior wall, is improved with the use of attenuation-corrected MPI.

Case 8.9.5 SPECT/CT—NORMAL PERFUSION AND CORONARY ANATOMY (FIG. 8.9.5) MYOCARDIAL SPECT, SINGLE ISOTOPE (Tc99m-MIBI) STRESS/REST AND 64–SLICE CT

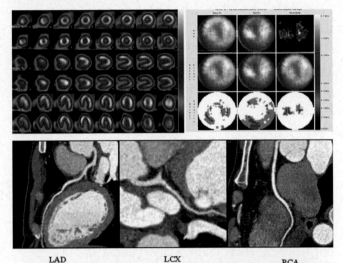

LAD   LCX   RCA

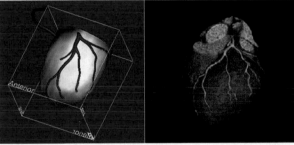

Brief History
A 55-year-old patient with hypertension and hyperlipidemia was assessed for the presence of occasional chest discomfort.

Findings
Attenuation-corrected SPECT images (first row, tomographic slices, left; summed "bull's eye" images, right) show normal myocardial perfusion.

Sixty-four slice CT coronary angiography (middle row) shows a mild calcified plaque at the left anterior descending artery ostium and a mild noncalcified plaque in the mid–right coronary artery, with no significant coronary stenosis. Total calcium score was 11.3 representing the twenty-fifth percentile for age.

Coregistered images (bottom row) demonstrated an essentially normal study.

Coronary catheterization showed diffuse luminal irregularities in the left and right coronary arteries, without significant stenosis.

Main Teaching Point and Summary
1. Registration of myocardial SPECT perfusion and multislice CT angiography coronary anatomy data is feasible either by coregistration of separately performed studies, as in this case, or, recently, with the use of integrated hybrid SPECT/CTA imaging devices.

(Courtesy of Dr. Tracy Farber, Emory University, Atlanta, Georgia.)

Case 8.9.6 SPECT/CT—MYOCARDIAL ISCHEMIA AND CORONARY LESIONS (FIG. 8.9.6)
MYOCARDIAL SPECT, SINGLE ISOTOPE (Tc99m–MIBI) STRESS/REST AND 64–SLICE CT

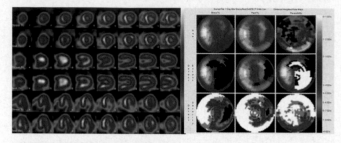

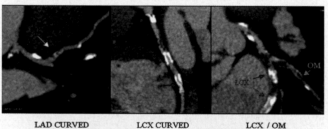

LAD CURVED   LCX CURVED   LCX / OM

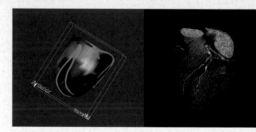

Brief History

A 62-year-old male patient with hyperlipidemia and stents previously placed in the proximal right coronary artery and distal left circumflex (LCX) presented with shortness of breath on exertion.

Findings

Attenuation corrected SPECT images (first row: tomographic slices, left; summed "bull's eye" images, right) show large, significantly reversible perfusion defect in the anterior, lateral, and inferolateral walls, suggestive of three-vessel coronary artery ischemia.

CT angiography (middle row) shows significant noncalcified plaque in proximal left anterior descending artery and 50% large calcified and noncalcified plaque near the origin of LCX. There is also a large noncalcified plaque that appears to occlude the OM2 and the LCX.

Coregistered images (bottom row) demonstrate the relationship between the ischemic territories on MPI and the occluded vessels on CT.

Coronary catheterization found a 30% stenosis in proximal left anterior descending artery, 90% stenosis in mid-LCX involving the origin of OM1, and patent stent in LCX. Based on the fused data, percutaneous transluminal coronary angioplasty and stenting were performed to the mid-LCX.

Main Teaching Points and Summary

1. The use of the registered SPECT and CT data can improve detection of hemodynamically significant coronary lesions in patients with ischemic heart disease.
2. Hybrid SPECT/CTCA devices may play a growing role in noninvasive diagnosis of coronary artery disease, introducing an objective decision-making tool regarding the need for interventions in each vessel.

(Courtesy of Dr. Tracy Farber, Emory University, Atlanta, Georgia.)

Index

A

Abdomen, 143–187
  abdominal wall, 144–149. *See also* Abdominal wall
  aortic aneurysm, 182
  aortic graft infection, 183
  aortic wall calcifications, 181
  bowel, 163–164
  colon, adenoma, 163
  colon cancer, 164
  gastric cancer, 161–163
  gastric uptake, 160
  gastrointestinal stromal tumor, 162
  kidneys and adrenals, 170–176. *See also* Kidneys and adrenals
  liver, 149–157. *See also* Liver and spleen
  lumbar spine, 184–187. *See also* Lumbar spine
  lymph nodes, 177–180. *See also* Lymph nodes
  normal pattern, 144
  pancreas, 158–159
  peritoneum, 165–169. *See also* Peritoneum
  psoas muscle abscess, 183
  small intestine, metastasis, 164
  spleen, 149–157. *See also* Liver and spleen
  stomach, 160–163
  vascular, 181–183
Abdominal wall, 144–149
  brown fat, 145, 146
  colostomy, 144
  rib fracture, 147
  surgical scar, 146
  tumor—metastasis, 148

Abscess, leg, 233
Acne, 54
Adrenals, 170–176. *See also* Kidneys and adrenals
Adrenal uptake, 261
Alzheimer's disease, 35–37
Aortic aneurysm, 182
Aortic graft infection, 183
Aortic vascular graft, 224
Aortic wall calcifications, 181
Aortobifemoral bypass, 223
Aortocaval lymph nodes, 180
Aortopulmonary window lymph nodes, 124
Arm. *See* Extremities

B

Bacteremia, infected aortic plaque, 278
Bilateral pheochromocytoma, 262
Bladder diverticulum, 206
Bladder herniation, 207–209
Blood clot, 130
Bone—lumbar spine, 184–187. *See also* Lumbar spine
Bone marrow, 248–249
Bowel, 163–164
Bowel and kidney uptake, 252
Bowel uptake, 255
Bowel uptake, infection, bone and soft tissue, 264
Brain, 13–37
  Alzheimer's disease, 35–37
  benign abnormalities, 19–21
  epilepsy, cerebellar diaschisis, 30–32
  epilepsy, congenital encephalomalacia, 19

Brain *(Coninued)*
  epilepsy, decreased cerebellar uptake, 33–34
  epilepsy, interictal pattern, 28–34
  lung cancer, metastases, 22–23
  neurological disorders, 28–37
  normal pattern, 14–17
  perfusion defects, 18
  pituitary adenoma, stroke, 27
  postsurgical changes, 20, 24
  radiation necrosis, 21, 25–26
  residual tumor, 24
  tumors, 21–27
Breast, 87–91
  cancer, 84, 87, 89–91
  granuloma, fracture of scapula, 88
  postradiation changes, 89
  saline implants, 87
  seroma, 88
Breast cancer, 84, 87, 89–91
Brown fat
  abdominal wall, 145, 146
  chest wall, 85
  head and neck, 47, 48, 70
  mediastinum, 129
Bulky disease, 131

C

Cancer
  breast, 84, 87, 89–91
  cervical, 215–217, 222
  colon, 164
  distal esophagus, 134, 135
  endotracheal recurrent lung, 131
  esophageal, 83
  gastric, 161–163
  lung, 22–23, 107, 108, 111, 113, 131

Cancer *(Continued)*
  prostate, 269
  proximal esophagus, 133
  rectal, 195, 199–202
  rectosigmoid, 199
  thyroid, 79, 257–259
Cardiac SPECT/CT, 278–282
Cardiac uptake, 260
Cardiovascular, 136–141
Cervical cancer, 215–217, 222
Cervical esophagus, 69
Cervix, 212–217. *See also* Ovary,
      cervix, uterus
Chest, 81–141
  blood clot, 130
  breast, 87. *See also* Breast
  brown fat, 129
  bulky disease, 131
  cancer of distal esophagus, 134, 135
  cancer of proximal esophagus, 133
  cardiovascular, 136–141
  coronary calcifications/pericardial
      effusion, 136
  endotracheal recurrent lung cancer,
      131
  esophagitis, 133
  esophagus, 132–135
  gastric pull up, 132
  hiatal hernia, 132
  lungs, 103–118. *See also* Lungs
  mediastinal lymph nodes, 123–129.
        See also Mediastinal lymph
        nodes
  mediastinum, 129–131
  myocardium, 137–140
  normal pattern, 82
  osteophyte, thoracic vertebra, 93
  pleura, 97–102. *See also* Pleura
  postradiation "cold" vertebrae, 94
  rib, metastasis, 94
  rib fractures, 92
  sternum, fracture, 93
  Takayasu's aortitis, 136
  thoracic lymph nodes, 119–123. *See
        also* Thoracic lymph nodes
  thoracic vertebrae, metastases, 96
  thymus, 130
  wall, 83–87. *See also* Chest wall
Chest wall, 83–87
  asymmetric muscular uptake, 83
  axillary postinjection uptake, 84
  breast cancer, 84, 87
  brown fat, 85
  esophageal cancer, 83
  gynecomastia, 83
  postsurgical changes, 86
  tumor—chest wall recurrence, 87
Cholecystitis, 152
Colon, adenoma, 163
Colon cancer, 164
Colostomy, 144, 191
Cul-de-sac peritoneal nodule,
      metastasis, 196

D
Dental and uterine inflammatory
      process, 256
Diabetic foot, 276, 277
Dilated prostatic urethra, 206
Disseminated carcinoid, tumor, 254

E
Ectopic parathyroid adenoma, 271
Ectopic pelvic kidney, 203
Ectopic stomach, update, 257
Endotracheal recurrent lung cancer,
      131
Epidural space, 227
Epilepsy
  cerebellar diaschisis, 30–32
  congenital encephalomalacia, 19
  decreased cerebellar uptake, 33–34
  interictal pattern, 28–34
Epitrochlear lymph nodes, 241
Esophageal cancer, 83
Esophagitis, 133
Esophagus, 132–135
Extremities, 229–249
  abscess, leg, 233
  arm, metastasis, 240
  bone/bone marrow, 244–249
  epitrochlear lymph nodes, 241
  femur, bone metastasis, 246
  femur, multiple myeloma, bone
        marrow, 248
  hip, infection, 239
  hip, metal-induced periprosthetic
        activity, 236
  humerus, bone metastasis, 245
  joints, 236–239
  knees, synovitis, periarticular uptake,
        237
  lymph nodes, 241–242
  lymphoma, humerus, bone marrow/
        soft tissue, 248
  lymphoma, humerus/soft tissues, 247
  lymphoma, tibia/leg, bone marrow/
        soft tissue, 249
  melanoma, thigh/legs, 232
  muscles, 239–240
  osteomyelitis, foot, 244
  popliteal lymph nodes, 241, 242
  sarcoma, hand, bone involvement,
        235
  scapula, bone metastasis, 245
  skin, 230–232
  skin ulcers, legs, 231
  soft tissue, 233–235
  subcutaneous lymphoma, nodule in
        arm, 233
  subcutaneous melanoma, nodule in
        thigh, 234
  surgical scar, thigh, 230
  tenosynovitis, tendon tear, foot/leg,
        238
  thigh, metastasis, 240
  thigh, tense muscles, 239

Extremities *(Continued)*
  trochanteric bursitis, periarticular
        uptake, 237
  vascular graft, 243
  vascular uptake, 242

F
Facet joint disease, 272
Femur
  bone metastasis, 246
  multiple myeloma, bone marrow, 248
Fibrous dysplasia, 274
Focal peritoneal nodules, metastases,
      196
Foot. *See* Extremities

G
Gallbladder uptake, 252
Gastric cancer, 161–163
Gastric pull up, 132
Gastric uptake, 160
Gastrohepatic ligament lymph nodes,
      177
Gastrointestinal stromal tumor (GIST),
      162, 169
Gastrointestinal tract, 197–202
  aortic vascular graft, 224
  aortobifemoral bypass, 223
  bone, 225–228
  focal uptake, bowel, 197
  iliac nodes, 202
  inflammatory bowel disease, 198
  lymph nodes, 220–222
  lymphoma, involvement of ischium,
        228
  metastasis, ilium and soft tissues,
        227
  metastasis, sacrum/epidural space,
        227
  orchiepididymitis, 218
  ovary, cervix, uterus, 212–217. *See
        also* Ovary, cervix, uterus
  Paget's disease, 226
  pararectal nodes, 199
  prostate and testes, 218–219
  prostatic hypertrophy, 218
  radiation-induced "cold" sacrum,
        225
  rectal cancer, 199
  rectal cancer, recurrence, 201, 202
  rectal cancer, response to treatment,
        200
  rectal polyp, 198
  rectosigmoid cancer, 199
  sacral fracture, 225
  testis, lymphoma, 219
  urinary tract, 203–211. *See also*
        Urinary tract
  vascular, 223–224
GI tract. *See* Gastrointestinal tract
GIST, 162, 169
Gluteal mass, metastatic melanoma,
      222

Goiter, 78
Gynecomastia, 83

H

Head and neck, 39–79
  acne, 54
  brown fat, 47, 48
  FDG-negative parotid, 51
  goiter, 78
  infection and inflammation, 53–56
  lymph node compartments, 72–77
  maxillary sinusitis, 55
  misregistration, 40
  missing orbit, ethmoid, extraocular,
      52
  missing salivary gland, 50
  neck, unilateral muscle uptake, 43
  normal pattern, 40
  physiologic artifacts/pitfalls, 40–52
  posttreatment changes, 49–52
  reconstituted lymphoid tissue and
      muscles, 49
  rheumatoid arthritis, atlanto-
      odontoid joint, 56
  thyroid, 77–79
  thyroid adenoma, 79
  thyroid cancer, 79
  thyroiditis, 77
  tongue, muscle uptake, 41
  torticollis, metal artifact, 44
  tracheostomy, 53
  tumors. *See* Tumors—head and
      neck
  vocal cord paralysis, 45, 46
Hematoma at prior injection site, 275
Hepatic hilum lymph nodes, 177
Hepatocellular carcinoma, 153
Hiatal hernia, 132
Hilar lymph nodes, 127
Hip
  infection, 239
  metal-induced periprosthetic
      activity, 236
Humerus, bone metastasis, 245

I

Iliac nodes, 180, 202, 216–217,
    220–221
Inflammatory bowel disease, 198
Inguinal hernia, focal uptake, 191
Inguinal lymph nodes, 222
Inhomogeneous cardiac uptake,
    pheochromocytoma, 260
Intracholedochal stent, 149

J

Joints, 236–239

K

Kidneys and adrenals, 170–176
  distorted renal pelvis, 173
  ectopic kidney, 172
  horseshoe kidney, 173

Kidneys and adrenals *(Continued)*
  regional lymphadenopathy near
      renal pelvis, 170
  single kidney, pitfall, 171
  tumor, bilateral adrenal involvement,
      lymphoma, 176
  tumor, multiple renal lesions,
      lymphoma, 175
  tumor, single adrenal metastasis, 176
  tumor, single renal metastasis,
      174–175
Knees, synovitis, periarticular uptake,
    237

L

Larynx, 66, 67
Leg. *See* Extremities
Lip, 62
Liver abscess, infection, 265
Liver and spleen, 149–157
  cholecystitis, 152
  hepatocellular carcinoma, 153
  intracholedochal stent, 149
  lesions at liver-lung interface,
      150–151
  liver metastasis, recurrence at site of
      surgery, 155
  metastasis, right liver lobe, 154
  metastasis, spleen, 156
  multiple lesions, spleen, nodal
      involvement, 156
  multiple liver metastases, 155
  splenomegaly, lymphoma, 157
Lumbar spine, 184–187
  articular facets, degenerative
      changes, 184
  intervertebral disc, degenerative
      changes, 185
  tumor, bone and soft tissue
      metastasis, 187
  tumor, lytic FDG-avid metastasis, 185
  tumor, sclerotic FDG-negative
      metastases, 186
  vertebral body, degenerative changes,
      184
Lung cancer, brain metastases, 22–23
Lungs, 103–118
  bronchioloalveolar lung cancer, 108
  endotracheal recurrent lung cancer,
      131
  FDG-negative lung nodule/interval
      shrinkage, 106
  FDG-negative small lung nodule, 106
  mesothelioma, postsurgical changes,
      112
  metachronous lung cancer, 111
  misregistration, 103
  multiple FDG-negative lesions,
      metastases, 117
  multiple lesions, lymphoma, 114, 115
  multiple lesions, metastases, 116
  multiple lesions, multifocal primary
      lung cancer, 113

Lungs *(Continued)*
  multiple lesions, treated and new
      metastases, 118
  Pancoast tumor, 109
  pneumonia, 105
  postradiation changes, 104
  pulmonary sarcoidosis, 105
  response to treatment, nodal
      metastases, 110
  single lesion, primary lung cancer,
      107, 108
  single lung nodule, granuloma, 107
Lymph node compartments, 72–77
Lymph nodes
  abdomen, 177–180
    aortocaval, 180
    gastrohepatic ligament, 177
    hepatic hilum lymph nodes, liver
        metastases, 177
    iliac, 180
    mesenteric and retroperitoneal,
        178
    mesenteric nodes, region of root of
        mesentery, 179
    para-aortic, 179
    splenic hilum, 178
  epitrochlear, 241
  gastrointestinal tract, 220–222
  mediastinal, 123–129. *See also*
      Mediastinal lymph nodes
  popliteal, 241, 242
  thoracic, 119–123
Lymphoma
  head, neck, and mediastinum, 265
  humerus, bone marrow/soft tissue,
      248
  humerus/soft tissues, 247
  involvement of ischium, 228
  kidneys, 175, 176
  lungs, 114, 115
  muscle, rib fracture, lung infiltrate,
      267
  ovary, 214
  pelvic mass, 266
  splenomegaly, 157
  stomach, 161
  subcutaneous, nodule in arm, 233
  testis, 219
  tibia/leg, bone marrow/soft tissue,
      249
  urinary tract, 211

M

Maxillary sinusitis, 55
Mediastinal lymph nodes, 123–129
  anterior mediastinal/paratracheal,
      123
  aortopulmonary window, 124
  hilar, 127
  paraesophageal, 126
  paratracheal, 127
  pre-/subcarinal, 125
  pretracheal, 127

Mediastinal lymph nodes *(Continued)*
  prevascular, 124
  retrocaval-paratracheal/response to
    treatment, 128–129
  tracheobronchial, 127
Mediastinum, 129–131
Melanoma, thigh/legs, 232
Menstruation, 212
Mesothelioma
  lungs, 112
  pleural masses, 102
  pleural thickening, 100
Metastatic carcinoid, tumor, 253
Misregistration
  patient movement, 40
  respiratory movement, 103
Muscles, 239–240
Myocardial perfusion/ischemia,
  278–282
Myocardium, 137–140
Myositis ossificans, 275

N
Neck. *See* Head and neck
Neuroblastoma, bone marrow
  involvement, 262
Neurological disorders, 28–37

O
Orchiepididymitis, 218
Osteoarthritis in hip, 273
Osteomyelitis, foot, 244
Osteomyelitis, infection, 263
Ovarian carcinoma, 214–215
Ovary, cervix, uterus, 212–217
  cervical cancer, 215–217
  iliac nodes, 216–217
  lymphoma, ovary, 214
  menstruation, 212
  myoma, 213
  ovarian carcinoma, 214–215
  ovulating ovary, 212
Ovulating ovary, 212

P
Paget's disease, 226
Pancoast tumor, 109
Pancreas, 158–159
Para-aortic lymph nodes, 179
Paraesophageal lymph nodes, 126
Parathyroid adenoma, 270, 271
Paratracheal lymph nodes, 127
Paravertebral abscess, infection, 264
Pelvic abscess, infection, 194
Pelvis, 189–228
  colostomy, focal uptake, 191
  cul-de-sac peritoneal nodule,
    metastasis, 196
  focal peritoneal nodules, metastases,
    196
  gastrointestinal tract, 197–202. *See
    also* Gastrointestinal tract
  inguinal hernia, focal uptake, 191

Pelvis *(Continued)*
  normal pattern, 190
  pelvic abscess, infection, 194
  pilonidal sinus, infection, 193
  psoas muscle, metastasis, 195
  rectal cancer, presacral recurrence,
    195
  skin granuloma, 192
  tumor—diffuse peritoneal
    involvement, 197
  urinary catheter, focal uptake,
    192
Peritoneum
  granulomatotic nodule, 165
  multiple nodules, metastases,
    166–167
  single nodule, metastasis, 166
  tumor, diffuse pattern, peritoneal
    seeding, 168
  tumor, peritoneal masses, GIST,
    169
PET/CT
  abdomen, 143–187. *See also*
    Abdomen
  brain, 13–37. *See also* Brain
  chest, 81-141. *See also* Chest
  CT component, 2–3
  extremities, 229–249. *See also*
    Extremities
  head and neck, 39–79. *See also*
    Head and neck
  integrated system, 3–4
  patient preparation, 5–7
  pelvis, 189–228. *See also* Pelvis
  performing the study, 7
  PET component, 2
  purchase choice, 1
  quality assurance, 4–5
Pharynx, 65
Pilonidal sinus, infection, 193
Pituitary adenoma, stroke, 27
Pleura, 97–102
  malignant effusion and tube
    insertion, 99
  malignant implant, pleural nodule,
    101
  mesothelioma, pleural masses, 102
  mesothelioma, pleural thickening,
    100
  pleurodesis, 97, 98
Pleurodesis, 97, 98
Pneumonia, 105
Popliteal lymph nodes, 241, 242
Positron emission tomography/
  computed tomography. *See*
  PET/CT
Pretracheal lymph nodes, 127
Prevascular lymph nodes, 124
Prostate and testes, 218–219
Prostate cancer, abdominal
  lymphadenopathy, 269
Prostatic hypertrophy, 218
Psoas muscle abscess, 183

Psoas muscle, metastasis, 195
Pulmonary sarcoidosis, 105

Q
Quality assurance
  PET/CT, 4–5
  SPECT/CT, 9–10

R
Radiation-induced "cold" sacrum, 225
Radiation necrosis, 21, 25–26
Rectal cancer
  presacral recurrence, 195
  primary, 199
  recurrence, 201, 202
  response to treatment, 200
Rectal polyp, 198
Rectosigmoid cancer, 199
Remnant thyroid, 255
Renal calculus, uptake, 272
Renal transplant, 203
Renal uptake, 261
Residual carcinoid, tumor, 253
Rheumatoid arthritis, atlanto-odontoid
  joint, 56
Rib fracture, 92, 147
Rib, metastasis, 94

S
Sacral fracture, 225
Sacrum, 225, 227
Salivary gland uptake, parathyroid
  adenoma, 270
Sarcoma, hand, bone involvement,
  235
Scalp, 57–59
Scapula
  bone metastasis, 245
  fracture, 88
Single photon emission computed
  tomography/computed
  tomography. *See* SPECT/CT
Skin granuloma, 192
Skin ulcers, legs, 231
Small intestine, metastasis, 164
SPECT/CT, 251–282
  acquisition protocols, 8–9
  adrenal uptake, 261
  bacteremia, infected aortic plaque,
    278
  bilateral pheochromocytoma, 262
  bowel and kidney uptake, 252
  bowel uptake, 255
  bowel uptake, infection, bone and
    soft tissue, 264
  cardiac procedures, 10–11
  cardiac SPECT/CT, 278–282
  cardiac uptake, 260
  dental and uterine inflammatory
    process, 256
  diabetic foot, 276, 277
  disseminated carcinoid, tumor, 254
  ectopic parathyroid adenoma, 271

SPECT/CT (*Continued*)
ectopic stomach, update, 257
facet joint disease, 272
fibrous dysplasia, 274
Ga67 scintigraphy, 263–267
gallbladder uptake, 252
hematoma at prior injection site, 275
I123-MIBG scintigraphy, 260–262
I131 scintigraphy, 255–259
imaging devices, 7–8
In111-pentetreotide scintigraphy,
    252–254
In111-capromab pendetide, 268–269
In111-WBC scintigraphy, 276–278
inhomogeneous cardiac uptake,
    pheochromocytoma, 260
liver abscess, infection, 265
lymphoma, head, neck, and
    mediastinum, 265
lymphoma, muscle, rib fracture, 267
lymphoma, pelvic mass, 266
metastatic carcinoid, tumor, 253
myocardial perfusion/ischemia,
    278–282
myositis ossificans, 275
neuroblastoma, bone marrow
    involvement, 262
nuclear medicine procedures, 10
osteoarthritis in hip, 273
osteomyelitis, infection, 263
parathyroid adenoma, 270, 271
paravertebral abscess, infection, 264
prostate cancer, abdominal
    lymphadenopathy, 269
quality assurance, 9–10
remnant thyroid, 255
renal calculus, uptake, 272
renal uptake, 261
residual carcinoid, tumor, 253
salivary gland uptake, parathyroid
    adenoma, 270
Tc99m-MDP, 272–275
Tc99m-MIBI, 270–271
technical staffing, 11
thymic uptake, 256, 263
thyroid cancer, bone metastasis,
    259

SPECT/CT (*Continued*)
thyroid cancer, cervical/
    supraclavicular nodal
    metastases, 258
thyroid cancer, lung metastasis, 258
thyroid cancer, mediastinal nodal
    metastasis, 257
vertebral metastasis, neuroendocrine
    tumor, 254
Spleen, 156–157. *See also* Liver and
    spleen
Splenic hilum lymph nodes, 178
Sternum, fracture, 93
Stomach, 160–163
Subcutaneous lymphoma, nodule in
    arm, 233
Subcutaneous melanoma, nodule in
    thigh, 234
Supraclavicular lymph nodes, 119
Supradiaphragmatic lymph nodes, 123
Surgical scar, thigh, 230

T
Takayasu's aortitis, 136
Tenosynovitis, tendon tear, foot/leg,
    238
Thigh. *See* Extremities
Thoracic lymph nodes, 119–123
    axillary, 121
    axillary/pectoralis, 120
    internal mammary *vs.* sternal lesion,
        122
    supraclavicular, 119
    supradiaphragmatic, 123
Thoracic vertebrae, 93, 96
Thymic uptake, 256, 263
Thymus, 130
Thyroid, 77–79
Thyroid adenoma, 79
Thyroid cancer, 79
    bone metastasis, 259
    cervical/supraclavicular nodal
        metastases, 258
    lung metastasis, 258
    mediastinal nodal metastasis, 257
Thyroiditis, 77
Tongue, 41, 62, 63

Tonsil, 64
Torticollis, metal artifact, 44
Tracheobronchial lymph nodes, 127
Tracheostomy, 53
Trochanteric bursitis, periarticular
    uptake, 237
Tumors—head and neck
    auditory canal, 59
    bone, vertebral metastasis, 71
    cervical esophagus, 69
    larynx, 66, 67
    lip, 62
    nasopharynx, 61
    neural sheath and brown fat, 70
    parotid, 60
    parotid and peri-parotid nodes, 60
    pharynx, 65
    scalp, benign FDG-negative, 59
    scalp, melanoma, 57, 58
    tongue, 62, 63
    tonsil, 64
    vocal cord, 68

U
Ureter, carcinoma, 210
Urinary bladder, carcinoma, 211
Urinary catheter, focal uptake, 192
Urinary tract, 203–211
    bladder diverticulum, 206
    bladder herniation, 207–209
    carcinoma of bladder, 211
    carcinoma of ureter, 210
    dilated prostatic urethra, 206
    ectopic pelvic kidney, 203
    focal uptake, ureter, 204–205
    lymphoma of bone, 211
    renal transplant, 203
Uterus, 212–217. *See also* Ovary, cervix,
    uterus

V
Vascular graft, 243
Vascular uptake, 242
Vertebral metastasis, neuroendocrine
    tumor, 254
Vocal cord, 68
Vocal cord paralysis, 45, 46